JESSE VENTURA'S
MARIJUANA MANIFESTO

T0039991

JESSE VENTURA'S
MARIJUANA MANIFESTO

HOW LIES, CORRUPTION, AND PROPAGANDA KEPT CANNABIS ILLEGAL

JESSE VENTURA

WITH JEN HOBBS

Foreword by **STEVE KUBBY**

Skyhorse Publishing

Skyhorse Publishing books may be purchased in bulk at special discounts for sales promotion, corporate gifts, fund-raising, or educational purposes. Special editions can also be created to specifications. For details, contact the Special Sales Department, Skyhorse Publishing, 307 West 36th Street, 11th Floor, New York, NY 10018 or info@skyhorsepublishing.com.

Skyhorse® and Skyhorse Publishing® are registered trademarks of Skyhorse Publishing, Inc.®, a Delaware corporation.

Visit our website at www.skyhorsepublishing.com.

10 9 8 7 6 5 4 3 2 1

Library of Congress Cataloging-in-Publication Data is available on file.

Cover design by Brian Peterson
Cover photo credit Lauren B Photography © 2015

Print ISBN: 978-1-5107-2376-4
Ebook ISBN: 978-1-5107-2378-8

Printed in the United States of America

Dedication

To my dear friend Tommy Chong, who has taught me
a great deal about cannabis, and to all those like him who have
been unjustly persecuted because of a plant.

Table of Contents

Note to the Reader from Jesse Ventura

When Donald Trump was announced the winner of the 2016 presidential election, I said I was going to wait and see what happens. People promise all kinds of things when they run for office. President Obama vowed to close Gitmo. President HW Bush said "read my lips, no more taxes." So I gave President Trump a chance. But he and Attorney General Jeff Sessions have stated they'd like to see the DEA come into states like Colorado where marijuana is legal and tell *legal* recreational marijuana users that they are breaking federal law and therefore must be prosecuted. It is completely wrong, unethical—not to mention unconstitutional—to reverse state law just because you feel like it. Shame on President Trump for even *considering* this.

Now, I'm writing this when we're about one hundred days into Trump's presidency. Our country is in a strange state of flux right now. In the 2016 elections, eight states voted to legalize marijuana—for either medical or recreational purposes—which brings the total to thirty-three states. That means more than half the states in our country have legalized marijuana in some way.

According to the latest CBS News poll[1] (the results were revealed coincidentally on April 20th, 2017), 61 percent of the country is now in favor of marijuana legalization! This is a five-point increase from 2016, and the highest percentage ever recorded.

The poll also found that:

- 88 percent of Americans *favor* medical marijuana use
- 71 percent *oppose* Jeff Session's plans to stop marijuana sales and the use of marijuana in states that have already legalized it
- 65 percent think marijuana is less dangerous than most other drugs
- 69 percent think drug abuse should be treated as an addiction and mental health problem rather than a criminal offense

So what should we do with this information? Act! If you can pick up a phone to answer polling data questions about marijuana, you can use it to call your representatives and put their feet to the fire.

Congressman Tom Garrett introduced the Ending Federal Marijuana Prohibition Act 2017 on February 27th, so when Sessions told legislatures to change the laws if they don't want the Feds coming after legal recreational marijuana users, our legislatures were listening.

If passed, the Ending Federal Marijuana Prohibition Act 2017 would take marijuana off the federal controlled substances list (which is what makes it such a dangerous, supposedly addictive substance) and place it in the same category as the alcohol and tobacco industries.

This bill was originally introduced by Senator Bernie Sanders in 2015, and there was not enough bipartisan support to see it go anywhere. Actually, that bill was previously introduced in 2011 and again in 2013—you'll read more about the bill's unsuccessful history in this book.

If you want history to stop repeating itself, then pick up the phone and call your representatives. They might not even be aware that 61 percent of the country wants this bill to be passed!

When I originally wrote my marijuana manifesto, I wanted it to serve as not only my philosophy on marijuana, but also as a reference book for all things cannabis. You'll notice not much is updated in the paperback edition because quite frankly, I'm still waiting for the world to change to a point where I can say, yes, there's something completely new to add to America's history with this plant.

Canada's Prime Minister Justin Trudeau introduced legislation in April 2017 so that recreational marijuana will be legalized nationwide by 2018—which means our neighbors to the north will be the second nation (after Uruguay) to completely legalize marijuana as a consumer product—but when it comes to America, we're still doing this uncomfortable dance between states' rights and federal law. Yes, cannabis has become more socially acceptable, now that it is becoming a major industry with incredible growth potential, but it's still illegal on the federal level.

This book presents all the reasons why it's time to accept marijuana into our culture once and for all. It doesn't matter if you're for marijuana legalization or not. It doesn't matter if you consume it or not. This plant has been part of our country since the British colonized America, and the time has come to accept the facts—and if you've been fed the government's alternative facts, prepare to have your eyes opened.

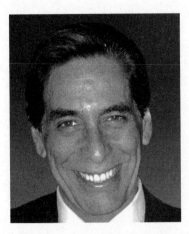

Foreword by Steve Kubby

My life journey has included studying the amazing medical benefits of cannabis firsthand, then dedicating myself to cannabis policy reform, and, now, developing new products and technologies for overall health and wellness of every human being.

I was born in El Paso, Texas, and in 1968 and at age twenty-three, I was diagnosed with malignant pheochromocytoma, a fatal form of adrenal cancer that required surgery.

Following my diagnosis, I began to consume cannabis to alleviate the symptoms, and eventually I experienced personal proof of remission of one of the most deadly forms of cancer. Dr. Vincent DeQuattaro, a professor of medicine at University of Southern California who treated me with various operations, chemotherapy, and radiation, said this in his *Inside Edition* interview about me and my experiences: "For him to survive this long with a tumor is a miracle." I attribute that miracle to cannabis.

In 1975, my cancer returned. I had my second tumor surgery, and then another in 1976. In 1981, I had further surgery and was given radiation treatment at the Mayo Clinic. Prior to my 1981 treatments, the cancer had spread to my liver and beyond. The diagnosis had a 100 percent mortality rate within five years.

After thirty-five years of continual cannabis treatments, I am now entirely cancer free. No one else in the world can make the claim to have beaten my form of cancer. That is why when I look at medical data, I believe that my recovery is entirely due to cannabis.

During my recovery years, I studied the unjust marijuana laws in the United States that threatened the freedom and the very lives of so many Americans. I learned how to advocate and organize those who had the vision to change these laws. I met people who would make considerable personal sacrifices to protect the rights of others, and people who were willing to take whatever actions were necessary to prove it. I knew I had to take action as well.

For years the police told my wife, Michele, and me, "We don't make the laws, we just enforce them," and, "If you don't like the law, then change it." So in 1996, I played a key role in the drafting and passage of California's Proposition 215 (otherwise known as the Compassionate Use Act of 1996), the first ballot initiative to legalize medical marijuana in the country. Now, twenty years later, twenty-four states have followed suit and now six or more will soon allow full adult use. But back in 1996, it felt like we were dreaming when voters ultimately approved the use of medical marijuana by a stunning 55.6 percent to 44.4 percent.

In 1996, when law enforcement officials were well aware that Prop 215 would legalize marijuana, these officials pulled together to announce that Prop 215 was "only an affirmative defense" for seriously ill people. I was outraged by law enforcement's efforts to gut 215, and I decided to run for governor and speak out publicly about this terrible assault on our American values and principles. Fortunately, the Libertarian Party was anxious to help and even gave me their first-ever unanimous nomination.

From that point, I campaigned for Governor of California, hounding my opponent, Attorney General Dan Lungren, faulting him as a Republican who ignored states' rights and refused to uphold the results of the election.

Lungren and his buddies were not amused, however, and my wife and I soon found ourselves under surveillance. We would learn later that the four agencies investigating us were doing so based upon an unsigned letter that alleged something we were already admitting publicly, that we were growing our own medical marijuana. Our friends warned us to be careful, because the word was out that the police intended to punish us. Angry that such tactics were being used against us, we vowed to turn the tables and create the perfect test case to uphold 215 and expose these rogue police and prosecutors who were attempting to overthrow it.

With the help of our attorneys and activist friends, we carefully documented the medical marijuana garden my wife and I had started and even sent a notice to the police, via our garbage. We knew we were under surveillance and we knew they were picking through our garbage and would find the note. In the notice, we informed them that I had cancer, and that my wife and I both had doctor recommendations, and that we were growing our own medical marijuana as specifically provided by the new law. Our "trash note" even invited the police to come to our home and inspect our crop.

Although the police later admitted receiving this letter from us in our garbage, our status as bona fide patients meant nothing to them, and they continued to go through our garbage and peek through our windows until January 19, 1999, when twenty heavily armed SWAT team members raided our house with laser-guided assault weapons and body armor. You may wonder why such a brute show of force was required against an unarmed third-party politician and his wife attempting to lawfully assert their rights, but we can only speculate that the police were afraid we would flush our entire garden down the toilet in the few minutes gained by an armed invasion of our home.

Our garden met the standards adopted by the City of Oakland, California, which in turn were based upon the 7.1 lbs of medical marijuana the US government gives every year to each of the eight federal medical marijuana patients. Under the Oakland Guidelines, we were allowed 144 plants each, or a total of 288 indoor plants, which were expected to produce a one-year, seven-pound supply. Along the walls leading to our garden we posted a copy of 215 and the Oakland Guidelines, as well as a recent notice from the attorney general that if patients presented credible evidence of a physician's recommendation, the police should just take some samples and photos and leave the garden intact.

None of this meant anything to the police or prosecutors who arrested both my wife and me, treating us as common criminals and demanding $200,000 in bail. Suddenly we found ourselves guilty until proved innocent and stripped of virtually every protection guaranteed by the Bill of Rights to every American. Remember, we were not disobeying any law, but attempting to uphold lawfully the rights won in a democratic election. Unless we defended our right to grow our own medical marijuana, as specifically granted in our new law, those cultivation rights would quickly be lost.

All this took place a mere two months after losing the 1998 election for governor. When my wife and I were finally released from jail, I was a contender to become the Libertarian Party VP candidate in 2000, losing the nomination 418 to 338 (by only 80 votes), and I was a 2008 candidate for the Libertarian Party Presidential nomination.

However, you might want to know what Michele and I faced when twenty heavily armed narcs arrive at our house early in the morning on January 19, 1999, informing us that we were under arrest.

Welcome to the War on Drugs, with a cancer victim like me forced to be on the front lines. I found it outrageous that a nonviolent man and his family were being held at gunpoint. That day, I explained to the narcotics task force that I personally wrote and passed Prop 215 and we were legally entitled to grow medical marijuana. The head of the task force told me that Prop 215 may apply to those "faggots" in San Francisco, but not to me in Placer County.

The cops forced us to open our wallets and give the cash we had in our possession. Imagine being sick with needs for expensive high blood-pressure medicine, and then they took the very money used to buy that medication. This is how the system worked to wear the defendant down. Upon release, we later found that the Christmas card to my daughter from her grandparents was also confiscated and they never returned the money the card contained. I realized that just passing a law isn't good enough with people who want to drag me away, keep me from my medicine, and kill me.

The police thought they were going to come in and scare me into silence, but I was going to teach them a lesson they would never forget.

Riding down to Auburn Jail under arrest, my wife and I didn't know the police were secretly recording us in the back of the SUV. Michele was terrified that our life was over. I just laughed and told her that they were the ones who were in trouble. This was only the beginning. They were the ones who would end up being scared because I didn't even have to go to the media because they all chased after me. Just about every national and local media source, from *Inside Edition* to the *LA Times,* had contacted me in jail, which empowered activists and created sympathy for my cause.

When we were carted off to jail, we were detained in a poorly heated cell and we were denied blankets. I was not allowed to use my medication, and as a result, my health began to deteriorate rapidly. Without access to medical marijuana, I became blind in one eye, I was urinating blood, and I was suffering from blood pressure attacks. Doctors testified that if I wasn't released from jail soon, I would die. But the courts went so far as to say my wife and I couldn't use the Compassionate Use Act as a defense for why we had marijuana in our home. Can you believe that? I of all people knew I could, because I helped get Prop 215 passed! We found ourselves facing nineteen criminal counts and forty years in prison for something that was completely legal in the State of California.

Fast-forward to our trial where we were found innocent of all marijuana charges. There were also other minor charges of minuscule amounts of peyote and mushrooms. I was ordered to accept a five-year felony in return for no further time in court. I told them to forget it. I told them that I had a job waiting in Canada on the Sunshine Coast, but they said I had to go to jail. Then the jail said they couldn't take me because I was too sick for the staff to care for. I was allowed to appeal the conviction for peyote possession and obtained the court's permission to move to Canada, with Michele and our two children.

So after two and a half years and a quarter of a million dollars in legal expenses, a jury acquitted us of the initial marijuana charges, and we regained our freedom, but little else. Even though we had proved our innocence, none of the terrorists involved were ever punished for this illegal raid, nor was any of the property stolen from us returned, not even the data off of our computers. But we survived and sought an escape from such terror in the freedom and wildness of British Columbia, because the court agreed to let me go to BC for my job opportunity. Little did they know my wife and I would be the new co-anchors for *Pot TV News*.

I arrived in Canada as an American cannabis refugee in 2001. I saw my Canadian doctor, who confirmed that cannabis was the best treatment for my malignant pheochromocytoma, a fatal form of adrenal cancer. I had been growing the cannabis for about six months in Canada, and once again I was arrested for growing my medicine, but this time it was the RCMP who showed up. The Canadian government required me to see a doctor to confirm that I really was sick. Cancer specialist Dr. Joseph Connors of the BC Cancer Agency said that I had a large malignant tumor resulting from the cancer and that pot helps lower the excessive level of a chemical called catecholamine in my blood. He said I would die within four days of not smoking marijuana. The court affirmed his recommendation.

In September 2002, I was given authorization by the Canadian government and Health Canada to grow fifty-nine plants, travel with 360 g (12 oz.), and hold 2655 g (under 6 lbs.). A stunning victory! After a review a year later, my doctor increased my dose.

While I was in Canada, a California state appeals court ruling changed my mescaline possession misdemeanor to a felony without my knowledge or consent; suddenly, I was wrongly reclassified as a fugitive, which put my refugee status in jeopardy. I spent the next five years appealing this fugitive status through Canada's legal system, but I was eventually asked to leave the country under a "conditional departure order."

When I returned to the United States in 2006 after losing my Canadian refugee status, I had to face pending charges. Upon arriving in San Francisco, in order to shield me from the public and media, I was taken off the plane and escorted away by SF police to a waiting car. When I was pulled off the plane, I was handcuffed so tight that I bled. I was paraded by frog-walk past every government agency you ever heard of while all these officers high-fived each for succeeding in capturing this international refugee cancer patient.

Then, one of the most revealing and touching moments in my journey occurred during my 2006 arrest at the San Francisco airport. It was certainly one of the clearest examples of the sheer hypocrisy of my situation and society itself at that moment in time. As soon as I sat in the patrol car, the deputy told me I was a hero! I held my hands up showing him I was under arrest, with blood dripping from my wrists. "Lucky me!" I said.

He immediately replied, "No! You don't understand!" He said I had hundreds, if not thousands, of supporters, and all the news organizations—even *Fox News*—were on my side. He got choked up and began to tell me his story. His father was diagnosed with cancer and they got him a cannabis card. The deputy told of the years gifted to his family by his father's extended life. They made fishing trips and outings; more than two years' life expectancy they attributed to his use of medical marijuana. He told me he wanted to take me home as a hero but instead he had to take me in.

As we left the airport, I realized that even the police suffer from this War on Drugs. They have parents and relatives that need help who are being abused by this process.

While in jail, I was tortured by the system, denied my medicine, left to sleep on icy cold cement while puking blood and sick from my cancer symptoms for three days. Then, suddenly, everyone started treating me nicely. I was allowed to take Marinol, a prescription drug containing THC, to help to control my blood pressure, which I was thankful for. On the other hand, I lost thirty-three pounds in sixty-two days while on Marinol, and suffered from almost constant nausea while on the drug.

I later learned from the Placer County Sheriff that the San Francisco City Board of Supervisors passed formal resolution No. 060153 on my behalf, "reaffirming the right of Steven Wynn Kubby, who requires medicinal use of marijuana to remain in good health while in custody in the Placer County jail." This is why I was allowed Marinol.

I was eventually freed due to my doctor sending in pleas based on the medical efficacy cannabis provided me, and also by the formal resolution passed by the San Francisco City Board of Supervisors.

On April 14, 2006, I wrote a letter to my supporters because without their help, I would have never received any medication at all, and my life would have probably ended in that San Francisco jail cell. In the letter, I wrote about how grateful I was to receive Marinol, as it was better than nothing at all, but I did list the symptoms I experienced on the drug:

During that time I experienced excruciating pain, a vicious high blood-pressure crisis, passed blood in my urine, and I lost thirty-three pounds. However, there was also good news. I learned that Marinol is an acceptable, if not ideal, substitute for whole cannabis in treating my otherwise fatal disease. Now I am a free man and I am profoundly grateful to be alive and to have friends and supporters such as you.

I later discovered that in July 2007, the Office of National Drug Control Policy (ONDCP—the drug czar's office) used this letter to misrepresent me during congressional hearings on medical marijuana. In written testimony before the House Judiciary Subcommittee on Crime, Terrorism and Homeland Security, Dr. David Murray, ONDCP's chief scientist, stated that Steve Kubby no longer supports medical marijuana! He took what I said about Marinol out of context by never stating all the side effects. He misrepresented me by saying I wrote, "Marinol is an acceptable, if not ideal, substitute for whole cannabis in treating my otherwise fatal disease," and nothing further.

Of course, I had to squash his deceptive and dangerous misrepresentation. Whole cannabis is not only the best medicine for me, it is the only medicine that has kept me alive *and* in relatively good heath, despite a terminal diagnosis of malignant pheochromocytoma.

Currently, the FDA says there is no effective cure for the form of cancer I had. I was supposed to die within five years of my initial diagnosis, which was over thirty-five years ago. And yet, for the past thirty-five years, I've either been in remission or cancer-free. Today, I am completely cancer-free and I attribute that to my continued use of cannabis. I am now dedicating my years of experience and knowledge to develop proprietary processes combined with a patent-pending cannabis strain to offer everyone the same benefits from cannabis that I have achieved. There are untold secrets of life-changing characteristics in the cannabis plant that must be researched and discovered.

For example, using cannabis helps my conditions, but I still suffered each day from terrible blood pressure. I started reading about research being done in Israel by Dr. Raphael Mechoulam about all of the different strains of cannabis that were damaged by how they were dried or prepared for usage, and it occurred to me that nobody was trying whole-green cannabis, used to create cryogenic extracts. I decided to try one-third of a teaspoon a day for two months and didn't notice too much effect until I vomited nonstop for four days with constant convulsions. After the fourth day, it cleared. I had no daily symptoms of high blood pressure, and that's when I realized I had been cured. My cryogenic raw plant extract cured my cancer, and in 2011, it had cured my high blood pressure. This is when I knew I wanted to spend the rest of my life making this life-saving medicine to help others.

As I move to the next phase of my journey to better health, I continue my vision under the simple name of KUSH. Our mission is to create a new beginning for cannabis, a new beginning for a healthier way of life, and a new beginning for freedom, long life, and happiness for all. Obama spent trillions of dollars to create a government health program, but I have a far simpler plan that will genuinely help patients and save the government all those trillions of dollars: reschedule marijuana to reflect reality, and authorize its use for medical purposes nationwide.

—Steve Kubby, founder of the American Medical Marijuana
Association, activist, author, political candidate, consultant,
public speaker, cannabis warrior, policy advisor, and cancer survivor.

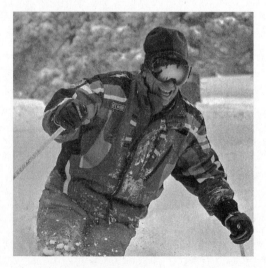

Introduction

"The greatest service which can be rendered any country is to add a useful plant to its culture."

—Thomas Jefferson, *Memorandum of Services to My Country*

I know what you're thinking. This is another one of those pro-pot books written by a liberal hippie, and he's calling for decriminalization and full legalization of marijuana because he's breaking the law right now by smoking it. Well, think again.

People probably think I'm a hippie because I like wearing tie-dyed shirts or because I grew up in the '60s or because to this day one of my favorite bands is the Rolling Stones. When I was eighteen years old in 1969, I enlisted in the US Navy. I am a Vietnam veteran and hardly a hippie. I don't drink alcohol and I've long since given up my vices of chewing tobacco and smoking cigars. I'm not an alcoholic, and I have nothing against drinkers, but it's a personal preference of mine not to drink. I choose not to drink, not to use tobacco, and guess what? It happens to be healthier for you in the long run if you don't do either of these activities. I also don't drink coffee or caffeinated beverages. Again, personal preference. More on that later.

So have I rolled a joint and smoked it before? Yes. Absolutely. And I've always been up front about this.

I've smoked pot before—not while I was governor—but I have used it in the past in a recreational capacity. If I someday require it for medical reasons, I wouldn't be opposed to using it. In fact, I would prefer to use it, especially if it keeps me from relying on prescription pills with all those awful side effects. My friend Tommy Chong says there shouldn't be a distinction between medical and recreational marijuana because any way you look at it, it's a medical plant. Instead of going to a doctor to get a prescription of Prozac or an antidepressant, those who are smoking it specifically for the euphoric feeling are doing it for mental health reasons.

I believe in marijuana's medicinal uses because I've seen it significantly benefit people I know. A dear and very close member of my family, who has suffered from seizures, is now seizure-free due to medical marijuana. She takes a few drops of cannabis oil twice a day and now she's seizure-free and off of all her medication. I'm so glad to see she's off all those pills that had to be constantly adjusted, each with a long list of side effects that sometimes seemed like a worse trade-off from the seizures. She no longer has to take those pills because she now lives a normal life with taking just drops of cannabis oil per day. I am fully convinced of the medicinal benefits of marijuana because I've seen the positive effects it has had on her quality of life.

The fact is Big Pharma just can't duplicate what this plant is capable of doing. And the fact that our government continues to deny sick people access to this plant is truly a crime against humanity. Who knows when you might need medical marijuana? How do you know what the future has in store for you? You don't.

Every month and every year that goes by, we find out more positive things about marijuana. The list is getting longer and longer and longer to the point where I question why they kept all this information from us. Why was marijuana demonized all those years when obviously this plant has a great deal of positive attributes—not only medical. It's also a renewable resource! That's the part that troubles me the most.

How did we go down this road to ruin about marijuana? Well, marijuana is a cash crop, and that means it's bad for the pharmaceutical industry. Marijuana is also competition for the energy people because it's an alternative source of energy. And now there are studies proving it can help our veterans with post-traumatic stress disorder. So when are we going to take the blinders off and do what's right for humanity and legalize this stuff once and for all?

At this point, to get the DEA to declare the end of the war against marijuana means that they are going to decide to quit their jobs for the betterment of society. Yeah, that ain't gonna happen. Marijuana will remain illegal because it creates more jobs and puts more and more people in prison (which in turn, creates more jobs). Our national anthem states American is "the land of the free," yet we have more people locked up in prison than any other industrialized nation. So those who are benefiting off of the drug trade aren't just drug lords—remember that. Our government won't do the right thing and legalize marijuana unless we the people demand it because there are many people within our own government on the payroll all thanks to the War on Drugs.

Yes, this book calls for ending the War on Drugs. This book calls for ending the marijuana prohibition. I'm not an anarchist. I believe in laws and regulations, but I also believe in common sense, and the government hasn't been doing a good job in that department when it comes to cannabis. Before she passed away, my mother often told me that the prohibition of alcohol is identical to the War on Drugs. And she should know because she lived through both. You can either read and study history or you'll find you're destined to repeat it. Alcohol prohibition is what started all the trouble in Mexico. Mexican border towns like Tijuana became cesspools of crime, corruption, prostitution, and drugs all because of the prohibition of alcohol. Americans would go across the border to drink in towns like Tijuana, and then once the ban on alcohol was lifted, the criminals just strengthened their stronghold on the supply of marijuana until it became a major industry.

I've said it a million times: just because something is illegal, that doesn't mean it goes away, it just means criminals now run it. Take the Mexican drug cartels. They're now more powerful than the government. Guns are illegal in Mexico, yet they have guns. They have the money and they have the power. It's not rocket science. If we end the War on Drugs, then the cartels no longer have the power. It just takes politicians with the courage to do the right thing. Remember, as I said before, it's not just the drug lords who are getting richer off of the War on Drugs. Our politicians in Washington are making big money by keeping drugs illegal. As Deep Throat in *All the President's Men* said, "Follow the money. Always follow the money." It will take you to the answer.

To all the parents out there who are worried about how marijuana legalization will impact their children, I say, parent. It's as simple as that. I've been for the legalization of marijuana for years. Neither one of my adult children are drug addicts. It's that simple.

Think about it this way: what does marijuana actually do to you? You can't overdose on it. You might gain a couple of pounds, you know, from eating too much once the effects kick in and you get the munchies. You might have to work out a little bit harder the next day to compensate, but other than that, what's the downside? Oh yeah, it makes you high and it makes you feel good. That's a negative? Ha! Give a guy a joint, some Jimi Hendrix music, and a pizza, and that guy will be entertained for hours. Give the same guy alcohol and he might drink and drive or get violent and hurt someone.

I say legalize marijuana because we have a chance to leave this world a better place for our children. Marijuana legalization is job creation, tax dollars, something to rejuvenate our pathetic economy. This is a multibillion-dollar industry. This is about jobs; this is about economics; this is about freedom. This is about taking our country back. This is about getting out of these useless wars and getting back to what matters most to Americans: taking care of our own economy and our own citizens.

Cannabis is a plant that grows abundantly, that has been around long before laws existed, before our country even existed, and has a multitude of modern-day uses—aside from getting hippies high. If you read this book, you'll find out that this plant can literally cure cancer. This plant can literally end our dependence on foreign oil and fracking. This plant can literally rebuild our economy—we can make everything from car parts to airplane parts to paper to clothing to nutritious meals cheaply from it, but only if the American people are smart enough to recognize the truth from the bullshit.

The truth is, none of those uses for cannabis that I just mentioned is new. They might seem groundbreaking, almost too good to be true, but there are other countries taking advantage of those uses right now, and the United States is falling behind again. We've known about these and many other unique benefits of cannabis for generations, yet we continue to dig a hole deeper and deeper into the sand and stick our heads in it. Why? All because of a ridiculous movie called *Reefer Madness*? All because the DARE program says marijuana is a "gateway drug"? All because our government doesn't want us to believe there are more uses for this plant other than just hippies getting high?

The conspiracy against this plant is one that dates back hundreds of years. Our country was founded on this plant. I bet you didn't know that. I bet you didn't know that when the thirteen colonies paid their taxes to the British crown, the colonists had the option of paying for it in hemp because hemp was more valuable than money. Yet, our country has been successful in morphing a negative connotation of this plant for a select few people's political gains and for a select few corporations' profits. The select few in both cases just happen to be powerful enough to create a propaganda campaign that is still in existence today . . . primarily because those same forces from our history books have changed hands over the years, but they still carry the same agenda.

This book presents the facts and evidence from primary sources, such as scientific research documents and medical studies, to prove the greatest cover-up of all time: We've been at war with a plant for generations.

And for what purpose? You'll soon find out.

This book will also show you the practical, everyday applications of this plant. From biodiesel fuel to cooking and baking recipes to nutrition facts, this book will show you what this plant can do to change your every day life for the better.

And for all those religious people reading this book, remember this: God supposedly created the earth and everything in it . . . including cannabis. So if God created everything on earth for us to use, how dare we try to eradicate a plant that He put here for countless uses? Think about it. It's here for a reason. Let me prove to you how valuable that reason is through this book.

When I was governor, I tried to legalize hemp. I would have done anything to do it, but the legislature wouldn't even give the people of Minnesota the opportunity to vote on it. Well, I left office in 2003, and I find it ridiculous that today there is only limited medical marijuana legislation in my home state. Hemp makes the best biodiesel fuel on the planet. Medical marijuana helps people who are sick from chemotherapy eat. I challenge anyone in government: What right do you have to tell someone what they can or cannot use if they have cancer? Do you have a medical license? What right do you have to turn sick people into criminals so that they can eat?

There was a time when I was proud to be an American. There was a time when I looked at the United States and looked at the future of my country with hope. I don't necessarily have that feeling today. Most days I don't recognize my country or the American values that my parents fought so hard to uphold in World War II. I wrote this book with the hope that this might change in my lifetime. When it really comes down to it, you're reading a book written by a veteran, a former mayor, a former governor, and a former Harvard (yes, the Ivy League university) professor. I am pro-freedom, I am pro-marijuana, and I've written this book to show you how we can take our country back.

1

Mexico Says *Sí* to Recreational Weed

I 've said it before and I'll say it again: marijuana is to rock 'n' roll what beer is to baseball. If you took away beer from a baseball game—or really any sporting event—you'd have some fans in the stadium ready to riot. Well, as far as I'm concerned, it's the same way with marijuana and music. For many people who go to concerts, marijuana is just part of the whole experience. It's a recreational activity, just as drinking beer is at a baseball game.

There are many legal activities we can partake in that aren't exactly healthy decisions, but our government has no say in how frequently we do them or if we're doing them to excess. For instance, as Americans we can buy and consume as much alcohol as we want, we can smoke as many cigarettes as we want, and we can eat as much fast food as we want. All of these decisions aren't exactly good decisions for our health. Take alcohol, for example. If you drink too much, it can cause liver damage, addiction, even death. According to the CDC, in 2014 alone, more Americans died from alcohol-induced causes (30,722) than from overdoses of prescription painkillers and heroin combined (28,647).[1] As an American citizen, you have the right to literally drink, smoke, and eat yourself to death, but when it comes to consuming marijuana, that's off the table, even though it is impossible to die from smoking too much pot.

Here's the way I see it: every person on the planet should be allowed the freedom to use his or her judgment when it comes to what's best for his or her life and well-being, as long as it doesn't infringe on anyone else's rights. If you want to go into cardiac arrest from eating five Big Macs three times a day, then that's your prerogative. If you want to use marijuana to alleviate a migraine headache, be my guest.

Oddly enough, this philosophy of "do what you want as long as it doesn't infringe on anyone else's rights" now applies to marijuana use in Mexico. Get this: According to the Mexican constitution, the government cannot pass any law that prohibits the free development of a Mexican citizen's personality.[2] In fact, the Mexican Constitution states that all Mexican citizens have the right to develop their own unique personalities without government restriction or intervention. How does one develop a unique personality? By doing what you want as long as it doesn't infringe on anyone else's rights!

Under their constitution, Mexicans have the fundamental rights "to personal identity, self-image, free development of personality, self-determination and individual liberty, which arise from the same recognition of human dignity, and the right to health."[3] Which is why in November 2015, the Mexican Supreme Court ruled in a 4–1 decision that personal recreational use of marijuana is covered under the constitutional right of "free development of personality."[4] Just as the Mexican government can't prohibit its citizens from drinking as much beer as they want simply because it's bad for their health, it now can't prohibit its citizens from using marijuana. How's that for freedom of expression?

Now before all you marijuana enthusiasts dreaming of the opportunity to fully develop your own unique personalities start googling "how to apply for Mexican citizenship," you should know that this ruling only affects the four people who challenged the law and won the Supreme Court case. The court ruled that the four plaintiffs—two lawyers, an accountant, and a social activist—are allowed to "sow, grow, harvest, prepare, possess, transport, and consume marijuana for recreational uses." [5] However, they are not allowed to sell or distribute the drug or smoke it in the presence of children or anyone else "who hasn't given consent."[6] As long as they don't hinder anyone else's rights, they're free to light up a joint wherever and whenever they'd like.

So how did four people get the Supreme Court to allow them to produce, possess, and consume marijuana when it is illegal for anyone else in Mexico to do so?

In 2013, four members of the activist group known as the Mexican Society for Responsible and Tolerant Consumption (*la Sociedad Mexicana de Autoconsumo*

Responsable y Tolerante, or SMART, as the acronym reads in Spanish) started a petition to grow, own, and use marijuana.[7] The petition was initially denied, but the four members then appealed to the Supreme Court, and the rest is history.

The usual argument for Mexico to legalize marijuana is that if drugs were legalized, then that would end the drug cartels and the overwhelming death tolls from the War on Drugs. SMART is the first activist group to ever try to change the law by stating it is against the Mexican constitution, and they certainly succeeded. Meanwhile, in America, the same argument would probably never even see its day in court!

After the four members of SMART won their case, more individuals have come forward citing the same reasoning—that "using marijuana is just one way for individuals to differentiate themselves from the rest of society, and that since the Mexican constitution protects the individual's right to be unique and independent, the state cannot infringe upon that right."[8] Currently, there are five Supreme Court petitions pending, and if the court rules the same way on those five petitions, it would then establish the precedent to change the law and allow general recreational use for all Mexican citizens.[9] When that happens, all Mexican citizens would have a basic human right under their constitution to get high. Could you imagine?

Some people may think this decision is insignificant because only four Mexicans have the right to use pot as they see fit, but I see the Supreme Court's decision as the way marijuana should be legalized. The court recognized that Mexicans have a constitutional right to use the plant, regardless of the fact that marijuana legalization isn't a popular issue among the majority of Mexicans. Keep in mind, the Mexican Supreme Court made this decision even though President Enrique Peña Nieto has repeatedly stated he opposes legalization,[10] and the number of Mexicans who consume marijuana or approve of its use is extremely small in comparison to their American neighbors. Exactly one day after the Mexican Supreme Court ruling, the newspaper *El Universal* published a poll showing that two-thirds of Mexicans still oppose legalizing marijuana.[11] Meanwhile in America, Pew Research complied data in April 2015 from various surveys and Gallup polls to determine that at least 53 percent of Americans want marijuana to be legalized.[12] And our federal government continues to classify marijuana and heroin as equally addictive and equally dangerous. How's that for democracy?

So in one instance, a country is ensuring that all citizens can express their individuality, regardless of what the president or the majority might believe, because it is against the law to deny anyone the right to individuality. Yet, here we are in the "Land of the Free," where the majority of the citizens want marijuana to be legalized and we can't get our federal government to grant us that same right. Hell, even President Obama has admitted to smoking marijuana. So has George W. Bush. So have the majority of 2016 presidential hopefuls—and smoking marijuana was one hundred percent illegal at the time they all did it. Did you notice how none of them have a criminal record for consuming an illegal substance?

Yes, it is one hundred percent legal for only four people in Mexico to grow and consume marijuana, but marijuana isn't one hundred percent legal for even one American, even though the drug has been "legalized" in some way, shape, or form in twenty-three states. In every state, there are huge restrictions on every aspect of marijuana "legalization." No one can grow it without getting a license from the state or without paying excessive taxes. No one can sell it without paying excessive taxes. No one can consume it without paying excessive taxes. (Are you seeing a theme here?) Plus, consumers have limits as to how much they can buy at one time and how much they can carry on them at any given moment. Meanwhile, the Mexican Supreme Court hasn't made any of these stipulations for the four members of SMART. They can grow as much as they want, carry as much as they want, and even smoke as much as they want. That's true legalization as far as I'm concerned.

Take Colorado, for instance. If you're a Colorado resident, you can buy up to 1 oz. of marijuana at one time, but if you're visiting from another state, you can only purchase up to 1/4 oz. at a time.[13] Name one other legal substance that is regulated in this manner. Like I said before, I can buy as much alcohol as I want because it is a legal substance. So if marijuana is truly legal in Colorado, why can't I max out my credit card in a retail marijuana shop if I so choose to? As I said earlier, there were more alcohol-related deaths in 2014 than heroin-related deaths and we keep hearing that there's a national heroin epidemic in this country. So why am I not limited to the amount of alcohol I can purchase if it's such a deadly substance? Could you imagine if the government did such a thing? Let's limit the amount of beer to a six-pack per person per day and see how much rioting there'd be in the streets! If a substance is legal to purchase, then I should be allowed to purchase as much of it as I so desire. To me, that's the definition of a legal substance.

Just as a side note, I will be presenting marijuana laws throughout this book, but I won't be going into all the fine print when it comes to what states have and haven't legalized marijuana. Whenever a state legalizes medical or recreational marijuana, that state's lawmakers write a whole litany of stipulations as to what is and isn't legal in the state's constitution; Colorado's limitations on how much pot an individual can purchase is just one example. Needless to say, each state is different, and comparing each state's individual marijuana laws is another book for another time. If you aren't sure which states have legalized marijuana or if you aren't sure to what degree marijuana has been "legalized" or decriminalized, the answer is just a few clicks away. Websites like *NORML* and *Leafly* list that information and update it accordingly as laws change. Anyway, back to Mexico.

Sure, Mexico isn't allowing the four people to sell their pot, but there aren't any stipulations on how much they can grow or consume, and it's being treated just like any other crop. If they want to have a vegetable garden in their back-yards, they can plant as many cucumbers, tomatoes, and marijuana plants as they'd like. Before you get all up in arms about cannabis not being a vegetable, there's roughly 10 g of vegetable protein in three tablespoons of hemp seeds.[14] Shelled hemp seeds (also known as hulled hemp seeds) are actually considered the most nutritious superfood on the planet (more on this later). Those four SMART members could very well become the healthiest human beings in a country of approximately 120 million people if they decide to grow hemp.

And just as a side note, for those of you who don't know, hemp doesn't flower or grow buds like the marijuana plant, which means it can't get you high. It just produces seeds and abundantly strong fibers that can be used to make practically anything. Hemp is being used to make airplane parts, car parts, clothing, lotions, paper, biodiesel fuel—did I also mention it's nutritious? But all that doesn't matter, because America has yet to cash in on the true value of cannabis, and we probably never will. I hope that won't be the case. I hope I'll see true marijuana and hemp legalization within my lifetime, but I'm afraid that goes against our basic, capitalistic principles.

Let me put it to you this way: if marijuana is legalized in America, it won't be because "it's the right thing to do." We won't be going the way of the Mexicans on this one. Pot will be legalized because of the vast amount of money that can be made off of it. When enough politicians, corporations, and the general public realize how much money is on the table, marijuana will become legal in America very quickly. However, it will never be one-hundred-percent legal, as it is for the four Mexican citizens, because then we couldn't regulate it and tax it and make ridiculous amounts of money off of it. For me, that's the most surprising takeaway from this Mexican Supreme Court case: those four Mexicans don't have to pay any additional taxes in return for the right to grow and consume weed.

I also find it interesting that after the Supreme Court's marijuana decision, I have yet to hear from any American politician on whether or not this could potentially change the drug trade or end the War on Drugs completely. I'm sure we'll be quick to point the finger when something bad happens that we can somehow link to this decision, but could crime go down if marijuana were legalized in Mexico? Let's say, hypothetically, that this one decision did open a can of worms and Mexico does decide to legalize marijuana nationwide. Would this stop the drug war killings and kidnappings and put the Mexican cartels out of business? Yes and no.

2

How to Win the War on Drugs

I believe there is a way to win the war against the drug cartels: America and Mexico would have to legalize all drugs that have the potential for substance abuse, just like we do with tobacco and alcohol. Legalizing marijuana alone isn't enough.

Even if we just decriminalized all drugs, we could significantly help addicts get the care they need in clinics and hospitals. Drug addiction should be treated medically because addiction is a medical condition. Putting drug addicts into jail doesn't solve the root cause of the problem.

As the famous quote goes, "Insanity is doing the same thing over and over again but expecting different results." This type of insanity describes the so-called War on Drugs perfectly. We continue to treat drug addiction criminally. However, if we treat it as a medical condition, I think you'd see our incarceration rates drop dramatically due to the fact that we are not putting these people in jail but in hospitals and rehab facilities. I think you'd see the drug war death tolls drop dramatically too.

In 2009, Mexico did decriminalize the possession of small amounts of all major narcotics, from marijuana, to cocaine, to heroin, to ecstasy, to crystal meth.[1] Instead of arresting people caught with drugs, the police advised them to get clean and even gave them the addresses to the nearest rehab clinics. When I say *small* amounts of drugs, however, I mean *really small* amounts, what I would consider a nearly insignificant amount of drugs: cocaine was set at 0.5 g, heroin at 50 mg, methamphetamines at 40 mg, and marijuana at 5 g. These amounts are all considered acceptable "personal use" amounts—meaning if a person is caught with this amount, it is clear that person isn't intending to sell it (which is still illegal) but that the person is intending to use it. I'd like to know, however, how the courts arrived at these particular quantities as the exact amount for "personal use." For instance, in Washington state and Colorado, it is legal to have up to 28 g (about 1 oz.) of marijuana on you, and that is considered "personal use."[2] See what I mean by 5 g of marijuana being an insignificant amount? In any case, this decriminalization law has yet to lower arrest rates because officers rarely arrested people caught with those small amounts of drugs in the first place. They typically used the opportunity to get a bribe out of someone. Again, it still remains illegal to sell drugs in any capacity, so clearly that isn't stopping anyone from buying them.

Unfortunately, the law didn't achieve very much because the police wanted the drug dealers all along, not the small quantity buyers. Case in point: 60 percent of the 254,108 people in Mexico's prison system are incarcerated due to drug-related crimes.[3] In Mexico, there is also a huge disparity between the sentences for small-time drug dealers and violent criminals. For example, a 2012 Center for Research and Teaching in Economics (CIDE) study revealed a drug dealer can receive a maximum of twenty-five years in jail, but the maximum for armed robbery is fifteen years, and it's just fourteen years for a convicted rapist.[4] Does that sound like justice to you? A rapist could be out of jail and on the streets eleven years earlier than a drug dealer!

Now, don't get me wrong. I am well aware of the drug-war death tolls and the strong arm of the Mexican cartels. I understand that a drug dealer could also be a violent criminal. Six months out of the year, I live completely off the grid in Mexico on the Baja peninsula. I live in a solar-paneled house. I'm about an hour from paved roads and any building powered by Mexico's electrical grid. I can't speak much Spanish (and the Spanish I can speak, I admittedly don't speak very well), but I can get across what I need to say through pantomiming. If you ask a local down there, you might be surprised to know that the majority of Mexicans think it's shameful to admit to or be accused of drug use. Being called a *marijuano* (pronounced "marihuano") or pot head is actually considered an insult. That's part of their culture, probably because if you're a Mexican citizen caught with too much of any illegal drug, including marijuana, you could be subject to prosecution, heavy fines, and even jail time. And probably because the drug trade and the cartels have done such horrible things to the Mexican people that no Mexican would want to be associated with them in any way.

Consider these facts: In July 2015, the Mexican government released data showing that between 2007 and 2014, more than 164,000 people were victims of homicide due to the drug war[5] and in 2007 alone, 2,837 people were killed.[6] To put those numbers into perspective, let's compare War on Drugs casualties to casualties from two other American wars that were being fought between 2007 and 2014, also on foreign soil. The United Nations and the Iraq Body Count website estimate that there were 103,000 civilian deaths in Afghanistan and Iraq over that same seven-year time period.[7] That means there were approximately 61,000 more civilians who died in Mexico due to the War on Drugs in comparison to the War on Terror.

Also worth considering are the fatalities of our troops in the Iraq and the Afghanistan wars: 2,379 US soldiers died in the Afghanistan War (from 2001 to January 2016). In the Iraq War, 4,495 US soldiers died from 2003 to 2015.[8] That means more people died in Mexico in 2007—in one year—compared to the amount of US troops that died throughout the entire span of the Afghanistan war. And when it comes to the 4,495 US soldiers who died throughout the entire span of the Iraq war? In 2008 alone, the Mexican government reported there were 6,844 people killed in Mexico's drug war. In 2009, there were 9,635 people who died due to the drug war. Again, that means more people died in one year in Mexico than the number of service men and women in the entire span of the Iraq war (and the entire span of the Afghanistan war, for that matter). Go ahead, reread that and let it sink in a little.

The War on Drugs has also resulted in thousands of people being kidnapped. Over twenty-six thousand people have gone missing in Mexico between 2006 and 2012.[9] Hundreds of villages have been devastated, and families have been forced to abandon their homes out of fear for their lives. That is the tragic cost of the War on Drugs. As long as we continue this war, the death toll will continue to climb. As I've said before, just because you make something illegal, that doesn't mean it goes away. That just means criminals now run it. And as long as drugs are illegal, the cartels will stay in business, and they're doing quite well for themselves too, if I might add. According to a bi-national study conducted by our government agencies and Mexican government agencies (including Homeland Security's Office of Counternarcotics Enforcement, US Immigration and Customs Enforcement, Mexico Secretaría de Hacienda y Crédito Publico, and Unidad De Inteligencia Financiera), the Mexican drug cartels reap between $19 billion and $29 billion, approximately, in profits from US drug sales each year.[10] So will legalizing marijuana in Mexico put a dent in the cartels' profits? I think the greater question is: Why does America insist on fighting wars it cannot win?

When it comes to marijuana in particular, the United States has—to put it lightly—a very sensitive relationship with Mexico. Our government is constantly putting the blame on our southern neighbors when it comes to our illegal drug problem. Our politicians say Mexico is lax in confiscating illegal drugs that are produced in the country and then shipped into the United States. We're also constantly pointing out the corruption within the Mexican government (because there's zero corruption in DC, right?) and claiming there are back-channel bribery deals between Mexican politicians, law enforcement, and Mexico's drug cartels. We claim the drug war will never go away because the Mexican drug cartels are part of the Mexican economic infrastructure. Talk about a conspiracy theory!

Meanwhile, Mexico is quick to respond to these accusations with the obvious: there would be no illegal drug problem between our borders if the demand from American drug users didn't create this lucrative market in the first place. And I agree. This is about supply and demand. If American drug users didn't want Mexican drugs, they wouldn't buy them. Again, just because you prohibit something, that doesn't mean it goes away. People will always find a way to get what they want, if they want it badly enough.

To further this point, when marijuana was "legalized" in the United States, demand for illegal Mexican weed actually decreased and is continuing to decrease. The Drug Policy Research Center at the RAND Corporation states that in 2008, Mexico was responsible for as much as two-thirds of the marijuana consumed in America each year, [11] but because it is now legal for people to grow pot in the United States, Mexican marijuana accounts for less than a third of the total amount consumed in the United States today. Less than a third! Like I said, supply and demand. If I can purchase weed legally from a store, why on earth would I risk getting arrested to purchase it illegally from another country? We're not putting the cartels out of business yet, but as Bob Dylan said, "the times, they are a-changin'!"

There isn't much reliable data right now to determine how much marijuana is being produced in Mexico—or rather how much *less* weed is being produced—due to the limited legalization of marijuana in America. But we do know that the amount of weed that is being confiscated at the US border has decreased.

So has the amount of weed that has been found and destroyed in fields by the Mexican government.

According to the Mexican attorney general's office, in 2015, the Mexican government eradicated about twelve thousand acres of illegal marijuana, which is down from more than forty-four thousand acres in 2010.[12] And although drug seizures at the border only represent a tiny fraction of what actually gets imported into the United States, the US Customs and Border Protection seized about 1,085 tons of marijuana at the border in 2014, which is less than the previous four years with 1,500 tons confiscated each year.[13] And when it comes to arrests, the US Drug Enforcement Administration (DEA) is seeing declining numbers as well. The *Los Angeles Times* reports that the number of US arrests by DEA agents involving foreign-grown marijuana dropped from 4,519 in 2010 to 2,367 in 2014.[14] I suspect that these numbers will continue to decrease as Americans continue to buy homegrown, legal marijuana.

Also interesting to note is that the price of Mexican marijuana has decreased dramatically, which again follows the typical economic principles of supply and demand. Within the last four years, since there hasn't been as much of a demand for Mexican marijuana, the amount that Mexican farmers receive per kilogram has fallen from $100 to $30![15] Stay with me here, people. I'm proving to you that by legalizing drugs we will loosen the grip of the cartels!

There's one more thing that no one seemed to anticipate when weed was legalized in certain parts of the United States: quality of product. US and Mexican growers now compete not only on price, but also on quality. My good friend Dan Skye, the editor-in-chief of *High Times* magazine, would be able to vouch for me on this statistic: Mexican weed is without a doubt the bottom of the barrel when it comes to quality. First of all, it's not as fresh as what you'd get in your local smoke shop. Secondly, it's typically pressed tightly together due to the way it's transported—and it's full of seeds. When you're looking for quality weed, look no further than cannabis grown in the USA because our legal weed distributors take great pride in their products! Legalization has also created demand for unique strains of weed, not to mention more specialized strains with higher concentrations of THC.

Think of American marijuana like craft beer: When it comes to beer, there's always Budweiser, which will do the trick, but there are also local microbreweries that specialize in various flavors and higher alcohol contents. If you drink beer, what are you going to go with if you have a choice? Something in a can, that's been sitting on a shelf for months—and before it got there, it went through several forms of refrigeration, and at some point wasn't even refrigerated—or something fresh from the tap that was brewed with great emphasis on the quality, flavor, and brewing technique? Sure, Budweiser might be cheaper, but they also skimp on flavor and the freshness of ingredients.

So, back to our hypothetical scenario from Chapter 1: If Mexico and America legalized marijuana, would it make the Mexican cartels go the way of the dodo bird? Well, if Mexicans are allowed to grow it in their own backyards and Americans are allowed to do the same, then who needs to purchase pot illegally? If I can go to a store and buy it legally, why would I take the risk to get it on the black market, especially since I don't know exactly what I'm getting? Now that marijuana is being regulated in the states where it is legal, it is being inspected and tested for pesticides and other harmful chemicals, just like any other consumer good. In December 2015, marijuana products from over one hundred thousand plants in Colorado were recalled when independent lab testing by the *Denver Post* showed that they contained high levels of banned pesticides.[16] Luckily, no one reported any illness from partaking in pot grown with pesticide treatment, but that raises a very interesting question: Would you trust a Mexican drug lord to be up front with how the plant was grown? How would you even verify that information? I know people cringe when I say legalize all drugs, but when something is legalized, you take the power away from the criminals, and you know the purity of the substance because it's being regulated. If people no longer have to rely on Mexican drug cartels for their weed, then there will be one less illegal substance responsible for all the death and destruction the drug trade has caused. It's as simple as that.

To go back to why we should be legalizing *all* drugs, let's not forget that the Mexican drug cartels do not make all of their money from marijuana, and they are already adapting to the changing markets. It's no secret that Mexican cartels make more money selling heroin and meth than they do pot.[17] A 2010 RAND study claimed that marijuana only accounted for 15 percent to 26 percent of cartel revenues.[18] I'm sure that percentage has decreased even more now that America is busy growing the Rolls Royce of weed strains. Even though poppy plants (what heroin is made from) are a more labor-intensive crop than weed, require more water, take longer to mature, and the seeds are overall are more expensive and difficult to acquire, the profits are greater. There is a heroin epidemic in America, and we are driving up the prices for the underground market yet again. The Mexican cartels are already shifting from marijuana fields to poppy fields due to the principles of supply and demand. You know, it's no accident that the world's biggest consumer of illegal drugs and the world's biggest supplier of illegal drugs just happen to be neighbors.

Now, there are benefits and setbacks from switching gears from the marijuana market to cocaine, heroin, and meth. There's a reason why coke and heroin cost so much more than pot on the street. See, addicts aren't paying for the drugs; they're actually compensating everyone along the distribution chain for the risks they took in getting the drug into the neighborhood. According to *New York Times* magazine, the value-to-weight ratio of heroin is better than any other drug, but moving it is a "capital-intensive business."[19] Mexican drug cartels typically subsidize the cost of heroin with their ready source of easy income: marijuana. Even though Mexican pot is cheap to buy, it's often considered the "cash crop" for Mexican cartels because it is grown abundantly in the Sierra mountain region and requires no processing.[20] However, pot is bulkier to carry and it has a very particular smell, which makes it difficult to conceal no matter how it is transported. So moving away from the "cash crop" of marijuana to plant more poppy fields might mean profits could initially go down, but they'll eventually go back up again as heroin will ultimately bring back a better profit margin. Also, there's a huge difference between those who smoke pot and those who use heroin. Heroin is extremely addictive—just one use and a person could be hooked for life—whereas marijuana isn't an addictive substance at all. In fact, pot can be used in rehab situations to help a person kick heroin addiction. So when it comes down to it, by focusing on heroin rather than pot, the Mexican cartels will be able to secure repeat customers. Many Americans will unfortunately be invested for life. It's true that more Americans use marijuana than heroin, but remember—the profit is bigger from heroin than marijuana. And if the drug cartels need another "cash crop" to replace marijuana, they can just start cooking more meth.

When Mexican drug cartels first started producing meth, they stashed the product in cocaine and marijuana shipments to the United States and they let their usual customers try it out for free.[21] Today, the drug sells for so much money in the United States that the cartels don't even bother shipping it to Europe. Compared to pot, meth is much easier to smuggle into the United States because it isn't bulky, it doesn't smell, and it sells out instantly. Meth is more addictive than cocaine, and it is much more expensive to purchase than marijuana.

For instance, in 2002, the Office of National Drug Control Policy (ONDCP) reported that 1 g of pure meth could sell for as much as $330 in Chicago, but only $60 in Seattle.[22] Today, an ounce of meth costs nearly ten times as much as an ounce of gold.[23] There are approximately 1.4 million meth users in America;[24] needless to say, this is a booming market for Mexican drug cartels. In fact, the DEA's 2015 National Drug Threat Assessment noted that the cartels are shifting away from the cocaine business and moving toward building more meth "super labs."[25] In 2015, the DEA saw that the amount of cocaine caught by law enforcement dropped in nearly every significant smuggling corridor along the entire US–Mexico border. There was a 20 percent drop in South Texas's Rio Grande Valley and a 12 percent drop in San Diego—the two places that are known to be hot spots for cocaine trafficking. Meanwhile, meth seizures are climbing by 90 percent in the Rio Grande Valley and 245 percent in El Paso. That's just in one year.

Another reason why meth is on the rise is because it is much more addictive than coke, which means the drug cartels have an even better consumer base. Animal studies conducted at UCLA show that cocaine releases 350 units of dopamine (what creates the high), while meth releases almost four times as much—about 1,200 units.[26] Now, your brain produces dopamine naturally and when you have that much more dopamine in your system, it actually causes your body to produce less dopamine until it stops producing it entirely. The more a person uses meth, the more the drug changes the brain's wiring until it actually destroys the brain's dopamine receptors. This is why the drug is so addictive. Once the dopamine receptors are destroyed, meth users can never experience pleasure again unless they artificially put more dopamine into their bodies by using more meth. Although dopamine receptors can eventually grow back over time, chronic meth use can also cause other permanent brain damage, including declines in reasoning, judgment, and motor skills.[27] Needless to say, I'm against meth use one hundred percent, but just because I'm against it, that doesn't mean people won't use it. All we're doing by making it illegal is helping the Mexican cartels get more rich and powerful.

So just how powerful are the Mexican cartels today? *New York Times* magazine reports that the cartels bribe a host of senior officials—from mayors and prosecutors to governors, state police and federal police, to the army and the navy.[28] To give you an example of how high up the chain of command this bribery extends, in 2008, President Felipe Calderón's own drug czar, Noe Ramirez, was charged with accepting $450,000 each *month* from the drug cartels![29] But the bribery doesn't end there. Our guards at the US border are also pawns in the system. *New York Times* magazine reports that US border security guards have been known to wave cars through checkpoints—without doing any of the procedural searches—for a few thousand dollars.[30] How's that for your tax dollars at work? From 2004 to 2012, there have been 138 convictions or indictments in corruption investigations involving members of the United States Customs and Border Protection,[31] and don't get me started on what the DEA has been getting away with—more on that in chapter 3. True to our capitalistic nature, our government employees are certainly not above being bribed by the cartels in the so-called War on Drugs!

In the interest of preserving life, I think it's high time we consider some alternatives to whatever our strategy has been in the never-ending War on Drugs. We've been at "war" with drugs since President Nixon proclaimed us to be in 1971. As of 2016, that's forty-five years ago! The *Associated Press* reports that in the past forty years, we've spent $1 trillion on the drug war.[32] I say *we* because our taxpayer money is what's footing the bill. On average, we're spending about $51 billion a year trying to eradicate drugs from our country. Meanwhile, the DEA has been successful in capturing less than 10 percent of all illegal drugs that enter the United States. How much more money do you think it will take to stop the other ninety percent? Too much. Does $51 billion a year for a 90 percent failure rate seem like a good investment of our tax dollars to you? I know that $51 billion per year has done nothing to change the fact that illegal drugs are readily available and people are continuing to use them nationwide. I also know that we spent over $900 million in the first week of 2016 alone on the War on Drugs! For what? We might never know! You can check for yourself to see how much we are spending each day on a second-by-second basis at the drug war clock: http://www.drugsense.org/cms/wodclock.

What is wrong with our country? How can the war on drugs possibly be worth it? Addiction is a mental health issue. It should not be treated criminally. That's why we have prisons that are full, and that's why we're paying hundreds of millions of dollars for these people to stay in jail instead of getting them the help they need.

My final thought is simply this: the drug war is not working. We have to start looking at all drugs as a necessary evil, not just select drugs like tobacco and alcohol. The only way to fight back is to educate and treat people. Incarceration doesn't work. Allowing drugs to be managed by criminals doesn't work. Allowing drugs to be legal? We haven't tried that yet. Maybe Mexico's Supreme Court decision will allow marijuana to be fully legalized. Government officials are already looking into the benefits of medical marijuana, and 79 percent of Mexican citizens are in favor of its medical use.[33] Who knows, maybe if Mexico loosens its marijuana laws, it will also update its decriminalization laws so more people wind up getting treatment instead of jail time. Any way you look at it, the United States is the biggest consumer of drugs from Mexico, which means we're the major root of the problem, which means we have to change our policies as well. Too many lives are being destroyed.

There's a lot of money to be made from the legalization of marijuana. If we legalize marijuana nationwide, then we'll create more jobs than the Keystone Pipeline ever could. But not everyone sees it that way. Remember: always follow the money! The War on Drugs is happening because Democrats and Republicans are getting paid to keep it going.

Forget for a minute how much the United States stands to gain by ending this so-called war. Forget for a minute that we can make massive amounts of money off of the legalization of marijuana. Think for a minute: Who is making money off of the War on Drugs right now? Do you really think the DEA is going to turn around and say, yes, let's end this war? Why on earth would they? They'd all be out of a job! Think of all the committees and task forces too. Hillary Clinton is running for president, claiming it's time for prison reform, but in case you forgot, when her husband was president he did a great job of creating today's prison problems—like increasing mandatory minimum sentencing for minor drug offenses—and I'll be giving you a refresher course on that and more a little later on in this book.

If we want to end the War on Drugs, we need to elect the right people who truly want to reduce government. The people who truly want us to pay less in taxes. This war is happening because the people in power right now are being paid off to keep it going. Could you imagine how many people would be out of a job if the war on drugs ended today? People in high places are making money by keeping drugs—including marijuana—illegal, and it isn't just the cartels and the Mexican authorities.

3

Ross Ulbricht and the Silk Road Conspiracy

Before we get into marijuana's historical significance and how America turned from hemp production to the war against weed, you should know what we're up against when we all come together to demand that marijuana be legal once again, from sea to shining sea. Our government itself is the biggest obstacle standing in the way of marijuana legalization, and if you read Steve Kubby's foreword in this book, then you already know that. Over the past forty-five years, our politicians and presidents have thrown billions of tax dollars into the corrupt monster they created, known as the US Drug Enforcement Administration (DEA). Many of the "successes" from the War on Drugs do not make the six o'clock news because those who are taking down the drug lords and criminal masterminds do so through extortion, bribery, and a litany of illegal activities.

The last major publicized "victory" for the DEA was the takedown of Silk Road and the arrest of the site's creator, Ross Ulbricht, in 2013. However, the federal government hasn't tooted its horn about this recently and probably wants us to forget the whole operation ever occurred. An entire book could be written on Ross Ulbricht's takedown, subsequent trial, and his recent appeals process, especially because most articles about his case present false or misleading information. Maybe news sources were looking for clickbait headlines, but they definitely got the information wrong, and to this day, the majority of those articles haven't been corrected. When I first started looking into Ross Ulbricht's case, I wasn't comfortable with the discrepancies in facts, so I read through the court documents and corresponded with Ulbricht's legal team to get to the truth.

If you missed the whole Silk Road phenomenon and its downfall, here's a refresher:

- Silk Road was referred to as a "darknet" marketplace because it was tucked into another realm of the Internet that was completely inaccessible by any of the typical search engines like Google.
- The website was only accessible through a browser called Tor.
- Silk Road connected buyers and sellers completely anonymously so that they could buy and sell narcotics, false documents, and legal items that could be considered controversial, like raw milk. However, the site was mostly used for drug trafficking, and there were some items you couldn't sell or purchase, such as child pornography. You couldn't hire a hit man either. Remember that for later.
- All users paid with Bitcoin, which made all transactions completely anonymous.
- Ulbricht was accused of being the site's head honcho, whose username was the Dread Pirate Roberts (or DPR). DPR earned a commission on each transaction, which is how the jury considered him guilty of what the users were doing on the website: drug trafficking, money laundering, and hacking.
- Ulbricht was arrested in a San Francisco library in 2013.
- On the day he was arrested, Ublricht was downloading the *Colbert Report* on an open-source network at the library. At Ulbricht's trial, an undercover agent testified that he logged into Silk Road under his alias Cirrus and messaged DPR to log into his account. When DPR logged in to chat with Cirrus, the DEA arrested Ulbricht.
- The prosecution claimed Ulbricht was DPR, and that's why he was arrested. However, after looking through Ulbricht's trial documents, I've come to find out that there were others who had access to DPR's account as well, and that this was common knowledge. More on that later.
- On May 29, 2015, Ulbricht was sentenced to double life without parole, plus 40 years, which is virtually a triple life sentence.

- The federal judge didn't hide her intention of making an example of him. She stated at his trial hearing: "What you did was unprecedented, and in breaking that ground as the first person you sit here as the defendant now today having to pay the consequences for that."[1]
- Ulbricht's family, defense counsel, and supporters started a public campaign through the website FreeRoss.org and they filed an appeal in mid-January 2016.

Ulbricht is currently appealing his case,* not only because the government suppressed key exculpatory evidence, but also because his Fourth Amendment rights were violated when evidence was gathered against him. According to Ulbricht's appeal and an amicus brief—submitted by the National Association of Criminal Defense Lawyers (NACDL) and joined by Electronic Frontier Foundation (EFF) (which you can read in their entirety on FreeRoss.org)—the initial case against him should have been thrown out of court based on the fact that the government did not use constitutional warrants to search and seize Ulbricht's laptop, email, and social media accounts.[2]

Instead, the Secret Service obtained a court order directing Comcast to install—without any warrant—pen registers and trap and trace devices (known as pen-traps) on Ulbricht's routers, IP addresses, and MAC (Media Access Control) addresses. Then the government abused what the pen-trap is intended to be used for.

Now, I'm not all that technically inclined, but to put it simply, a pen-trap court order is only allowed to be used to verify identifying information (such as to verify a computer's IP address), but Ross's appeal asserts that these pen-traps had an ulterior purpose: "to track Ulbricht's Internet activity and his physical location, in an effort to connect him" to the Silk Road Servers as DPR.[3] In other words, the government used this basic pen-trap court order to monitor everything Ulbricht did online as well as where Ulbricht was when he accessed his computer. Well guess what? These additional purposes fall into violation of the Fourth Amendment because they require a warrant, which is a specific document that only allows monitoring a suspect based on probable cause. Since the government didn't have probable cause and obtained all evidence to implicate Ulbricht from this illegal pen-trap search, Ulbricht should have never gone to trial in the first place.

Yes, the pen-traps were acquired legally, but under the law, they were used *illegally* by the Secret Service. You can't put someone under surveillance like that without the proper warrant to do so. The FBI, Secret Service, and DEA were monitoring Ulbricht in his house, and wherever he used his laptop, and they also were monitoring his cell phone. Ulbricht's appeal brief lists previous cases where this type of monitoring requires a separate and specific warrant, which these government agencies never obtained in the Silk Road takedown.[4]

In their amicus brief, EFF and NACDL state that the court "ignored the limiting principles enshrined in the Fourth Amendment's protection against unreasonable searches and seizures,"[5] and my personal hero Edward Snowden took this a step further. Even though the NSA has ignored accusations of any involvement in the gathering of evidence against Ulbricht, Snowden has stated it is "unthinkable to him" that the NSA didn't play a role in extracting this information.[6]

What makes me think there is even more to this story is the convenient timing of "developing" information. Get this: Approximately two months *after* Ulbricht was convicted, news broke that two of the federal agents who took him down were actually under federal investigation for the past nine months for stealing and extorting funds from Silk Road.

The lead undercover agent at the core of the Maryland Silk Road investigation—DEA agent Carl Mark Force IV—and Secret Service agent Shaun Bridges pled guilty to a massive corruption scheme. Here are the details of their illegal activities:

- DEA agent Carl Mark Force IV pleaded guilty to extortion, money laundering, and obstruction of justice.
- Force was with the DEA for fifteen years; two of those years he worked as an undercover agent in an interagency team tasked with identifying the owner of Silk Road.
- He used his position to swindle at least $700,000 in Bitcoin money.[7]
- Once he and Bridges figured out how to manipulate the administrator platform on Silk Road, he seized more than $300,000 in assets from Bitcoin users and transferred it into his account. He also siphoned Bitcoin given to him by the government to aid in the investigation into personal accounts and his own personal Bitcoin investment fund, Engedi LLC.[8]
- He extorted more than $200,000 from DPR in exchange for (fake) inside information on the federal investigation, and without notifying his supervisors, he signed a $240,000 contract with Twentieth Century Fox Film Studios for a film about the Silk Road takedown.[9]

- Shaun Bridges also pleaded guilty to money laundering, obstruction of justice, and pocketing 20,000 Bitcoins from the accounts of Silk Road users, which was worth $300,000 at the time.[10]
- Before he was brought up on charges, Bridges was able to create a shell company—Quantum International Investments LLC—and raise the value of his stolen Bitcoins to $820,000.[11]

In October 2015, Force was ordered to pay $340,000 in restitution to one of his victims, and he was given a paltry six-and-a-half-year sentence for thinking he was above the law and abusing his position as a public servant. In December 2015, Bridges received a seventy-one-month prison sentence. He was ordered to forfeit $475,000 and pay $500,000 in restitution.[12]

Then, the day before Shaun Bridges was scheduled to begin his prison sentence, he was arrested at his home in Laurel, Maryland. Court documents state that officers found several Secret Service–issued bulletproof vests—stolen from the government—as well as bags containing Bridges's passport, a notarized copy of his passport, and corporate records for three offshore "entities" in Nevis, Belize, and Mauritius.[13]

Here's the kicker though: Ross Ulbricht's defense team learned about the federal investigation into Bridges and Force only five weeks prior to his trial, but they were blocked from referring to documents from that federal investigation because the documents were sealed pending completion of the federal investigation![14] The defense requested that Ulbricht's trial be postponed until Force's and Bridges's investigations were concluded, so that they could have access to all the files and so that the jury could know the entire story, but the judge denied the request.

I find it oddly coincidental that the federal investigation on Force and Bridges concluded a mere two months *after* Ulbricht's trial. Impeccable timing, wouldn't you say?

To this day, there is still evidence from Force's and Bridges's investigations that are sealed or encrypted, such as email conversations that could possibly implicate them (and others). So Ulbricht's defense team still couldn't present the full story when they appealed his case in January 2016!

According to the correspondence I had with Ulbricht's attorneys, there is still material that remains fully encrypted. They told me, "As a result of these considerable gaps in knowledge of the misconduct with respect to what has been disclosed to us, and what the government doesn't even know, there is every reason to believe this is merely the tip of the iceberg." I'd like to paraphrase it in non-legal terms: To this day, no one knows the full extent of the grand jury's investigation into these agents. No one knows the full range of misconduct or if there were more people involved. No one knows what the government knows (or doesn't know) either! And unfortunately for Ross Ulbricht, we probably never will.

I ask you this: why would the federal government continue to protect a DEA agent and a Secret Service agent who are both serving time in prison right now? These two disgraced their agencies and made hundreds of thousands of dollars doing it, so why are their documents still sealed? And come on, these guys get a six-and-a-half-year sentence and almost a six-year sentence? Their sentences are a joke! They took oaths to support and defend the Constitution—oaths that they willingly violated—whereas Ulbricht did not. Why didn't they get the maximum sentences for their crimes—which was still only about twenty years?[15] And why did Ulbricht get the maximum sentencing for each count even though none of the charges accuse him of actually selling an illegal substance, laundering money, hacking into a computer, or selling fake IDs? Clearly, there are people at the top who wanted him to go down. He was charged because he ran a website that permitted these actions, all of which I might add are nonviolent and didn't cause anyone direct harm. No terrorist bought a fake ID from Silk Road, and no one got stabbed or beaten or shot as a result of a drug deal.

Set aside for a moment that the goods and services on Silk Road were illegal. The actual operations of the web-based marketplace were legal and reputable. Members bought what they paid for; no one was in a situation where they were ripped off by a customer or a seller, and DPR certainly didn't steal from any of them either, even though clearing out their Bitcoin bank accounts was something he could have easily done at any time.

Yes, selling an illegal drug is illegal, but Ulbricht created a site that allowed drugs to be sold in an incredibly safe capacity. Buyers knew exactly what they were getting. Before a buyer could make another purchase on the site, he had to leave feedback on the seller's page regarding the purchase. This allowed for community verification of a product, and since it was all done anonymously, no one had any reason to lie. Customers received their drugs through the mail, so Silk Road also shielded people from the violent interactions that the drug trade is known for. It was like a darknet Amazon, complete with reviews and great customer service. Since it was a marketplace beyond government control, using a made-up currency called Bitcoin, you can bet those who took Ulbricht down were the ones threatened the most by it. I'm sure the federal government wanted him to go away for life as a warning to anyone else who wanted to replicate the same concept, but the only problem with that logic is that others have created similar sites, and those sites are still up and running. And guess what: many of those sites are far bigger *and* more popular than Silk Road ever was!

It is also interesting to note that Ulbricht wasn't the only person who faced criminal charges in the Silk Road takedown, but he did receive the harshest sentencing. Jan Slomp, the site's leading drug seller, received ten years; Steven Sadler, the most successful heroin and cocaine dealer, received five years; and Peter Nash, who was the forum moderator and site administrator when Silk Road had its highest sales volume, got a mere seventeen months. So why did Ulbricht get the short end of the stick?

Here's why I think there was more to this federal corruption than two rogue, compromised agents: When Ulbricht was originally arrested, he was charged with ordering six assassinations through Silk Road. Then, two months after those charges were used to deny Ross Ulbricht bail, five of the six murder-for-hire charges were dropped completely without explanation, even though Ulbricht allegedly paid a total of $730,000 for these executions.[16] All we know is that DEA Agent Force and Bridges are behind the fake murder of Curtis Green, a Silk Road employee, which is the only murder-for-hire charge left.[17] The two claimed that DPR hired them to kill Green and paid them the Bitcoins necessary to do so. Keep in mind that ordering hit men through Silk Road was against the site's policies. DPR knew this better than anyone, so why would he break his own rules? There's also the fact that when someone pays an assassin to murder someone, there's a dead body. In this case, there wasn't any missing persons report filed and "there were no known deaths."[18]

Think about it: If you hired someone to *kill* another person, wouldn't you be suspicious if there was absolutely *no* news coverage? Even if the assassin disposed of the body somewhere where no one would ever find it, there would still be some kind of investigation into this person's disappearance. Even if these federal agents posing as hit men provided photos or some kind of "evidence" that they took Green out, wouldn't DPR wonder why no one had reported Green missing? Wouldn't that have raised a red flag that maybe the murder was staged, and that this could even cause DPR to go on the run or disappear, therefore compromising the entire investigation?

When federal agents started investigating this further in 2014, Force admitted to lying about the staged murder of Curtis Green.[19] Force and Bridges also admitted that they had the power to change aspects of Silk Road—including the ability to access administrator platforms and passwords, change PIN numbers, commandeer accounts—including the account of DPR—as well as to manipulate logs, chat room conversations, private messages, user posts, account information, and bank accounts,[20] so who knows what else they cooked up to implicate Ulbricht.

When the multiagency task force started to figure out the scale of the corruption Force used to take down Dread Pirate Roberts, upper management probably realized they had to come clean about something, or they could lose the entire case. That final sixth murder-for-hire charge was still on the table and now the agent who put forward the allegation said he lied! Think about it: How could the federal government drop the other five murder-for-hire charges without any explanation and then drop this last charge too? Wouldn't that put into question all of the other evidence that Force and his team collected?

Personally, I think Force and Bridges were thrown under the bus to cover everyone else involved in this takedown. Why else would their documents be concealed if they don't implicate anyone else, such as those who are farther up the chain of command? Force was probably ordered to do whatever it took to find Dread Pirate Roberts, and he certainly did what he was told and then some. I'd like to quote Lord Acton about what happens when you give someone total control: "Power tends to corrupt and absolute power corrupts absolutely."[21] This could be said about the DEA in general (more on that later) but in this situation, it is definitely what happened to the fifteen-year veteran in charge of the Silk Road takedown.

Think about it: Ulbricht was denied bail when he was arrested due to the six murder-for-hire charges. He was considered a flight risk. Hell, if he could get someone to kill for him six times, he could easily get out of the country, right? Well, shortly after his bail hearing, five of those six murder-for-hire charges were no longer on the table, and the sixth was based on the word of a corrupt agent. But by that time, every news source in the country had already run the fascinating story about this libertarian anarchist who didn't believe any laws applied to him. In the end, Ulbricht was never charged at trial with murder for hire, even though he was indicted in Maryland with planning the murder of Curtis Green the day he was arrested (October 1, 2013). This indictment was based on corrupt Agent Force's testimony, and, to this day, it has yet to be proven at trial that Ulbricht hired anyone to assassinate anybody. Unfortunately, because those articles about Ulbricht hiring assassins were never updated to reflect the truth, to this day the public has many grave misconceptions about him, unless, of course, people are willing to go to the primary source of the information—the trial documents—instead of a news article, and learn the truth.

Just because Ulbricht wasn't charged with murder for hire at his trial, that didn't stop the prosecution from liberally referring to how the DEA and Secret Service set him up by creating false user accounts on Silk Road and claiming to be hit men who will take out whoever DPR wanted for the right price. But let's put the pieces of the puzzle together in the right order:

1. Murder for hire wasn't allowed on Silk Road.
2. Force said he could manipulate DPR's accounts.
3. Maybe the *real* way the task force set Ulbricht up was fabricating the entire "hit men for hire" conversation by simply typing whatever "evidence" they wanted to collect on DPR.

When the intent-to-murder charges were officially taken off the table, six overdose death charges suddenly appeared at sentencing. The government claimed that six drug overdose deaths were the result of drugs sold through Silk Road, and in the end, these allegations also greatly contributed to Ulbricht's life sentencing.[22] Defense expert Mark L. Taff, MD, a board-certified forensic pathologist, reviewed the evidence behind the overdose deaths and "concluded the information was utterly insufficient to attribute any of the deaths to drugs purchased from vendors on Silk Road."[23] After reviewing the evidence, Dr. Taff disagreed with the official versions of the causes of death because "critical information was missing."[24]

In some cases, Taff couldn't make a determination whether the drugs came from Silk Road at all, and in one case, he couldn't determine if the primary cause of death was actually a drug overdose or due to a preexisting heart condition because the information was incomplete or unreliable.[25] The court barely acknowledged these discrepancies, and although the overdose deaths weren't even mentioned at Ulbricht's trial, this didn't stop the prosecution from exploiting the bereaved parents at his sentencing hearing to ultimately provide justification for the harsh punishment of a triple life sentence.

Excuse me, but even if people did overdose and die from drugs they bought through Silk Road, did Ulbricht force these people to buy the drugs? Did Ulbricht force these people to take the drugs in the quantity that they did? It stands to reason that these questions will be addressed again during Ulbricht's appeal, but it also stands to reason that the government will have a hard time backing down from being wrong about so many aspects of this case.

On May 29, 2015, the prosecution won in convincing the judge that Ulbricht was a dangerous man, capable of anything, when to this day they haven't been able to prove how he—a guy who previously owned a bookstore in Austin, Texas that donated its profits to charity[26]—somehow had the knowledge to create an encrypted global marketplace specializing in illegal drugs. We'll have to wait and see if Ulbricht's legal team prevails in the appeals process, which could take years. Meanwhile, Ulbricht is serving double life without parole, plus forty years in New York City's Metropolitan Correctional Center.

As much as this sounds like the makings of a new crime drama, conspiracies and corrupt practices aren't anything new for DEA agents. If you want to know more about Silk Road, I urge you to watch the documentary *Deep Web*, which presents a balanced view of what happened to Ulbricht. Whether the media was misled or got it wrong on purpose to bait people into reading, the majority of "reliable" sources got the facts wrong time and time again. I didn't even know until I watched the documentary that it was common knowledge on Silk Road that there were *multiple* DPRs running the site! During his trial, Ulbricht admitted to creating the site and to running it for a time, but there is evidence that there were others who also used that same log-in name to run the site. Those people are still out there, along with millions of dollars worth of Bitcoin unaccounted for, and no one is looking for them.

During his trial and throughout his appeal brief, Ulbricht's defense team reasoned that because multiple people have used that same DPR login, then the login is vulnerable to hacking, manipulation, and complete fabrication of evidence (including by corrupt agents), so anything the DEA pulled from that login and linked to Ulbricht can't possibly be reliable. Yet during Ulbricht's trial, the court ruled to prevent the jury from hearing that evidence too. Doesn't that make Ulbricht the definition of a patsy?

What is unique about the Silk Road case is that it is extremely rare for any DEA agent to be prosecuted for his crimes. It is also nearly impossible to fire an agent, let alone imprison an agent. The agency has allowed its employees to stay on the job despite internal investigations that prove they had distributed drugs, lied to authorities, and even paid for prostitutes with stolen Colombian drug lord money.[27] Why is that? Because the DEA is the darling child of the Justice Department's War on Drugs. They can do no wrong.

---

* Ross Ulbricht lost his appeal in May 2017 and will serve his original sentence.

4

Why and How the DEA
Is Rigging the Drug War

President Richard Nixon established the Drug Enforcement Administration under the Department of Justice on July 1, 1973,[1] just two years after the War on Drugs was established. In 1973, the DEA's budget was $75 million.[2] As of 2015, the DEA's annual budget was set at $2.88 billion.[3] It might interest you to know that the actions of DEA agent Carl Mark Force IV during the Silk Road investigation were minor compared to what his peers get away with on an everyday basis. He probably thought there was no way in hell he'd ever get caught, and if he did get caught, there was no way in hell he'd ever be reprimanded.

Recently, the Justice Department's inspector general made an inquiry into how federal law enforcement agencies handle sexual misconduct and harassment reports. In March 2015, the Justice Department's review was finalized, and it determined that from 2008 to 2012, DEA agents that were assigned to Colombia engaged in sex parties involving prostitutes supplied by local drug cartels.[4] In fact, while the agents attended the parties, a local Colombian police officer often stood guard to protect the agents' firearms and property. That puts a whole new meaning to the term "fraternizing with the enemy," doesn't it?

The report also found that three supervisors in the DEA were also "provided money, expensive gifts and weapons from drug cartel members."[5]

Okay, I get the money and the expensive gifts part, but weapons? What kind of weapons do these Colombian drug cartels have that a DEA agent can't get his hands on? And "provided" is about the loosest term I've ever heard for bribery. Who are they trying to fool here? They weren't *provided*! They were *bribed* with money, expensive gifts, and weapons!

That's not even the worst of it. Apparently, even though this misconduct jeopardized the three agents' security clearances, the matter was never reported to the DEA's Office of Security Programs for review. Instead, the agents were issued suspensions, ranging from two to ten days.[6]

Again, that's not the worst of it. The report stated "most of the sex parties occurred in government-leased quarters where agents' laptops, BlackBerry devices, and other government issued equipment were present . . . potentially exposing them to extortion, blackmail, or coercion."[7]

And again, *that's* not even the worst of it. After doing whatever they did with these prostitutes, and doing it in government-leased rooms—where all the paperwork for their investigations was available for that taking—two of the agents allegedly assaulted one of the prostitutes during a payment dispute.

USA Today reports that in 2010, this misconduct was reported in an anonymous letter to the DEA's Office of Professional Responsibility (OPR), but nothing happened. The OPR was also notified of at least four complaints involving loud parties attended by prostitutes in a government-leased apartment from 2005 to 2008, but the agents' supervisors and managers never forwarded these allegations for investigation.[8]

So why didn't the DEA supervisors ever investigate the misconduct? Because they were in on it! The *Washington Times* states that during a farewell party for a high-ranking DEA official, the money to pay prostitutes was included in the "operational budget."[9] People, "operational budget" means government funds. So yes, DEA agents use your tax dollars to pay for prostitutes. See what I mean about being unable to be fired?

The Justice Department's report on the DEA was prompted by the Secret Service prostitution scandal in 2012, also in Colombia. After Secret Service agents prepared for President Obama's arrival in Cartagena, Colombia, they brought several prostitutes back to their hotel. One of the agents became involved in a dispute over payment to one of the prostitutes, which led to the woman alerting authorities, and the incident resulted in agent dismissals once it made national headlines. After that, there were inquiries by congressional committees and a separate investigation into allegations involving the DEA. The March 2015 DOJ Inspector General report was the result of the investigation.

So after the Justice Department gave its report to Congress, what do you think happened? In April 2015, Congress conducted more hearings. During the hearings, Congress found out that these sex parties might have included teenagers or underage prostitutes![10] Ultimately, Congress demanded that any DEA employee who purchased sex must be fired. So the DEA agents involved in the scandal were all punished and fired, just like Congress wanted, right? Wrong! Those agents received punishments that ranged from a letter of caution to a two-week suspension—and to this day, not one agent was ever fired! So to recap: Secret Service agents can be fired for paying for sex, but DEA agents cannot.

And get this: The agents under investigation were actually rewarded with year-end bonuses for 2015. Yes, those same agents identified for participating in sex parties with prostitutes (who may or may not have been underage) "received tens of thousands of dollars in bonuses, time off and other favorable personnel actions,"[11] even after Congress called for the bastards to be fired!

And guess who rewarded them with bonuses? We did, because they were paid with taxpayer money.

So let's "follow the money." Exactly how much did these agents receive after a DOJ Inspector General report and a congressional hearing? The *Washington Times* reports:

- Eight out of the fourteen agents involved in sex parties organized by Colombian drug lords received bonuses.[12]
- Three of the agents received performance awards ranging between $1,500 to almost $32,000.[13] That's more than some Americans in minimum-wage jobs make in one year.
- A DEA regional director received four performance awards, three senior executive service bonus awards, and one SES Meritorious Executive Rank award over a four-year period, a total of $68,600. Again, that's not his salary. That's in addition to his salary.
- One agent who was suspended for ten days received one monetary and one time-off award of forty hours. So essentially he was suspended for ten days (with pay) and then paid another bonus the equivalent of one week's worth of work.

- A supervisory special agent received $2,000 in just two months after being named the subject of an OPR investigation. The agent later received other awards bringing the total to $8,400.

No wonder the DEA needs a budget of nearly $3 billion dollars! Clearly, money well spent, huh?

Some of you might be thinking, okay, the DEA has a few bad apples. One rogue agent on the Silk Road case, fourteen agents on the prostitution scandal, that's not too bad for an agency of eleven thousand employees, right? Wrong! These guys aren't the exception, they're the norm.

The Freedom of Information Act has proven time and time again that those who are enforcing the law continue to feel they are above it—here are just a few more examples from a DEA internal review log:

- In one case, the review board recommended that an employee be fired for "distribution of drugs," but a human resources official imposed a fourteen-day suspension instead.[14]
- The log shows officials also opted not to fire employees who falsified official records (this is also known as committing fraud).
- Employees also aren't fired for "improper association with a criminal element"—people, this means agents of the Drug Enforcement Administration are not fired for using drugs![15]
- They also aren't fired for "misusing" government vehicles, sometimes after drinking.[16] You read that right: DEA agents can drink and drive without any consequences.
- The DEA's Board of Professional Conduct recommended that fifty employees be fired for misconduct investigations from 2010, but as of today, only thirteen were terminated.
- Then the DEA was forced to take some of those thirteen employees back into the agency after a federal appeals board intervened.[17]
- Records from the DEA's disciplinary files show that agency typically gives a letter of caution—the lightest form of discipline—or a brief unpaid suspension instead of firing its agents.[18]
- DEA managers recommended firing an employee in less than 6 percent of all disciplinary cases; most often, either the employee is allowed to quit or they settle on a lesser punishment.[19]

- DEA records show that the agency hasn't even finished some of the misconduct cases it opened in 2011, including two cases involving agents that the DEA's Board of Professional Conduct recommended firing.[20]
- Even when employees are fired, they can be reinstated by the federal Merit Systems Protection Board, an independent body that reviews federal disciplinary matters.[21]
- This Merit Systems Protection Board stopped the DEA from firing an agent who left a voice mail for his girlfriend threatening "to give the couple's consensually made sex video" to her eight-year-old daughter as a birthday present.[22]
- It also ruled another agent could not be fired "after he accidentally fired his gun during a foot chase," threw away the shell casing evidence, and told an investigator that "the shooting never happened."[23]

In 2015, the Justice Department opened an inquiry into whether the DEA is able to adequately detect and punish wrongdoings by its agents. Really? An inquiry! Because we still can't determine if DEA agents are treated as if they are above the law! What a dog and pony show. If the Justice Department really cared about whether DEA managers impose penalties on their agents that are too lenient, then they should abolish the Merit Systems Protection Board.

Are you pissed off about the DEA yet? Well, I haven't even gotten into how DEA agents confiscate items from people who haven't committed a crime! Get a load of this: The DEA is allowed to take anything it wants from any law abiding American citizen if it wants to. This is something called asset seizure or civil asset forfeiture and it happens more often than the DEA would want you to know. Forget the term "probable cause." The DEA and any law enforcement agency, including local police, are legally allowed to seize any property they want if they suspect the property is related to criminal activity. They don't have to charge you with anything, they don't need a warrant, and they don't need any evidence whatsoever. They can just take it—and by "it" I mean cash, jewelry, cars, and houses—and then they have the right to sell your property. Guess where the profits go? Right back into the department that made the seizure![24] How's that for an incentive? From 2001 to 2015, law enforcement agencies seized $2.5 billion in cash alone from people who were never charged with a crime.[25] And they did all this without ever issuing a single warrant. These folks are of course welcome to go to court and prove their innocence and demand their property back—that is unless all their assets were taken and they don't have the funds to hire proper representation.

I could write volumes of books on the corruption of the DEA and what they've been doing with their nearly $3-billion budget. I could write a new book each year on the amount of crap they get away with on an annual basis. I could do the same with all the other law enforcement agencies in this country. But I'm more interested in getting back to the benefits of marijuana, so I'll leave you with the DEA's greatest hits of all time, so to speak. Here are twelve examples of the DEA's worst forms of corruption. I'm sure that after you read these, we can agree that the DEA does more harm than good, and they're just as corrupt as the Mexican federal police, or *federales*:

- Forget the NSA! The DEA has been spying on US citizens through a program called the Hemisphere Project, which gives the agency access to every call that passes through an AT&T switch. According to the *New York Times*, they have access to calls dating back twenty-nine years, starting in 1987![26] Some four billion calls are added to the database every day, including conversations from "burner phones." AT&T claims it doesn't share what's been recorded until the feds get a subpoena to listen to conversations,[27] a likely story!

- Get this: Any information acquired from the Hemisphere Project is then attributed to another possible source in the investigation. DEA agents are also instructed from time to time to conceal how their investigations truly begin, not only from defense lawyers, but also from judges and prosecutors.[28] So if an agent obtains information from wiretaps, informants, or other (illegal) surveillance methods, that agent can then lie about how the information was obtained by crediting it to a (legal) source. I believe this is how the DEA and FBI truly got their hands on Ross Ulbricht. Whether they coerced someone to give them access to the site or hacked into it, they had to have violated the Fourth Amendment along the way.

- In 2005, the DEA had around four thousand informants,[29] and these snitches are paid more than you could imagine. Court filings have shown some informants have made over $1 million in federal payouts. Some even get a cut of seized assets—up to $250,000 or 25 percent of the total value of confiscated drugs.[30]

- Andrew Chambers Jr., the highest-paid snitch in DEA history, made at least $4 million in government money from 1984 to 2000.[31] Today it's been proven that Chambers "perjured himself virtually every time he [sic] testified"[32] in the sixteen years he worked as an informant for the DEA. So far, not one of those cases has been overturned.

- The DEA's informants pay people to deal drugs to improve arrest records. I'll repeat that: DEA agents pay informants, who then pay "sub-informants" to set up drug deals, and then DEA agents arrest the people who purchase the drugs.[33] In May 2004, the *Los Angeles Times* reported that Guillermo Jordan-Pollito, one of the DEA's star drug dealers, was paid more than $350,000 for doing this.[34]

- The way in which the DEA acquires informants and "sub-informants" is questionable, to say the least. In 2014, a New Mexico man and DEA sub-informant named Aaron Romero filed an $8.5 million civil lawsuit against the US government and five members of the DEA. Romero, who had kicked his crack cocaine addiction in 2011, was given the opportunity to sell drugs by a DEA-sponsored informant. Instead of being paid with money, the DEA gave him as much crack as he wanted, for personal use.[35] All Romero had to do was provide the DEA informants with information on local drug dealers and users. Well, I guess Romero wasn't a good enough snitch once he relapsed into his crack addiction because in May 2012, the DEA arrested him and charge him with seven federal accounts of distributing crack cocaine near a school.[36] This is a forty-year prison sentence, which was dismissed once Romero filed his lawsuit.

- The DEA also promises citizenship for Mexican informants, but never gives it to them. One confidential informant was strung along since 1989, when she was nineteen years old. Although she upheld her end of the bargain and put her life on the line for the DEA for twenty years, the agency has yet to grant her citizenship and she now worries she'll be deported back to Mexico, where her life would be in danger for coming forward.[37]

- In January 2013, David Coleman Headley—a US citizen of Pakistani descent—was sentenced to thirty-five years in prison for a dozen federal terrorism crimes related to his role in planning the November 2008 terrorist attacks in Mumbai, India (essentially what is known as India's

9/11) and a planned attack on a newspaper in Denmark.[38] What connection does he have to the DEA? He was a confidential DEA informant between 1997 and 2005.[39]

- If you don't think the DEA would knowingly consort with a terrorist, then consider this: In the 1980s, the DEA and FBI took a fourteen-year-old from Detroit and turned him into a drug kingpin.[40] Richard Wershe became known as "White Boy Rick," a notorious American drug lord and valuable informant to the DEA. When the DEA decided they no longer had any use for him, they arrested him with 17 lbs of cocaine, which resulted in a life sentence.[41] Wershe was arrested in 1988 at seventeen years old, and he'll be behind bars for the rest of his life. You see, at the time, there was a "650-lifer" law in Michigan, which allowed the state to give life sentences to minors or anyone convicted of possessing, delivering, or intending to deliver more than 650 g of cocaine or heroin.[42] Most of the targets Wershe helped put in jail—drug dealers, murderers, and former police—have been released, and even though it is widely known that the DEA corrupted a young, impressionable teenager, he'll likely remain in jail for the rest of his life.

- In the past twenty-five years, the DEA has terrorized and killed innocent Americans through "no-knock raids." This can be said of other federal, state, and local law enforcement agencies that subscribe to the "no-knock raid" policy, where agents can force their way into a home in which drug use or drug dealing is suspected. The DEA and other agencies will never admit to how many times they've had the wrong house or the wrong person. We only find out about it when these victims file lawsuits. In 2003, the DEA shot a fourteen-year-old girl, Ashley Villareal, mistaking her for her father, whom they suspected of dealing cocaine. The girl died, but the agents responsible never faced charges.[43] During another no-knock raid in 2008, the DEA woke up the two daughters of Thomas and Rosalie Avina, ages eleven and fourteen, by pointing guns at their heads and handcuffing them.[44] When the Avina family sued because the DEA had raided the wrong house, the Obama administration said the DEA had done nothing wrong.[45] None of the agents faced disciplinary actions.[46] How's that for a police state?

- In 2015, the DEA had to be ordered by a federal court in California to stop busting legal pot shops in states that have legalized marijuana.[47]

How's that for thinking they're above the law? According to the Rohrabacher-Farr amendment,[48] which Congress attached to the 2014 spending bill, the Justice Department (namely the DEA) cannot use federal funds to prevent states that have legalized medical marijuana "from implementing their own state laws."[49] A leaked February 2015 memo from the DEA, however, shows that they had every intention of pursuing legal medical marijuana shops for criminal activities, since marijuana is illegal under federal law.[50] In October 2015, California Judge Charles Breyer ruled against the US Department of Justice[51] to uphold the Rohrabacher-Farr amendment, and now the twenty-three states that have legalized medical marijuana don't have to worry about being raided by the DEA.

- The DEA allows informants to break the law, even sell weapons to Mexican drug cartels, but there isn't any paper trail. Between 2006 and 2011, the ATF and DEA worked "gunwalking" tactics in missions like Project Gunrunner and Operation Fast and Furious. The idea was to have informants sell American guns to Mexican criminals in the hopes that the guns would wind up in the cartels' hands and the ATF and DEA could then track and recover the guns and arrest the cartels. Needless to say, this did not work. Remember how many Mexicans died in 2009 at the height of the drug war? More Mexicans died that year than the total number of US troops in the Iraq War or the total number of US troops in the Afghanistan War. How many of those Mexicans do you think were killed with American guns? By 2012, approximately two thousand US weapons fell into the hands of Mexican drug cartels[52] and only 710 guns were ever recovered! A report by the Justice Department's Inspector General determined that ATF and DEA agents knew their informants were selling guns to "suspected cartel operatives," but no one got authorization from their superiors to allow the sales to happen[53] and that means there is no record of the sales even taking place. Our federal agents are giving our drug war enemies firepower. They are purposefully doing so without putting a system in place to track the guns. And you're telling me they have every intention of catching these guys? I call bullshit!

I would go as far as to argue that the DEA doesn't actually enforce much. It seems their main responsibility is to make sure the War on Drugs continues forever, and they'll stop at nothing to make sure it does. As economist and Nobel

Prize winner Milton Friedman said in 1991, "If you look at the drug war from a purely economic point of view, the role of the government is to protect the drug cartel."[54] To me, the DEA is purposefully trying to increase the power of the drug lords. The DEA is doing what it can to increase the number of American drug addicts and criminals, which in turn increases US prison populations, which in turn helps out the prison lobbyists and the politicians on both sides of the aisle connected to them.

It's no wonder the DEA only confiscates about 10 percent of the drugs that cross our borders. They allow the rest of the drugs to come into our country on purpose! That's what's called job security. We've already determined they can't be fired, so they're rigging the drug war in their favor.

5

The American Historical
Significance of Cannabis

efore you go ahead and blame President Nixon and the Republican Party for the failure that is the War on Drugs, keep in mind that this war was upheld and strengthened by both political parties for the past forty-five years. Both Democrats and Republicans are to blame, especially when it comes to spending over $1 trillion[1] in taxpayer dollars.

President Nixon may have started one of the most useless, ongoing wars in the history of our great nation, but I have yet to find a Democrat who pledges to end it. If you want to know why, you should take a look at the Controlled Substances Act (CSA) of 1970, which classified marijuana as a Schedule I narcotic.[2] The main purpose of the CSA was to establish five schedules, or classifications, of drugs so that drug users and drug dealers could be "fairly" prosecuted depending on what kind of substance they were caught with. The CSA determined on a scale of one to five to determine what substances are the most dangerous, with Schedule I narcotics as the greatest potential for abuse. To this day, only two federal agencies can determine if any substances—including marijuana—can be added or removed from this list: the DEA and the Food and Drug Administration.

That's right. By passing the CSA, President Nixon and Congress crowned the DEA judge, jury, and executioner when it comes to the war on drugs. The DEA is more powerful than Congress in determining the true benefits of marijuana on the federal level. That's why this corrupt agency will continue to remain the nation's greatest obstacle when it comes to full legalization. How on earth can the DEA be objective about a plant's healing properties or its economic value when it's been the major focus of the drug war since 1990,[3] after President George H. W. Bush declared it was time for a "new" war on drugs! Forget medical studies that prove weed kills cancer tumors. When it comes to changing the classification of marijuana at the federal level, we are all at the mercy of the DEA and the Food and Drug Administration, and of course the pharmaceutical industry's lobbyists and every candidate's special interest groups and SuperPAC financiers. See? Equal blame across the aisle.

So how did we get here? Marijuana didn't just automatically become an object of national scorn and fear in the 1970s. After all, the propaganda film *Reefer Madness* was produced in 1936. Over the centuries, there have been politicians and American entrepreneurs who had something to gain from demonized weed or attempting to outright eradicate it. President Nixon was no different from the rest who wanted their names in the history books for doing something to "protect" the American people from ourselves and from a plant.

It might surprise you to know that cannabis wasn't indigenous to the Americas, but it played a huge role in founding the thirteen colonies and stabilizing the original American economy. Some sources say early Viking explorers were the first to bring cannabis here, but we know for certain that early Spanish and European settlers grew it here in 1545, and by 1611, it was a major commercial crop for British settlers in Jamestown.[4]

The first cannabis law in the New World was enacted in Jamestown in 1619, and it stated that all farmers must grow hemp.[5] Let me repeat: all farmers—and the majority of settlers in the New World were farmers—must grow hemp by law. Every colonist had to grow one hundred plants specifically to export to the British Crown.[6] You see, because hemp fiber is resistant to salt and rot, it was crucial in building all aspects of the ships in the British Navy. The British would rather have their colonists grow cannabis and give it to them (for free) than pay Russia for the amount of hemp they needed for the Empire. This is why Massachusetts, Connecticut, and the Chesapeake Colonies also had mandatory cultivation laws in 1630s. Meanwhile in England, foreigners who grew cannabis were rewarded with British citizenship, while those who refused to grow it were fined. Keep in mind: England is roughly about the same size as New York state, so there was only so much land available for growing food and cannabis, so the majority of hemp was imported into the country. Importing additional hemp fiber was a necessity, especially since Britain was the world's superpower at the time. Without hemp, they wouldn't have had a fleet of ships or soldiers' uniforms.

So what happened if a British colonist refused to grow hemp? From 1763 to 1769, the British hemp mandate was so serious that you could be jailed in Virginia if you did not grow it.[7] How do you like them hemp laws!

Back then cannabis was considered the cash crop of the New World, and for the entire world. It was in demand for all industries. It was the first crop to be grown in most of the colonies because hemp was not only a commodity; it was *the* commodity of the thirteen colonies. It was used for making rope, ships' sails, netting, textiles, clothing, linen, drapes, bed sheets, paper—even quality paints were made from hemp oil. If you owned a Bible during the time of the Founding Fathers, guess what it was made from? Hemp!

And since our Founding Fathers were once British colonists, they were no strangers to growing cannabis. In fact, Benjamin Franklin owned one of the first paper mills in America, and it processed hemp so that the colonists didn't have to request paper and books from England.[8] (If you recall, Britain taxed the hell out of anything it exported to the colonies, including tea.) In addition to Benjamin Franklin, our first president was also quite familiar with cannabis. George Washington wrote in his diary about tending to his hemp plants at Mount Vernon.[9] Also at that time, Chinese cannabis seeds were so valuable that it was illegal for anyone to export them, so Thomas Jefferson smuggled seeds from China to France then to America. That's right—America's third president was also one of America's first drug smugglers![10] Hell, you could even pay your taxes with hemp. In America, you could pay your taxes with hemp from 1631 to the early 1800s.[11]

The reason why hemp was more valuable than cash after the American Revolutionary War was simple: paper money held no value in the newly formed country. The American economy largely operated on the barter system, and anything and everything could be bartered for hemp. "For the first three or four decades," hemp was recognized "as the standard commodity" of the new American republic.[12] Here's a fun fact for you: when the early wagon-wheel settlers were heading out west during the days of "manifest destiny," they repurposed the sails from ships as the canvases for the top of their wagons. Canvas at that time was made out of cannabis.

Just to drive home how incredibly invaluable this renewable resource was, I'm going to test your knowledge of early American history: Did you know that the War of 1812 was fought because of hemp? If you recall, around 1793, France and England were at war (that's right, the war was taking place prior to 1812— we call it the War of 1812 because that's when the United States got involved). So what do you do to your enemy when you're at war? You cut off their supply chain. England's greatest resource, especially for her navy, was hemp. Remember, hemp was used to produce rope, uniforms, ships' sails, maps, you name it. It was as important back then as oil is today to the military. Since America was now an independent country, we were not supplying hemp to England for free, and the Brits had to go back to getting 90 percent of their hemp from Russia.[13] The War of 1812 escalated when Napoleon and the Russian czar signed the Treaty of Tilset, which cut off Moscow's hemp export to England. The United States was essentially neutral until 1812, when the British, who were commandeering our ships and forcing American traders to purchase hemp from Russia for them, instigated us into war.

It therefore stands to reason that once our ancestors were free and independent from England, they continued to cultivate and manufacture the world's most valuable commodity. The US census of 1850 counted 8,327 hemp plantations in America—with the majority of those farms being in Kentucky—each with at least two thousand acres. By 1910, hemp was called "the grand staple of Kentucky."[14] Even with an abundance of farms, America still imported about 80 percent of its hemp from Russia and other Eastern European states. So much for the history books claiming tobacco and cotton were the top two crops of the south!

So why on earth did we decide to stop producing hemp? There were three major blows to cannabis that caused its decline and led to its total prohibition: the cotton gin, federal medical classifications, and William Randolph Hearst's marijuana propaganda campaign. Newspaper tycoon Hearst was by far the biggest blow to cannabis. If it wasn't for him, we probably wouldn't have ever had the Marijuana Tax Act of 1937, which marked the beginning of the end of US cultivation and manufacturing of cannabis. So if you're looking for someone to blame for the War on Drugs, keep in mind: America's relationship with marijuana would be completely different today if William Randolph Hearst didn't own any newspapers and didn't own the forest that was used to produce paper (more on that later).

Let this sink in first: for over 160 years, cannabis was legal in America. It was grown for other purposes besides "getting high," and in fact, it wasn't widely used for this purpose, unless under medical assistance. The United States prospered and endured through tough times while having unlimited access to this plant—and I believe a great deal of our successes as a nation were because of this plant. Just think for one minute: our ancestors were able to build a nation with marijuana growing wild and free for over 160 years—and the nation not only thrived but even expanded.

So what does all this historical information tell me? Well, to begin with, if marijuana were truly as dangerous as the DEA says, and as addicting as our federal government claims, then how the hell was our nation able to prosper? How the hell were we able to even figure out the Louisiana Purchase? Or trick the Native Americans out of their land? Or do all those other things in the history books with marijuana readily available to pluck from the soil and smoke whenever our ancestors chose to do so?

Think about it: Why didn't every person back then who smoked pot become an opium and morphine addict? If pot is such a "gateway drug," then our great experiment of democracy would have never worked! Especially because there weren't as many distractions as there are today. The Founding Fathers had books, they had newspapers, but what did they do to unwind? Drink alcohol and smoke pot! The United States should have crashed and burned before 1937, when marijuana really started to become public enemy number one, if it truly is a dangerous Schedule I narcotic as the DEA claims it to be.

Well, here's another history lesson for you: marijuana was everywhere, but the vast majority of colonists-turned-Americans were growing hemp. Remember in chapter 1 when I mentioned there are actually two genetic types of cannabis plants? There's the plant that produces hemp—the "father" plant—and the plant that produces THC (that's the stuff that gets you high)—which is referred to as the "mother" plant because it flowers and produces buds. When our ancestors were farming marijuana, they were almost exclusively farming hemp.

So let's go back to the three major historical events that caused the decline of cannabis in America—first up is the cotton gin. Prior to Eli Whitney's invention of the cotton gin, cotton and hemp production were both highly labor intensive, but hemp fiber was preferred over cotton due to its superior quality and cheaper price. By the 1820s, the cotton gin changed the game by making it faster and easier and therefore cheaper to produce cotton. Cotton plantations began to surpass hemp plantations, and as the Industrial Revolution swept the nation, hemp production was swept under the rug.

Also right around that time, American pharmacies started to carry medical cannabis. The pharmaceutical industry extracted the THC from the buds of the mother plant and sold it as a liquid. In 1850, the *United States Pharmacopaeia* recommended liquid cannabis as an aphrodisiac.[15] It was also prescribed to increase the appetite, to relieve pain, to help people sleep, to stop muscle spasms, and to compose nervous or anxious people.

However, there was no way to regulate the strength of the product in the 1800s. Depending on how the plant was grown (more on this later), the THC from one batch of liquid medical cannabis could be much more potent than the next. Plus, the effects varied greatly from person to person. It was just too difficult back then to fig-

Cannabis indica fluid extract, American Druggists Syndicate, pre-1937. *(Credit: Public domain)*

ure out the correct dosage for each person because each individual had a different reaction based on the brand, if not literally the bottle, and the amount.

Once morphine and the hypodermic syringe were invented around 1853, cannabis wasn't as heavily relied upon for medical purposes. Morphine was easier to administer, worked faster, and had more universal effects because it could be injected (whereas cannabis couldn't). Patients could experience delays of up to three hours when cannabis was administered orally, so it was difficult to standardize the dosage. This wasn't an issue with morphine. Doctors were able to tell how much morphine to administer because it was a universal potency. They could prescribe the right dosage based on age, weight, and severity of injury or cause of pain. Morphine took the guesswork out of pain management; however, it also led to severe addiction (whereas cannabis did not).

The late 1800s also marked the beginning of the regulation of the pharmaceutical industry. Prior to this time, there weren't any mandatory labels on pharmaceutical drug bottles, so if something was labeled "cannabis fluid extract" or "liquid morphine," there was no way to tell if it was diluted in any way. The federal government encouraged states to pass regulation laws, but these regulations varied from state to state. Most states required a doctor's prescription for a bottle of cannabis fluid extract, and anything that required a prescription—from opium to marijuana—was labeled as a "narcotic" or a "poison." However, this didn't stop people from using pharmaceutical drugs recreationally, or from smoking them recreationally.

As early as 1853, recreational cannabis was considered a "fashionable" narcotic. By 1885, you could find opium dens and hashish parlors in every major city, from New York to San Francisco.[16] There was an estimated five hundred hashish clubs in New York City alone! Who would have guessed Americans in the 1800s loved to get high! An article in *Harper's* magazine in 1883 referenced these hashish houses as frequented by males and females of "the better classes."[17]

However, in southern states like Texas, the "better classes" saw marijuana as something only Mexicans smoked after a long day in the fields. A 1917 Department of Agriculture investigation noted that the Texas border town of El Paso passed a city ordinance banning the sale and possession of marijuana in 1914 because Mexicans, blacks, "prostitutes, pimps and a criminal class of whites" used it.[18] During the Great Depression, when jobs were scarce in farming communities, the "better classes" intertwined marijuana with racial stereotypes even further. Thanks to the pot propaganda William Hearst was printing in his newspapers at the time, the people who were most often categorized as potheads—from Mexican laborers to circus performers to black musicians—were considered violently dangerous. Flash forward to 2016, and the "better classes" are still blaming Mexicans and minorities for all our drug problems.

So why was William Hearst on a mission to eradicate and defame weed? Why couldn't he just put some in a pipe and relax a little? Because a German by the name of G. W. Schlichten had patented a hemp gin in 1917, and by the 1930s—as Schlichten's patent had expired—American inventors such as Anton F. Burkard, Robert B. Cochrane, and Karl Wessel came up with their own versions and mass-produced several hemp gins.[19] Needless to say, this rejuvenated the hemp industry. In February 1938, *Popular Mechanics* magazine called hemp the "new billion-dollar crop" and *Mechanical Engineering* magazine called it "the most profitable and desirable crop that can be grown."[20] This was wonderful news for hemp farmers in Kentucky, but shitty timing for the tycoons of the Industrial Revolution, like Hearst.

Remember how you can make practically anything out of hemp? That means that nearly every industry established through the Industrial Revolution was going to have to compete against the plant! This did not sit well with the cotton industry or the paper industry—namely William Randolph Hearst. The American entrepreneur was faced with major competition in an industry where he was practically the monopoly—both in the production of paper and in owning the nation's most popular newspapers, including the *San Francisco Examiner* and the *New York Journal.*

The rich and the powerful wanted to stay rich and powerful, and William Randolph Hearst knew exactly how to do it. You know the saying "don't believe everything you read?" Well, Hearst was notorious for printing whatever he wanted—without it being fact checked or even truthful—in order to sell his newspapers. He knew the best way to get people to buy his newspapers over his competition was to print salacious stories. He went down in history for instigating the Spanish-American War of 1898 after he ran several stories about the Spanish Navy sinking one of our ships called the USS *Maine.*

Here's what actually happened: In 1898, the USS *Maine* was anchored in the Havana harbor (back when Cuba was under Spain's jurisdiction) when it mysteriously blew up. An official US Naval Court of Inquiry ruled that a mine blew up the ship. The report didn't place blame directly on Spain, but it definitely led Hearst to build public support for war. In fact, subsequent studies have determined that the explosion came from the *inside* of the ship, and the explosion was actually an accident involving a spontaneous combustion in the coalbunker. This also correlates with the views of the Navy's Chief Engineer at the time, George W. Melville.[21] You see, many ships, including the *Maine*, had coalbunkers located next to magazines that stored ammunition, gun shells, and gunpowder. A bulkhead was the only thing that separated the bunkers from the magazines. If the coal overheated due to spontaneous combustion, the magazines could easily explode. In January 1898, an investigative board warned the Secretary of the Navy about spontaneous coal fires that could detonate nearby magazines, so it is likely that this was the cause of the *Maine's* explosion on February 15, 1898, which killed 260 crewmembers.

Hearst's newspapers contradicted these facts, however. His headline read, "The warship *Maine* was split in two by an enemy's secret infernal machine," and he offered a reward of $50,000 for the capture of the Spaniards who he claimed had constructed a submarine and executed this plot.[22] Needless to say, Hearst's propaganda campaign, combined with his war cry of "Remember the *Maine*, down with Spain!" led Congress and the American public to call for a declaration of war.

Even after the Spanish-American War (which ended on December 12, 1898), Hearst continued to denounce Spaniards, Mexican Americans, and Latinos in his newspapers. For the next three decades, "Hearst painted a picture of the lazy, pot-smoking Mexican," which is *still* in existence today.[23] During the Mexican Revolution, Pancho Villa's army seized eight hundred thousand acres of Hearst's Mexican timberland, and then the slurs got even worse. From 1910 to 1920, Hearst's newspapers were on a hateful mission: if you were brown, then you smoked marijuana, and that made you a dangerous person.

You see, to eradicate something from society, you need a scapegoat. Hearst needed to convince the general voting public—which was all white males at the time—that marijuana turns brown people violent. He wrote stories of "marijuana-crazed negroes"[24] raping white women. He claimed that jazz was "anti-white, voodoo-satanic"[25] music and anyone who played it was under the influence of marijuana. He portrayed Mexicans as "frenzied beasts."[26] He did a hell of a job inventing new ways for white Americans to be fearful of black people and Mexicans and marijuana. And, boy, did that propaganda campaign work. Here's a timeline of what went down:

- The Federal Bureau of Narcotics was formed in 1930, headed by Harry J. Anslinger, who was on a mission to outlaw all recreational drugs, with marijuana being priority number one.
- In 1932, the Uniform State Narcotic Act was passed to ensure that all narcotic drugs had the same safeguards and regulations in all states. By the mid-1930s, all states had some regulation of cannabis, but that wasn't enough for Anslinger.
- Anslinger used Hearst's propaganda campaign to prove that cannabis caused people to commit violent crimes, act irrationally, and behave overly sexually.
- In 1937, the Marijuana Tax Act Hearings were held to determine if Anslinger was onto something and if marijuana should be taxed or downright illegal.
- These hearings were orchestrated by Herman Oliphant, the chief counsel of the United States Treasury Department, who was looking for

ways to make a name for himself by increasing the taxing power of the federal government.

- Oliphant was the muscle behind the National Firearms Act, passed in June 1934, which was the first act to hide Congress's motives behind a prohibitive or exorbitant tax. If you wanted to buy a machine gun, you had to pay a $200 transfer tax. The federal government didn't have the constitutional authority to state it was illegal to purchase a type of gun, but it wanted to outlaw machine guns. Oliphant found a way to make it nearly impossible for someone to have the funds to purchase a machine gun and pay the tax on it. He recommended Congress do the same with marijuana, hence the Marijuana Tax Act.

- Oliphant chose to conduct the Marijuana Tax Act hearings with those who were part of the House of Representatives Ways and Means Committee instead of another more appropriate House committee, like the Food and Drug Committee or the Agriculture Committee.

- Herman Oliphant did this purposefully to avoid committee members who would have a more thorough understanding of cannabis.

- What did Oliphant have against cannabis? Oliphant was lobbied by William Randolph Hearst to make it illegal!

- Angslinger testified before the Ways and Means Committee, claiming, "Marijuana is the most violence-causing drug in the history of mankind." He added that Spaniards, Mexican Americans, Latin Americans, Filipinos, African Americans, and Greeks committed "50 percent of all violent crimes" in the United States and these crimes were a direct result of marijuana use.[27] He was able to pass these allegations off as facts, even though to this day no one has ever found statistics to back them up.

- Between Heart's newspapers "reporting" on violent crime waves caused by marijuana and the popular 1936 film *Reefer Madness*, the Marijuana Tax Act of 1937 was presented before Congress after the Ways and Means Committee hearings and it passed without delay.

- The Marijuana Tax Act made the possession or transfer of recreational cannabis illegal throughout the United States under federal law. This allowed the states and the federal government to collect revenue from heavy fines, as well as easily imprison pot-smoking brown people before they can commit the violent crimes they are now supposedly widely known for committing.

- To begin the process of eradicating cannabis completely, the Marijuana Tax Act also imposed a hefty excise tax for medical and industrial uses for marijuana. Hemp importers, manufacturers, cultivators, and anyone using marijuana for medical, research, or industrial uses had to pay a tax. See why Oliphant didn't want the House's agricultural committee involved in the initial hearings?
- Get this: the American Medical Association (AMA) *opposed* the Marijuana Tax Act! The AMA even testified during the Ways and Means Committee hearings and claimed that Angslinger's "evidence" was completely fabricated or based off of tabloid journalism.
- Dr. William C. Woodward, a physician and an attorney/lobbyist for the AMA, went so far as to state that the medical community was only just beginning to figure out which ingredients in cannabis were active, and the law would "deny the world a potential medicine."[28]
- Democrat House Representative Carl Vinson, of the Ways and Means Committee, asked Dr. Woodward to state medical benefits of cannabis, and Woodward stated, "Indian hemp is employed . . . as a sedative and antispasmodic."[29] (In case you didn't know, medical marijuana is used today to treat spasms associated with multiple sclerosis and seizures.)
- However, once the bill was introduced on the floor of the Congress, and the members of Congress asked Vinson if he consulted the AMA, he said, "Yes we have . . . and they [the AMA] are in complete agreement."[30]
- Roosevelt's administration didn't exactly see eye-to-eye with the AMA, so no one was about to go through the transcripts from the House hearings and call Vinson a liar.
- That's right, the initial steps to eradicate marijuana happened under a Democrat: President Franklin Delano Roosevelt.
- Democrat Carl Vinson was also not forgotten, as he served for more than fifty years in the House of Representatives and was awarded the Medal of Freedom by President Lyndon Johnson.[31] How's that for irony? The guy who helped make us less free received the Medal of Freedom? Only in America!
- And whatever happened to William Randolph Hearst? Prior to his war on marijuana, he used the power and influence of his newspapers to be elected twice as a Democrat to the House of Representatives and served from 1904 to 1907. He also used his power to influence elections in the

1930s—including FDR's—and he ran stories to get the public's support on controversial legislation, such as the New Deal. At the height of his power, he owned nearly thirty newspapers in major American cities and expanded his business to include magazines, some of which are still in existence today.

See what I mean about politicians trying to make a name for themselves, all at the expense of a plant?

You might be wondering what Harry J. Anslinger's angle was in all of this. Why was he picked to head up the Federal Bureau of Narcotics (what Nixon later renamed as the Drug Enforcement Administration)? And why was he so eager to eradicate marijuana? Family connections, of course!

Anslinger had married Andrew Mellon's niece and had Andrew Mellon to thank for appointing him. Mellon ran the Mellon Bank of Pittsburgh and served as President Herbert Hoover's Secretary of Treasury. Aside from being rich and powerful, Andrew Mellon was the chief financial backer of DuPont, a company that owned thousands of acres of trees. DuPont had just patented the processes for making plastics from oil and coal, as well as new chemical processes for making paper from wood pulp. The rise of the hemp industry was too intimidating to DuPont and Mellon's operations. So with Hearst at the helm of the court of public opinion, Mellon made Anslinger the assistant US commissioner for prohobition, and then appointed him to the Federal Bureau of Narcotics, where he would rule the bureau until 1962.[32] Anslinger drafted the Marijuana Tax Act of 1937, and Ways and Means Committee Chairman Robert L. Doughton—a key DuPont ally—introduced it to Congress.[33] And the rest as they say is history.

Like I said, Nixon's War on Drugs is just the tip of the iceberg. The war against marijuana has been going on in our country for quite some time. As our federal government continued to get bigger and more powerful, we the people got slapped with more regulation. And more regulation. And more regulation, until our government regulated marijuana right out of America.

See what I mean about needing to elect the right people, who actually want to decrease the federal government? We need to elect politicians who aren't bought by corporations! Corporate CEOs in the early 1900s determined the prohibition of marijuana. Don't you think the same corporate greed exists today? Could you imagine if hemp was once again an abundant industry? Could you imagine how many jobs a new industry would bring to the American economy! But those in power right now don't want that to happen.

Think about it: there's a reason why cannabis is illegal in almost every country. The hemp gin wasn't around for most of the world's Industrial Revolution, and corporations that were founded back then are still threatened today by what hemp could do to their industries. Case in point: in 2015, *Forbes* listed the Du Pont family as number fourteen on the list of America's Richest Families, and they're listed as our nation's oldest billion-dollar family fortune at an estimated $14.5 billion![34] Although the family no longer owns the DuPont Company, they do hold a substantial chunk of its shares. Furthermore, DuPont is now a global company. In 2014 the *Financial Times* listed it as the world's fourth largest chemical company.[35] DuPont is a two-hundred-year-old company, with corporate headquarters still in the United States, and it ended 2014 with $35 billion in net sales.[36] So again, unless corporations like DuPont find a way to make some serious money off of cannabis, they'll continue to see it as a threat, and they'll continue to put politicians in place to stop our access to it.

We might have improved the way businesses operate with the Internet and cell phones, but we certainly haven't progressed as a society since the early 1900s. Case in point: today's CEOs have seen their salaries increase by more than half (by 54.3 percent) since 2009, while ordinary wages for the average American have barely moved.[37] And thanks to tax loopholes, the list of companies that don't even pay taxes continues to grow.

Think about it: with today's globalization, it's not just American corporations that don't want hemp to come back, it's corporations in every corner of the earth. The antipoverty charity Oxfam found that in 2015, there were sixty-two people in the world with the same amount of money as the *combined wealth* of 3.6 billion people.[38] By the end of 2016, Oxfam projects that the richest 1 percent will own more than 50 percent of the world's wealth.[39] That means there's plenty of wealth to go around, but no one wants to share. People, you can't take it with you. And like I said earlier: as wealthy as those sixty-two people are, they don't know what the future holds. No one is exempt from cancer, no matter how wealthy or healthy. By killing the world's chances of accessing and studying medical marijuana, they could one day be killing themselves.

6

America's Marijuana Hypocrisy

What I brought up in chapter 5 about America's history with cannabis, for the most part, is common knowledge if you know where to look for the information. It is not taught in schools, but it should be. It is proof of how corporate CEOs have hijacked our government for centuries for their own personal gains at the American people's expense.

Here's something else the federal government has been hiding from you: it owns a patent on marijuana and it has been giving marijuana to select individuals for free under the Compassionate Investigational New Drug program. To this day, four Americans receive *free* joints from the federal government! Before I get into how that program started (lawsuits against the feds were involved) you should know what happened after the Marijuana Tax Act of 1937. I want to make sure you know just how far back the federal government's hypocritical stance on this so-called Schedule I narcotic goes.

In 1938, New York Mayor Fiorello LaGuardia appointed a scientific committee to study marijuana use in New York City because he didn't buy what Anslinger and Hearst were selling. Remember, New York had over five hundred hashish clubs at the time, and this law wiped out that industry completely. I'm sure LaGuardia had to deal with some pretty pissed-off businessmen! He formed the LaGuardia Committee to investigate if there was any way to justify amending the Marijuana Tax Act, perhaps at the state level. The result of that investigation was the 1944 LaGuardia Report—just look at what Mayor LaGuardia had to say in the foreword of this report:

> My own interest in marihuana goes back many years, to the time when I was a member of the House of Representatives and, in that capacity, heard of the use of marihuana by soldiers stationed in Panama. I was impressed at that time with the report of an Army Board of Inquiry, which emphasized the relative harmlessness of the drug and the fact that it played a very little role, if any, in problems of delinquency and crime in the Canal Zone.[1]

The LaGuardia Committee that compiled the report included pharmacologists, public health experts, psychiatrists, and other members of the scientific community, including experts from the New York Academy of Medicine.[2] The LaGuardia Report contained sociological studies, clinical studies, and different medical aspects consistent with a professional medical and scientific investigation. It proved beyond a shadow of a doubt that Anslinger and Hearst were liars.

The next time Hillary Clinton says to a live audience "we need to do a lot more research"[3] before making a conclusion on the benefits of medical marijuana, I'd like someone to throw a copy of the LaGuardia Report at her—just like the Iraqi journalist Muntadhar al-Zaidi threw his shoes at then-President George W. Bush at a press conference.

The 1944 LaGuardia Report proved "that marijuana caused no violence at all" and it actually cited "other positive results" for the medical community,[4] but Anslinger wasn't going down without a fight. He prosecuted doctors who prescribed cannabis for what he deemed as "illegal purposes." By 1939, he had prosecuted more than three thousand AMA doctors for writing "illegal" narcotic prescriptions.[5] Anslinger offered the AMA a single option for reversing these past and potential future convictions: if the AMA publicly denounced the LaGuardia Report, then Anslinger would stop convicting its doctors. The heads of the AMA then claimed that they reviewed the LaGuardia Report and they found that it had no medical or scientific value. Anslinger kept his word as well. He prosecuted only three doctors for illegal drugs of any kind from 1939 to 1949.

However, if you know your history, then you know that when the LaGuardia Report came out, America was already fighting a much bigger war known as World War II—and this war was depleting our nation's resources. The US

Department of Agriculture had already launched the "Hemp for Victory" program, which encouraged farmers to plant hemp. The US Department of Agriculture even went so far as to give out seeds and grant draft deferments to those who would stay home and grow hemp!

By 1943, a year prior to the release of the LaGuardia Report, the American farmers registered in Hemp for Victory harvested 375,000 acres of hemp.[6] Overall, sixty million pounds of hemp fiber were produced by 1944.[7] We could have very well won WWII due to this program, but as soon as the war was over, the US government canceled virtually all hemp farming permits.[8] All those hemp farmers in Kentucky were once again unemployed after completing their patriotic duty.

This also affected our auto industry. On August 13, 1941, Henry Ford displayed his plastic car at Dearborn Days in Michigan. The car ran on fuels derived from hemp and other agricultural based sources. People, this means Henry Ford invented the first car powered by biodiesel fuel in 1941! The fenders were made of hemp, wheat, straw, and synthetic plastics. Ford said his vision was "to grow automobiles from the soil,"[9] and to this day, one of the only car manufacturers that has come close to Ford's vision is BMW—they use hemp plastic in car door paneling of the BMW i3, an electric car that was introduced in 2013. The hemp fibers make the car lighter—it is larger in size but still weighs in at 800 lbs. lighter than the Nissan Leaf and the Chevy Volt—and therefore it can go farther on one electric charge.[10]

So, like I said, our government picks and chooses what it wants us to believe about cannabis, and the government's "official story" about the value of the plant contradicts itself time and time again. At least they're consistent about being inconsistent, I suppose.

And yes, Angslinger, Hearst, and DuPont were able to win their war against cannabis, but just because it was illegal to partake in the plant, that didn't mean people didn't have access to it. In 1945, *Newsweek* reported that over one hundred thousand people smoked marijuana and that number continued to climb as our nation marched forward in its war on marijuana.[11]

I'd really like to know, if marijuana is as dangerous as the DEA claims it to be and if marijuana is as useless as the DEA claims it to be, then what interest does the federal government have in patenting it?

Get this: after the DEA and nearly every federal official since the 1930s has denied time and time again that marijuana has any medical benefits whatsoever, it turns out that the feds actually hold the patents for the medical use of the plant!

Dr. Sanjay Gupta, who produced the CNN documentary series *Weed*, told Anderson Cooper something in 2013 that sums up my thoughts on the matter exactly:

> The US holds a patent [on marijuana] on one hand, and on the other hand, [the] same government says it has no medical applications. Journalists are trained to hate hypocrisy. This is hypocrisy. I've never seen it quite like this.[12]

Isn't that astounding? In case you missed the memo because the government didn't go out of its way to publicize what happened, on October 7, 2003, the feds issued US Patent 6,630,507 on cannabidiol—and the patent's estimated expiration date is February 2, 2021.[13] What is cannabidiol, you might ask? It's CBD. It's what puts the final nail in the coffin on the government's hypocrisy on marijuana.

US Patent 6,630,507 is titled "Cannabinoids as antioxidants and neuroprotectants." The patent claims that:

> Cannabinoids have been found to have antioxidant properties, unrelated to NMDA receptor antagonism. This newfound property makes cannabinoids useful in the treatment and prophylaxis of wide variety of oxidation associated diseases, such as ischemic, age-related, inflammatory and autoimmune diseases. The cannabinoids are found to have particular application as neuroprotectants, for example in limiting neurological damage following ischemic insults, such as stroke and trauma, or in the treatment of neurodegenerative diseases, such as Alzheimer's disease, Parkinson's disease and HIV dementia.[14]

Did you catch that? The US government patented CBD—a substance found in marijuana that doesn't get you high but has medical benefits. The US government admitted in the patent that CBD cannabinoids have the properties to help people in a medical capacity. People who suffer from several incurable diseases and conditions—including strokes, Alzheimer's disease, Parkinson's disease, and dementia—can be helped by CBD.

This means that the patent is a direct contradiction of the government's own classification of a Schedule I drug! The DEA defines Schedule I narcotics as "drugs, substances, or chemicals are defined as drugs with no currently accepted medical use and a high potential for abuse."[15] Again, I'd really like someone to explain to me how the government can say marijuana has no currently accepted medical use, and at the same time, patent a substance found exclusively in marijuana and state that it has medical merit.

The only possible explanation I can think of is the distinction between the "father" and the "mother" cannabis plants. You see, hemp doesn't get you high because it contains 0.3 percent of THC or less, but it does contain cannabidiol (CBD). The mother cannabis plants have THC, which is what gets you high—but they also contain smaller amounts of CBD. So even then, the mother plant can't be discounted for medical purposes either. Whatever way you want to look at it, there are eighty-five known cannabinoids in the cannabis plant, and the US government has a patent on some of those cannabinoids. See, the government clearly knows the difference between hemp and THC—if they didn't, then they wouldn't have patented CBD.

For Hearst, DuPont, and Anslinger to be successful in eradicating hemp, they had to classify cannabis as one type of plant—this is why the government to this day does not distinguish between industrial hemp and marijuana. Both are classified as Schedule I narcotics, even though hemp has no psychoactive elements. Hearst, DuPont, and Anslinger were really at war with the hemp plant, and to demonize hemp, they had to lump it in the same category as the mother plant that produced the psychoactive element THC. Once legislation was passed that didn't differentiate the hemp plant from the THC plant, the damage was done. But if you asked any hemp farmer, he'd tell you there's no value in smoking hemp because it won't get you high. Hell, even George Washington wrote about this in is diaries! In his diary entry on August 7, 1765, Washington wrote how he "began to separate the Male from the Female hemp"[16] when it was time to harvest them because he used them for different purposes. Yet, to this day, it serves in the government's best interest to continue as if it doesn't know the genetic difference between these two plants, even though it is clear through its patent that it does!

Here's further evidence that the government believes in the healing properties of CBD: The 1976 *Randall v. United States* lawsuit. This lawsuit took place after President Nixon declared his War on Drugs, and it resulted in the Compassionate Investigational New Drug Study program, or Compassionate IND. This was the first blow to Nixon's War on Drugs, less than five years after he established the DEA, and he essentially already lost his drug war due to the lawsuit because it gave certain Americans the right to legally smoke pot.

In 1976, Robert Randall became the first legal pot smoker in the United States since the Marijuana Tax Act of 1937. He had to sue the Food and Drug Administration, the Drug Enforcement Administration, the National Institute on Drug Abuse, the Department of Justice, and the Department of Health, Education & Welfare to establish the right to smoke pot, but he succeeded. So why did this pothead go to such great lengths to get his fix?

Randall was barely out of college when he was diagnosed with hereditary glaucoma. He told his doctor that he could actually see better after smoking pot, and his doctor encouraged him to grow marijuana at his home. In 1975, Randall's apartment was raided and he was arrested for growing and possessing marijuana, a Schedule I narcotic. However, science was on his side. Scientific experiments in 1971 confirmed that marijuana did indeed help people with glaucoma. So after his arrest, Randall took the feds to court and sued under the plea of medical necessity. On November 24, 1976, Judge James Washington ruled in his favor, stating,

> While blindness was shown by competent medical testimony to be the otherwise inevitable result of the defendant's disease, no adverse effects from the smoking of marijuana have been demonstrated. . . . Medical evidence suggests that the medical prohibition is not well-founded.[17]

After the criminal charges against Randall were dropped, he filed a petition in May 1976 to grant him FDA-approved access to government supplies of medical marijuana. That's right. This guy got the feds to ship him his own personal supply of weed because it was the only substance that treated his medical disorder! Don't ever tell me that a pothead is lazy or stupid!

Shortly after he started receiving weed from the government, he went public with what happened to him, and then the government tried to cut him off from his supply! Randall had to sue them again in 1978. To avoid a media firestorm, the feds requested to settle out of court within twenty-four hours of Randall filing the suit. Randall was then able to get prescription access to marijuana through a local pharmacy near his home. Henry J. Anslinger must have been rolling over in his grave!

The settlement in the 1978 *Randall v. United States* lawsuit became the legal basis for the FDA's Compassionate IND program.[18] Initially, the program was only available to patients afflicted by "marijuana-responsive" disorders, such as glaucoma. Then it was expanded to include HIV-positive patients in the mid-1980s. At its peak, the program had thirty active participants, but it stopped accepting new patients in 1992 due to President George H. W. Bush's desire to "get tough on crime and drugs." The Bush administration's public health authorities actually concluded that there was no scientific value to the program. Really? So that means Robert Randall's case—you know, the one he won against the federal government—had no scientific value? So the Bush administration apparently knew more than all those scientists who proved glaucoma is a "marijuana-responsive" condition?

I guess these public health authorities didn't anticipate that by closing the program during the height of the AIDS epidemic that they would actually spawn the medical marijuana movement in the United States. Initially, the movement for medical marijuana focused on anorexia patients and AIDS patients suffering from "wasting syndrome." At that time, cancer patients took up the torch, and today we're still trying to get our hands on this plant with healing qualities.

As of April 2014, there are only four patients from the Compassionate Investigational New Drug Study program that are still alive.[19] They receive about 9 oz. of pot from the government per month. What are their aliments? Glaucoma, multiple sclerosis, nail-patella syndrome, and a rare bone disorder.[20]

Now, as great as this all was for Randall and the thirty people accepted into the program, the whole chain of events angers me. There are more than thirty people in America with glaucoma, multiple sclerosis, nail-patella syndrome, and rare bone disorders. Couldn't more people have benefitted from government-approved marijuana? If smoking pot is medically proven to help people with glaucoma improve their vision, then what right does the federal government have to deny people the ability to see?

And let's not forget all the US citizens sitting in prison right now due to trumped-up marijuana charges. The truth is that the so-called "Land of the Free" has more people behind bars than any of the dictators we so despise. How can the federal government give certain people marijuana and then try to arrest everyone else who uses it?

When it comes to marijuana, we don't have a criminal justice system, we have a criminal injustice system:

- The number of Americans incarcerated in federal, state, and local prisons and jails was 2,220,300 in 2013 (or 1 in every 110 adults), which gives the United States the highest incarceration rate in the world.[21]

- As of 2015, 51 percent of America's federal inmates are in prison due to drug-related convictions.[22]

- In 2014, there were 1.5 million people arrested in the United States for nonviolent drug charges.[23]

- In 2012, police arrested one person every forty-two seconds for marijuana possession.[24]

- In 2009 alone, 1.66 million Americans were arrested on drug charges—which is more than were arrested on assault or larceny charges. And four out of five of those arrests were simply for possession.[25]

- The number of students who have lost federal financial aid eligibility due to a drug conviction is more than two hundred thousand.[26]

- $63.4 billion of taxpayer dollars were spent on the prison system in 2014 and it costs taxpayers at least $31,000 per inmate per year.[27]

- You can be arrested for marijuana possession in states that have "legalized" marijuana. For example, as of March 2015, if you have 8 oz. of weed or more on you, you could wind up with a felony charge in Colorado![28]

- And forget about amnesty for pot convicts! Colorado still hasn't proposed a bill to release people imprisoned for marijuana-related crimes.[29] As of 2010, there were 210,000 marijuana possession arrests in Colorado.[30] Not one of those prison terms has been adjusted due to the legalization of marijuana and none of those people have had their records expunged once they've served their time.

I'm so proud of my country. We won't raise the minimum wage so people can get above the poverty line, but we're happy to throw you in prison and pay $31,000 per year to have you sit on your ass! Hell, maybe you're better off going to jail. Maybe I'm on the wrong side of this drug war after all. Most of those folks can also get a college degree while they're serving time. So forget your plan to get public colleges fully funded, Bernie Sanders. We'll just continue the War on Drugs until we're all in jail. Then we can all get government health care too. It might not be the best health care, and the food might not taste all that great either, but hey, at least the government is paying for all of it!

Now of course, I'm being sarcastic here, but come on now. How many Americans have been denied relief from pain and sickness due to the war against marijuana? How many lives have been completely ruined due to trumped-up marijuana charges? And how many people continue to live with a criminal record, even after their state has legalized the substance that caused their arrests?

Is there any way to end the war on drugs when so much of America's prison system is invested in it? Take California, for example. If California taxed and regulated the sale of marijuana like Colorado does, it would raise an estimated annual revenue of $1.4 billion.[31] In 2011, California spent $9.6 billion on the prison system (that's roughly $50,000 per inmate per year).[32] This tells me that politicians would rather spend our money than make money for the state! If illegal drugs were taxed federally at rates comparable to alcohol and tobacco, we'd see $46.7 billion in tax revenue every year, yet we currently spend more than $51 billion on the War on Drugs every year.[33] Wouldn't the federal government rather see billions coming in? Oh yeah, that's right. If they cut the War on Drugs program, they'd be cutting all their buddies out of a paycheck.

First things first: we need to stop the marijuana propaganda once and for all. Cannabis should have never been labeled as a Schedule I narcotic.

7

Marijuana is NOT a Schedule I Narcotic

I have a simple question to ask you: Do you consider heroin and marijuana to be the same drug? For instance, if a police officer finds heroin in your car or marijuana in your car, should the consequences be identical? Will smoking a joint or shooting heroin result in the same addiction? If you work for the federal government, then your answer is yes.

The DEA classifies heroin, LSD (lysergic acid diethylamide), ecstasy (3,4-methylenedioxymethampetamine), methaqualone, peyote, and marijuana as the same drug category. I'll repeat that: in America, heroin and marijuana are considered the same drug by federal law enforcement. They are listed as Schedule I narcotics, which means they are the "most dangerous" of all drugs because they have the potential to inflict "severe psychological or physical dependence."[1]

Therefore, in the United States, marijuana is considered to be just as addictive as heroin, even though pot has been proven not to be addictive by medical studies. The feds also consider marijuana to be just as dangerous as heroin, even though pot users cannot overdose.

To date, there have been zero marijuana overdose deaths, but heroin-related overdose deaths have continued to increase drastically each year. The CDC reports that from 2002 to 2013, heroin overdose deaths in the United States have increased by 286 percent. [2] So why are marijuana and heroin classified as identical substances under federal law? I'll give you a history lesson on how President

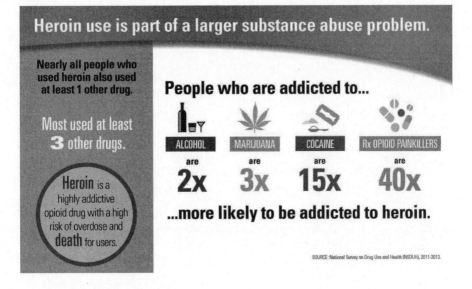

Heroin use is part of a larger substance abuse problem.

Nearly all people who used heroin also used at least 1 other drug.

Most used at least **3** other drugs.

Heroin is a highly addictive opioid drug with a high risk of overdose and **death** for users.

People who are addicted to...

ALCOHOL	MARIJUANA	COCAINE	Rx OPIOID PAINKILLERS
are	are	are	are
2x	**3x**	**15x**	**40x**

...more likely to be addicted to heroin.

SOURCE: National Survey on Drug Use and Health (NSDUH), 2011-2013.

Nixon allowed this to happen later, but first, there's more to the DEA's hypocrisy on the Schedule I narcotic classification you should know.

I have another simple question for you: What's the difference between a small cup of Pepsi and a Big Gulp cup of Pepsi? Isn't it just that one cup is a bigger size than the other? Heroin and prescription pain pills can be viewed in the same manner. Heroin is an opioid and pain pills are opioids—the only difference is that pain pills come in a smaller dosage. Because heroin and prescription pain pills are both opioids, they both bind to the same receptors in the central nervous system to give pain relief.[3] So why didn't prescription pain pills make the cut for the Schedule I classification if they have the same chemical make-up as heroin?

Even though oxycodone, hydrocodone, Vicodin, and heroin are essentially the same thing, the DEA classifies all opioid pain pills as Schedule II. Schedule II drugs include hydrocodone, Vicodin, cocaine, methamphetamine, methadone, hydromorphone (Dilaudid), meperidine (Demerol), oxycodone (OxyContin), fentanyl, Dexedrine, Adderall, and Ritalin. Here's where the hypocrisy really comes in: Schedule II drugs are labeled as drugs with a high potential for abuse, but less abuse than Schedule I drugs, so they can be prescribed by doctors. I find this laughable when doctors consider opioid pills "heroin lite" because addicts switch back and forth between prescription pills and heroin. Take the actor Philip Seymour Hoffman, for instance. He quit heroin more than twenty years ago, but struggled with addictions to medications like Vicodin, OxyCotin, and oxycodone, and he died of an overdose at forty-six years old. [4]

So essentially, prescription painkillers are the gateway drugs to heroin, yet they are classified as a Schedule II narcotic instead of a Schedule I—even though they are made from the same plant as heroin. Does that make any sense to you? Here's another head scratcher: the CDC states that people addicted to opioid painkillers (prescription medications) are forty times more likely to be addicted to heroin. [5]

So again, heroin and marijuana are identical under the law, but they do not have the same addictive properties. Heroin and prescription pain pills are opioids and are therefore classified as the same addiction by doctors (opioid addiction), yet the federal government considers prescription pain pills to be less harmful than heroin.

Just to really drive home the hypocrisy of these drug classifications, let's take a look at some statistics the American Society of Addiction Medicine (ASAM) has compiled about America's national opioid overdose epidemic:[6]

- Forty-six Americans die each day from prescription opioid overdoses, which is two deaths an hour and seventeen thousand people annually.
- Heroin poisonings increased by 12.4 percent from 1999 to 2002 in the United States, and the number of prescription opioid poisonings increased by 91.2 percent during that same time period.
- About 8,200 Americans die annually from heroin overdose.
- About 75 percent of opioid addiction disease patients switch to heroin as a cheaper opioid source.
- In 2012 alone, 259 million opioid pain medication prescriptions were written, which is enough for every adult in America to have a bottle of pills.
- Nearly one in twenty high school seniors has taken Vicodin and one in thirty has abused OxyContin.
- Over 50 percent of individuals twelve years or older has used pain relievers non-medically from a friend or relative.
- The number of opioids prescribed to adolescents and young adults (ages fifteen to twenty-nine) nearly doubled between 1994 and 2007.
- As of 2015, there are 1.9 million Americans living with prescription opioid abuse or dependence, while 517,000 Americans live with heroin addiction.

The ASAM also notes that any type of opioid can trigger "latent chronic addiction brain disease"[7]—which means if you take any type of prescription pain medication derived from opioids then you could become addicted to opioids.

This tells me that Big Pharma is in the lead when it comes to providing a gateway to heroin addiction. Have you heard of the painkiller called Zohydro ER? It is an opiate so powerful that it is referred to as "heroin in a capsule."[8] As of May 2014, twenty-nine states have demanded that the FDA overturn its decision[9] to approve Zohydro, a drug that releases the effects of pain pills like oxycodone at a higher dosage for a longer period of time.

So how do we cure the heroin and opioid pain pill epidemic in this country? Ladies and gentlemen, look no further than marijuana! Study after study after study proves that marijuana actually treats opioid addiction. Cannabis therapy has been used in all forms of addiction recovery for more than one hundred years. But hey, don't take my word for it:

- In 1889, Dr. Edward A. Birch reported his success in treating opiate and chloral addiction with cannabis in *The Lancet*.[10]
- In June 2003, the *Journal of Pain and Symptom Management* published a study for patients suffering from chronic pain. Those who suffer from chronic pain are most likely to become addicted to opioids due to the amount of prescription pain medication they must take. The study proved that when the patient smoked or ingested cannabis, that person reduced the dosage of opioids used to manage their chronic pain.[11] That's truly remarkable, considering that those who suffer from chronic pain develop a tolerance for opioid pills and must constantly up their dosages (which is what leads to opioid dependence and opioid addiction).
- A groundbreaking study published in *The Harm Reduction Journal* in 2007 looked at 4,117 marijuana smokers in California and found that those who regularly smoked weed decreased the desire to use tobacco, alcohol, and hard drugs.[12] In other words, weed isn't a gateway drug. Nearly 90 percent of those in the study claimed to have cut their drinking in half! Instead of enticing young people to use other drugs—including alcohol—weed has the opposite effect!
- In 2009, a study conducted by the Laboratory for Physiopathology of Diseases of the Central Nervous System proved that injections of THC eliminate morphine and heroin addiction in rats.[13]

- *The Harm Reduction Journal* published a 2009 Berkeley study that polled 350 cannabis users who were once addicted to a substance: 40 percent were alcoholics who used cannabis to control their alcohol cravings; 66 percent were addicted to prescription drugs and used cannabis to stop their addictions; 26 percent were addicted to more potent illegal drugs and used cannabis to end their addictions. [14]

- In September 2013, a study by the National Institute of Health showed that cannabis is an effective treatment for curing people of "hard drug" addiction, including cocaine, meth and amphetamines.[15]

- Did you know that drinking too much alcohol can lead to permanent brain damage? In October 2013, Pharmacology Biochemistry and Behavior published a study from scientists at the University of Kentucky and the University of Maryland that concluded cannabidiol (CBD) actually protects the brain from alcohol-induced brain damage and might be able to prevent it![16]

- A study published in October 2014 in *JAMA International Medicine* showed that states with legal medical marijuana had a 25 percent reduction in opioid overdose deaths.[17] What further proof do you need, people?

This is only a handful of studies that prove how marijuana can be used to treat addiction. As far back as the 1800s, doctors knew that "cannabis did not lead to physical dependence," and since it didn't have as many side effects as morphine, "it was found to be superior to the opiates for a number of therapeutic purposes."[18] To this day, all opioids including prescription pain pills have several side effects: constipation, dizziness, nausea, vomiting, tolerance (meaning your body builds up a tolerance to it and you have to increase the strength of the drug for it to be effective), and physical dependence (addiction).[19] Meanwhile, the prolonged use of cannabis does not lead to the development of physical dependence. Studies from as far back as the 1930s, 1940s, 1950s, and 1960s have proven this to be true.[20] In fact, reports commissioned by President Kennedy and President Johnson in the '60s found that marijuana use doesn't lead to violent acts or heavier drug use. This is why in 1968, the FDA merged with the Federal Bureau of Narcotics to form the Bureau of Narcotics and Dangerous Drugs—there was a policy shift to consider treatment instead of just criminal penalties for drug offenses.[21]

So why was marijuana labeled as a Schedule I narcotic in 1970, if it is not an addictive substance? Roger O. Egeberg, the Assistant Secretary of Health, advised Harley O. Staggers, the Chairman of the House Committee on Interstate and Foreign Commerce, to classify cannabis as a Schedule I narcotic until further testing could be done:

> Since there is still a considerable void in our knowledge of the plant and effects of the active drug contained in it, our recommendation is that marijuana be retained within Schedule I at least until the completion of certain studies now underway to resolve the issue. [22]

The only problem was that nothing was ever resolved. In 1972, the National Commission on Marijuana and Drug Abuse released a report favoring decriminalization of cannabis, but the Nixon administration ignored it. Also in 1972, the bipartisan Shafer Commission, appointed by President Nixon, recommended decriminalizing the personal use of marijuana.[23] Nixon again rejected this. And think about why he did: marijuana use was common in the '60s and '70s. If you want to start a War on Drugs, why would you decriminalize the one drug everyone knows about? Meanwhile, over the course of the 1970s, eleven states decriminalized marijuana and others reduced marijuana penalties.[24]

So as you can see, history again is repeating itself! Here's how the federal government has been at odds with a plant and at odds with the American people since the '70s:

- In 1972, the National Organization for the Reform of Marijuana Laws (NORML) petitioned to have cannabis transferred to a Schedule II drug so that it could be legally prescribed by physicians.
- This resulted in the Supreme Court ordering the government to start scientific and medical evaluations of cannabis in 1980.
- In the early 1980s, some members of Congress tried twice to reschedule the drug to a Schedule II through legislation—it did not get enough support either time, even though there was bipartisan support.
- On October 18, 1985 the DEA approved a pill form of synthetic THC to be classified as a Schedule II drug and sold under the name of Marinol and Cesamet.[25] Can you believe that? Big Pharma can sell you a pill made out of THC. But if you get your THC organically, straight from the source, you're going to jail.

Following this clearly hypocritical classification of Marinol, the DEA initiated public hearings from 1986 to 1988 on cannabis rescheduling. In a strange turn of events, DEA Chief Administrative Law Judge Francis L. Young declared cannabis in its natural form is "one of the safest therapeutically active substances known to man."[26] Clearly, Young wanted cannabis to be reclassified; however, John Law, the DEA Administrator appointed by President Ronald Reagan, overruled Young's determination. Keep in mind, these hearings were taking place during Reagan's administration—where the DARE drug education program, the "Just Say No" anti-drug campaign, and the country's first zero-tolerance drug policies were born.[27] In 1986, while the DEA hearings were going on, Reagan signed the Anti-Drug Abuse Act, which established mandatory sentences for drug-related crimes. Which goes to show you he did not learn from history. In the 1950s, there were mandatory minimum sentences for drug-related offenses, but Congress repealed those in the '70s because the laws "had done nothing to eliminate the drug culture that embraced marijuana use through the '60s."[28] With the Anti-Drug Abuse Act, if you possessed one hundred marijuana plants, you received the same penalty as 100 g of heroin.[29] See, what did I tell you? The federal government thinks heroin and marijuana are the same thing!

Unfortunately, DEA Chief Administrative Law Judge Francis L. Young was not successful in convincing Reagan's administration to reclassify weed. Reagan's appointed DEA Administrator John Law was backed up by the former DEA Administrator Robert Bonner, who said in 1992, "Those who insist that marijuana has medical uses would serve society better by promoting or sponsoring more legitimate research."[30] By 1994, the DC Court of Appeals sided with Law and Bonner.[31] Cannabis would remain a Schedule I narcotic. But by that time, we were already past President George H. W. Bush's new War on Drugs—which put a new spotlight on the "dangers" of marijuana—and onto President Bill Clinton's "tough on crime" policies, which is how we wound up with the prison system we have today. More on that later, but let's just say for now Clinton incarcerated more Americans than any of his Republican predecessors and his policies—which were completely out of proportion to the crime committed—had a small impact on actual crime rates or drug use.[32]

Even though it seemed like a losing battle, NORML and other vigilant activist groups kept coming at the federal government with more petitions and lawsuits demonstrating the need for weed. States also started passing their own medical marijuana laws, with California being the first in 1996.[33] Isn't that interesting? In the '70s, states decriminalized weed when Nixon classified it as a Schedule I narcotic and in the '90s through today, states are downright legalizing it—regardless if we have a Democrat or a Republican Commander in Chief!

What I find interesting about every petition, every lawsuit that was brought forward to the federal government concerning the medical necessity of marijuana is this: the outcome is the same. The courts determine there isn't enough research to justify reclassifying the drug. The courts also "demand" more studies, and the song and dance continues. Meanwhile in July of 1999, Marinol was rescheduled from a Schedule II to an even less restrictive Schedule III drug![34] That's right, folks: THC in a pill form is the same drug classification as testosterone, ketamine, anabolic steroids, and Tylenol cough syrup with codeine![35] THC—the psychoactive element in marijuana—is considered a drug with "a moderate to low potential for physical and psychological dependence"[36] if it's rebranded as Marinol.

Now do you see why corporations don't want marijuana to be legalized? Big Pharma had a monopoly on THC until California approved Prop 215 in 1996 to allow medical access, cultivation, and possession of marijuana. You know what the most astounding part of all this is? The number one side effect of Marinol (which you can now get as a generic known as Dronabinol) is feeling "high"— which is described as "easy laughing, elation, and heightened awareness" by the FDA—and the second side effect is "appetite stimulation."[37] But I could have told you that without looking at the results of the clinical trials!

So now that we've officially proven that marijuana is not the same as heroin, and it should not be classified as a Schedule I narcotic, especially when THC is available in a pill form as a Schedule III narcotic, let me tell you what the FDA has been up to recently in regards to justifying Marinol's classification because that hypocrisy is stranger than fiction. In June 2014, US regulators at the FDA started to conduct an analysis of whether the United States should downgrade the classification of marijuana as a Schedule I drug.[38] Remember what happened in 1980 after NORML petitioned to have marijuana reclassified as a Schedule II drug? The courts ordered the government to start medical and scientific evaluations to determine just that. Thirty-four years later, the FDA still needs to do more testing on weed? Bullshit! What kind of study still needs to take place? Don't they work with the scientific community, which has already determined time and time again the medical necessity of this plant?

And get this: the FDA's analysis on pot is at the request of the DEA! [39] We might as well be living in the 1940s when Henry J. Anslinger told William Randolph Hearst to run a story in his newspapers about the AMA debunking the LaGuardia Report because it sounds like the FDA is being tasked with "debunking" science and backing up the DEA's propaganda campaign that marijuana is a gateway drug and just as addicting as heroin.

So should we take this new FDA study seriously, whenever the results come out? Well, like I said earlier, the DEA isn't going to put itself in a position to be out of work. And like I mentioned earlier in this chapter, marijuana is effective in curing drug addiction. So if more people smoked pot, that means on a biological level, less people would feel compelled to drink or use hard drugs. Wouldn't that actually help end the War on Drugs, therefore putting the DEA out of a job? Wouldn't legalizing marijuana actually stop US drug users from wanting meth, coke, heroin, and all the other substances supplied by Mexican drug cartels? Science has proven that when marijuana interacts with our body, it works like the reverse of a gateway drug: we no longer want or desire those other harmful drugs from south of the border. Shit, do you think the DEA knows that? Well if it does, we're screwed!

The only reason I'm hopeful about the FDA study is that as of October 2014, there were roughly 1,137,069 people in the United States using marijuana legally as a medical substance.[40] This must be a huge thorn in the DEA's side because according to federal law, a doctor cannot prescribe a Schedule I narcotic under any circumstance. Thank goodness for states like California that have the courage to separate true medical studies from the government's propaganda campaign, or those more than one million people would still be suffering unnecessarily. In a country with a population of over 322.8 million people,[41] we still have a long way to go to get everyone the proper medication.

The first step in reclassifying marijuana is to stop referring to it as a drug. If Big Pharma can pass off THC in a pill form as medication, then weed is a medication. If the government owns a patent on CBD because it has medical benefits, then weed is a medication. It's that simple.

8

Marijuana Is a Medication

ince marijuana is a medication, let's take an honest look at weed from a medical standpoint. As of 2015, there has been some form of legal medical use for cannabis in twenty-three states as well as the District of Columbia. These countries have legalized or decriminalized medical marijuana in some way: Colombia, Czech Republic, Ecuador, the Netherlands, Israel, Canada, Norway, Peru, Romania, Spain, Uruguay, and Switzerland.[1] In 2001, Portugal became the first country in the world to decriminalize the possession and use of all drugs.[2] (More on that later.)

Today, doctors around the world are prescribing weed for many conditions, such as:[3]

- To dull pain
- To aid sleep
- To stimulate the appetite
- To de-stress the anxious
- To calm the aggressive
- As an anti-inflammatory, an analgesic, an antiemetic, a bronchodilator
- To cure a bad case of hiccups
- To protect the brain against trauma (like PTSD) and aids in "memory extinction" after catastrophic events
- To boost the immune system

- To treat ailments attributed to diseases, disorders and conditions such as multiple sclerosis, psoriasis, dementia, schizophrenia, osteoporosis, amyotrophic lateral sclerosis (Lou Gehrig's disease), glaucoma, Crohn's diseases, Tourette's syndrome, anorexia, nausea, mucous membrane inflammation, cough, leprosy, fever, urinary tract infections, hemorrhoids, and asthma
- To alleviate the side effects of chemotherapy
- To help AIDS patients recover from weight loss
- For use after kidney transplants to lessen the chance of transplant rejection[4]
- To treat neurological disorders, including epilepsy and seizures

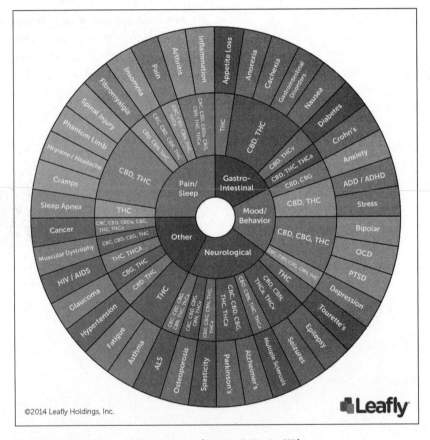

What a simple plant with strains of THC and CBD can do *(credit: Leafy Holdings Inc. 2014)*

However, none of these conditions are universally accepted by politicians as reasons to prescribe marijuana by law. Politicians can determine what medical studies they want to validate and which conditions still need more research. PTSD is one example of a controversial condition. Depending on what state you live in—or if you're a veteran—you may or may not be able to get a prescription for medical marijuana for PTSD (more on that later).

All I can tell you is the United States is falling behind when it comes to marijuana research. If you want to look at the future of cannabis medicine, you'll want to look into what Israel is doing. Since 1963, Israeli organic chemist Raphael Mechoulam has been conducting studies on the plant, and today he is widely known as the "patriarch of cannabis science."[5] And he isn't a pothead either. In fact, he doesn't smoke it at all. He's a respected member of the Israel Academy of Sciences and Humanities, and he's a professor at Hebrew University's Hadassah Medical School. He's authored more than four hundred scientific papers and holds about twenty-five patents on cannabis. His main claim to fame is isolating THC and CBD to research the medical benefits of each, and most of the modern uses for these two substances have come from his research.

So medically speaking, what does THC and CBD do to our bodies? Well, you've heard of the circulatory system, the skeletal system, the digestive system, the central nervous system, the reproductive system—but we also have what some refer to as the endocannabinoid system (or ECS). Remember cannabidiol (CBD) from chapter 6? Just like calcium strengthens our bones and omega-3 fatty acids help our brains function better, CBD and THC interact with our endocannabinoid system, which is located in our brains and throughout our central nervous system.

The ECS is what processes our sense of appetite and our sense of pain. It also plays a role in our mood and in short-term and long-term memory and in mediating the effects of cannabis. Dr. Mechoulam discovered how the ECS reacts to cannabis. The way he explains how it works is this: Have you ever heard an experienced runner talk about the "high" of jogging? Well, exercise elevates the endocannabinoid levels in our brains naturally—much the same way endorphins, serotonin, and dopamine do. According to Mechoulam, endocannabinoids play an important role in basic brain functions, such as memory, balance, movement, immune health, and neuro-protection. So essentially a plant that contains cannabinoids (weed) interacts with our ECS neurological network in much the same way jogging does for an avid runner. Exercise gives our ECS an extra jolt, as does weed. But that's how medication works—it's an artificial way of helping our bodies feel better or manage pain or trigger hunger.

Speaking of triggering hunger, mother nature provides mammals with endogenous cannabinoids ("endocannabinoids") in milk. In one of the papers Mechoulam published in 1998, he discovered that endocannabinoids are in cow's milk.[6] Other researchers have discovered endocannabinoids in human breast milk.[7] Endocannabinoids bind with receptors in the brains of newborns to trigger their desire to eat.[8] Therefore, endocannabinoids literally teach newborn mammals—including human infants—how to eat![9]

Now, let's circle back to our sense of pain. Bial, a Portuguese pharmaceutical company, attempted to artificially create a pain medicine that interacts with our endocannabinoid system to relieve pain. The goal was to create a substance—one without THC or CBD in it—to do what marijuana does naturally. The only problem was that the six folks who participated in phase one of the initial drug trial in January 2016 wound up severely injured for life due to the side effects—within four days of taking the recommended dosage.[10] One of the six participants is actually brain-dead. Bial's new drug was invented as a potential treatment for multiple sclerosis, leukemia, rheumatoid arthritis[11]—you know, those illnesses that weed already treats. It must be driving Big Pharma absolutely crazy to know that they have been entirely unsuccessful in duplicating what a plant can provide!

But what about Marinol? Didn't Big Pharma already create THC in a pill to alleviate pain? Lyn Nofziger—who served as Ronald Reagan's press secretary during his 1980 presidential campaign, then as Reagan's White House director of communication and chief speechwriter—has some personal experience with Marinol. When Nofziger's daughter was undergoing chemotherapy for lymph cancer, he explained:

> She was sick and vomiting constantly as a result of her treatments. No legal drugs, including the synthetic 'marijuana' pill Marinol, helped her situation. As a result, we finally turned to marijuana which, of course, we were forced to obtain illegally. With it, she kept her food down, was comfortable, and even gained weight. . . . Marijuana clearly has medical value. Thousands of seriously ill Americans have been able to determine that for themselves, albeit illegally. Like my own family, these individuals did not wish to break the law but they had no other choice.[12]

So let me get this straight—the guy who either wrote or approved all the speeches for Reagan's presidency, including those of the "Just Say No" campaign, was buying pot illegally for his daughter? At what point do you not bring the president to your daughter's bedside and say, "Look what your war on marijuana is doing—it has turned my family into criminals!"

I can completely understand how Marinol might not be effective for cancer patients. If you're vomiting and can't keep anything down, how the hell are you supposed to swallow a pill long enough for it to work? If you can breathe, you can inhale and exhale your medication, and guess what: It will actually stay in your system long enough to work. Weed has been known to calm the stomach, so why not smoke your medication? Weed will naturally induce hunger and stop the feelings of nausea so you can stop vomiting and put some nourishment in your body!

Of course there are side effects of nearly every medication, so what are the side effects of marijuana? That all depends on whom you ask. If you smoke it heavily, most studies state that you might wind up with a cough, wheezing, shortness of breath, or chronic bronchitis, but overall, today's studies state that there is no evidence that smoking pot will lead to "airflow obstruction or emphysema."[13] Yet again, if you ask a scientist, a member of the DEA, or a politician, they'll all have different answers about marijuana's side effects—and of course it depends on if you're talking about THC or CBD because the side effects are different.

Here's what we know about tetrahydrocannabinol (THC)—it gets you high:

- Early effects include light-headedness, dizziness, euphoria, and sometimes visual-perceptual changes (colors could be more vivid, etc).[14]
- Depending on the person and how much THC you take at one time, some people feel sedated, some people feel calm, some people can feel anxiety, panic, or paranoia.
- Most everyone experiences an increase in appetite due to THC.
- THC stimulates cells in the brain to release dopamine, which is what creates the high, euphoric feeling.
- The side effect of this is that it interferes with how information is processed by our hippocampus, the part of the brain responsible for forming new memories.
- THC can also affect your concept of time, speed, balance, thinking, problem-solving, and motion due to how it interacts with the brain.[15] That's why you shouldn't drive if you're high!

- THC can induce hallucinations, but I've never actually met anyone who has experienced this before. Hallucinations from mushrooms and acid? Yeah. Pot? Not so much. Well, unless you eat one of those really strong cookies. I would call a THC hallucination as close as you can get to overdosing on weed.
- THC can cause your heart rate and blood pressure to rise. It can also affect your body temperature.
- If you have a history of schizophrenia, THC can trigger an episode.
- There are contradictory studies about the effects of THC on pregnant women. Some women want to use it to relieve severe cases of morning sickness, among other symptoms brought on by pregnancy. Studies are still ongoing—some conclude weed affects fetal development in high dosages, others say there is no impact on birth size or infant development with moderate use.[16]
- As for long-term effects? Some studies say THC can impact brain development and memory because the human brain doesn't reach full maturity until you're twenty-five.[17]
- Some studies also state that adolescents who smoke a lot of pot can experience a decreased IQ and memory and cognition issues, but not enough research has been done on this to make it an official long-term effect.[18]
- In August 2015, the American Psychological Association (APA), the country's largest organization of psychologists, published findings from a new marijuana study in *The Psychology of Addictive Behaviors* that contradicted every other marijuana study. The APA discovered that "chronic marijuana use among teenage boys does not appear to be linked to later physical or mental health issues such as depression or psychotic symptoms."[19] So again, THC might not be as dangerous to teenage development as initially thought. Remember, until recently, many marijuana "studies" were done at the request of our government, and you can bet the outcomes were predetermined.

Here's what we know about cannabidiol (CBD)—it doesn't get you high:

- CBD is non-psychoactive and actually blocks the high associated with THC.[20]
- It has absolutely no psychoactive properties; it is not addictive whatsoever.

- The only negative side effect of CBD is that some people experience "wake promoting," which means if you take CBD too close to bedtime, it can keep you awake for hours.[21]
- It combats diabetes, tumor growth, and chronic pain. It's actually been known to shrink the cell tissue of tumors or even destroy tumors completely (more on that later).
- Studies have concluded that CBD does not alter embryonic development, so pregnant women can take it in certain dosages.[22]
- CBD doesn't have much impact on the appetite, but it does work as an antidepressant.[23]
- Studies in animals show that it does not affect blood pressure, heart rate, body temperature, or glucose levels—and get this: there is no short-term memory loss associated with CBD use (unlike THC). [24]
- If you have schizophrenia or bipolar disorder, CBD doesn't have any negative effects and can actually reduce psychotic episodes after two to four weeks of use![25]

Now, some studies state that marijuana *is* addictive. That approximately one out of every ten users can become addicted to marijuana.[26] Remember what meth does to the brain? It brings more dopamine to the brain than what the brain creates naturally, therefore causing the brain to produce less dopamine, which in turn means the person doesn't experience genuine "happy" moments without meth. It's easy to become addicted to meth because with more and more use, meth causes our bodies to stop producing dopamine entirely, and then the only way to feel happiness is by taking more meth. Well, THC causes our bodies to release dopamine, which is what give us that "high" feeling; so some studies conclude that THC can be addictive because it interacts with the brain's receptors to do this.[27] People who use THC heavily can go through "withdrawal"—which seems like a strong word for grouchiness, sleeplessness, decreased appetite, anxiety, and cravings[28]—but that's what the National Institute on Drug Abuse claims marijuana withdrawal symptoms to be.

I find it laughable that a Schedule I narcotic's "withdrawal" symptoms are worse than caffeine withdrawal. Get this: caffeine withdrawal is now a recognized disorder, according to the American Psychiatric Association.[29] Take a look at these withdrawal symptoms: intense headache, sleepiness, irritability, lethargy, constipation, depression, muscle pain (including stiffness and cramping), lack of concentration, flu-like symptoms (yes, that's right: stuffy nose, blocked sinuses, and sinus pressure), insomnia, nausea and vomiting, anxiety, brain fog, dizziness, and heart rhythm abnormalities.[30] According to Johns Hopkins Medicine, "caffeine is the most commonly used mood-altering drug in the world and in North America, between 80 and 90 percent of adults and children consume it" on a regular basis.[31] And guess what else? Because caffeine is a stimulant, it's not clear what the long-term effects of high dosages are to the adolescent brain![32]

Meanwhile, opioid withdrawal—from both heroin and pain pills—includes cravings, abdominal cramping, diarrhea, dilated pupils, goose bumps, nausea, and vomiting.[33] And methamphetamine—which is a Schedule II drug—has even worse withdrawals: depression, anxiety, fatigue, cravings, confusion, insomnia, mood disturbances, violent behavior, paranoia, visual and auditory hallucinations, and delusions (such as the sensation of insects creeping under the skin), weight loss, severe tooth decay, tooth loss (ever hear of the expression "meth mouth"? Google some photos—it isn't pretty), and skin sores.[34]

According to the National Institute on Drug Abuse, psychotic symptoms can last for months or even years after a person has quit abusing meth.[35] So that means you could have meth hallucinations and delusions for years after you've gone cold turkey! I'd really like to hear from the DEA on why this drug is considered a Schedule II narcotic when the withdrawal symptoms are so intense, not to mention how easily people get addicted to it. Remember, meth is the Mexican drug cartels' number one bestseller among American drug addicts—not weed, not coke, not heroin, but meth.

But let's go back to looking at some of those other legal drugs—like tobacco and alcohol. Which drug would you rather be addicted to, alcohol, tobacco, or marijuana? I mean, seriously, I crave a steak every now and then, but that doesn't mean I'm addicted to red meat. You can crave the effects of marijuana, but you can go on with your life if you can't get in touch with your dealer. You might be a little upset, but hey, life goes on! Could you imagine what would happen if caffeine disappeared off the face of the earth for one day? Or alcohol or tobacco? People would be murdering each other in the streets!

Clearly, everyone knows how bad tobacco products are and how addicting they are, but did you know that researchers have found that nicotine actually primes the brain for other addictions? In animal studies, the effect of cocaine was amplified for animals that were given nicotine first.[36] So tobacco products do something to our brains to make drugs even more intense and more addicting!

I've never seen a single study that says marijuana can do that, yet marijuana is the illegal drug.

Much to Big Tobacco's dismay, the United States is slowly catching on to the dangers of this very addictive substance. In 2014, CVS pharmacy stopped carrying tobacco products nationwide.[37] In 2015, Hawaii became the first state to raise the smoking age to twenty-one. You must now be twenty-one years of age or older to purchase cigarettes or any tobacco products in the Aloha State.[38] There are also over one hundred cities nationwide that have raised the legal age limit for tobacco products to twenty-one, including New York City, Cleveland, and Kansas City.[39]

Personally, I feel that if you're old enough at the age of eighteen to die for your country and kill people in war, you should be old enough to decide if you want to smoke a cigarette or drink a beer. Part of freedom is the ability to make smart decisions and stupid decisions. You can't have freedom without the ability to make stupid choices. Hell, I made some stupid choices in my day—including chewing tobacco and smoking cigars. And when I finally quit, the withdrawal symptoms felt worse than death at the time. Take it from me—as someone who has quit tobacco and someone who has smoked marijuana—anything with nicotine in it is more addicting and more harmful to your body than marijuana.

Hell, you can die from tobacco! It causes lung disease, cancer, and according to the CDC, cigarette smoking harms nearly every organ of the body.[40] Meanwhile, a study in the *American Thoracic Society Journal* in 2013 found that "habitual" use of marijuana alone does not cause lung or upper airway cancer.[41] And we've already established the fact that marijuana does not harm the body's organs in any way because it's a medicinal plant!

Take that a step further and think about the relationship between cigarettes and alcohol. When someone is buzzed from drinking and then smokes a cigarette, doesn't that person get even more drunk? There's a chemical reaction taking place to enhance the experience. In 2012, a Yale study published in the *Journal of Adolescent Health* found that people who used alcohol or tobacco in their youth were twice as likely to abuse prescription opioid drugs than those who only used marijuana.[42] So maybe if our country wants to stop prescription drug abuse and heroin addiction, we should be doing something about cigarettes and alcohol!

Here's something else our major corporations don't want you to know: alcohol and cigarettes are the real gateway drugs. In 2010, *The Lancet* published a study by the Independent Scientific Committee on Drugs that cited alcohol as the most harmful drug overall when compared with heroin, crack cocaine, and meth. [43] The study proved that the UK's drug classifications (which are almost identical to ours) are not based off of scientific data that shows how harmful a substance actually is. I found it astounding that the scientists in the drug study didn't even bother to include marijuana! Probably because they understand that weed isn't the problem when it comes to drug abuse or addiction.

In addition to this, a study published in the peer-reviewed *Journal of School Health* in August 2012 showed that among twelfth graders in the United States, alcohol was by far the leading gateway drug. Students who used alcohol "exhibited a significantly greater likelihood of using both licit and illicit drugs."[44] The study recommended that adolescence receive school-based substance abuse prevention geared toward alcohol use. Think that will ever happen?

Oh, and I almost forgot to reiterate one final point about marijuana being a medication instead of a drug. What does THC do? It curbs alcohol and tobacco addictions! That's right. Doctors and psychologists consider weed a recovery treatment for nicotine and alcohol addiction. The National Institute on Drug Abuse states that half the individuals who begin an addiction treatment program relapse within six months because of their chemical dependency to the drug.[45] Think about the withdrawal symptoms of alcohol: anxiety or nervousness, depression, fatigue, irritability, jumpiness or shakiness, mood swings, nightmares, clammy skin, headache, insomnia, loss of appetite, nausea and vomiting, rapid heart rate, sweating, delirium, hallucinations, and seizures.[46] Then think about the withdrawal symptoms of nicotine: tingling in the hands and feet, sweating, nausea and cramping, headache, cold symptoms, anxiety, insomnia, cravings, confusion, irritability, depression, temper tantrums, constipation, boredom, dizziness, and weight gain.[47] Then think about what marijuana does and how it could curb these symptoms entirely. Remember the study in the *Harm Reduction Journal* from chapter 7? Addicts who regularly smoked weed decreased their desire to use tobacco, alcohol, and hard drugs[48] without experiencing all those awful withdrawal symptoms.

But Big Pharma wants to keep all these benefits of cannabis under wraps. Hell, if you want to talk about drugs with side effects or drugs that are addictive, look no further than Big Pharma! Case in point: Take any drug commercial on TV. Don't the side effects seem worse than the symptoms of the condition that the drug treats? Take a look at the DEA's narcotic drug classifications—the majority of these addictive substances were invented in a pharmaceutical lab. So how does Big Pharma get away with all of this? It has friends in high places!

In September 2015, President Obama nominated Dr. Robert Califf to be the next commissioner of the FDA, to replace Margaret Hamburg, the outgoing commissioner.[49] The sixty-four-year-old cardiologist and clinical trial expert from Duke University hasn't gotten the job yet.[50] As of February 2016, Dr. Stephen Ostroff is the FDA's acting commissioner.[51] Ostroff is a scientist and a long-time official at the HHS, so he would seem to be a natural fit to replace Hamburg. So why did Califf get recommended by the president? Califf receives $100,000 a year in consulting fees from Merck & Co, Bristol-Myers Squibb, Eli Lilly & Co., and Norvartis.[52] Folks, if that doesn't tell you how much Big Pharma controls our government, I don't know what will. Califf is currently the deputy commissioner of the FDA. If he becomes the next commissioner, he'll hold the regulatory leash on food, drugs, tobacco, and just about any product sold across the United States. Remember, the FDA is the arm of the government that approves a pharmaceutical drug. If Califf gets the commissioner's position, you can bet we'll see more addictive drugs like Zohydro on the fast track for approval.

Meanwhile, in June 2015, the National Institute on Drug Abuse (NIDA) approved a $3 million grant to whatever pharmaceutical company can create of a pill to stop marijuana addiction![53] Folks, this is what our government is spending our taxpayer money on! If you go to the NIDA's website, it says that an estimated 9 percent of people who use marijuana will become dependent on it.[54] After offering Big Pharma $3 million to "cure" weed addiction, the NIDA claims an estimated 4.2 million Americans are addicted to cannabis.[55] Don't you wonder where these statistics come from? I sure as hell do.

So how many people abuse prescription drugs? According to the NIDA, an estimated fifty-two million people in the United States over the age of twelve have used prescription drugs for a "non-medical" purpose. On a monthly basis, an average of 6.1 million people use prescription drugs for non-medical reasons. And 2010, there were 5.1 million people who abused painkillers.[56] Take a look again at the side effects of marijuana and painkillers and you tell me which drug should get a $3 million grant to resolve addiction.

Did you know a severe side effect of pharmaceutical drugs is literally death? I'm not talking about overdosing. I'm referring to the harm your body takes on due to these drugs. The harm is so intense that it causes a certain percentage of the population to literally die due to a bad reaction. Take a look at these statistics from 2010: prescription drugs taken as directed kill one hundred thousand Americans per year. That's 270 people per day. That's one person every five minutes![57] In June 2014, Harvard University noted that prescription drugs—again, when taken as directed by a doctor—causes about 1.9 million hospitalizations a year due to serious adverse side effects.[58]

So of the 170 million Americans who take a prescription drug as directed by their doctors, approximately 1.5 percent will experience severe reactions—including death—due to the side effects.[59] But how do you know if you're one of those people who will have a life-or-death reaction to your cholesterol medication or your blood pressure medication? You might not know until it's too late because there's no way for a doctor to test how the drug will interact with your body before you take it.

Remember in chapter 5 when I mentioned that in the 1800s the pharmaceutical industry had to put a poison label on substances prescribed by a doctor? Well, maybe they should bring that warning label back. Something like "consume at your own risk." It's astounding to me that we outlaw a plant with healing properties and practically no adverse side effects, and then we artificially create medications that can cause irreversible harm to our bodies. Yet that's the world we live in, folks.

9

The Truth about Marijuana and Big Pharma

hat I've been telling you about marijuana being a medication isn't new. There is evidence as far back as 2737 BCE that proves people knew how to use weed as a form of medicine. That's right—in 2737 BCE, Chinese Emperor Shen Neng was prescribing *ma* (the Chinese word for cannabis) tea for the treatment of gout, rheumatism, malaria, and poor memory.[1]

So how did marijuana get labeled as the "gateway drug" in the first place if people knew of its healing properties for centuries? From the federal government, of course! Even Hearst and DuPont's partner-in-crime Harry Anslinger had previously rejected the idea of marijuana being a stepping-stone to harsher drugs. However, Anslinger quickly endorsed this philosophy in 1951 as a way to justify increased penalties for marijuana use.

From 1951 to 1956, the Boggs Act and the Narcotics Control Act were passed, which set mandatory sentences for drug-related offenses including marijuana. If you recall, by 1951, we were ending all production of hemp, and Anslinger needed some form of national drug enforcement to guarantee this happened. Here's another first in American history: as of 1952, someone caught possessing marijuana as a first-time offense received a minimum sentence of two to ten years and a fine of up to $20,000.[2]

To get this legislation passed, Anslinger told a congressional committee, "Over 50 percent of those young addicts started on marijuana smoking. They started there and graduated to heroin; they took the needle when the thrill of marijuana was gone."[3] Does that sound familiar to you? This argument also became the main justification for putting marijuana in the same category as heroin.

And we've been hearing that argument for years. Even in 1999, the Center on Addiction and Substance Abuse stated that "twelve-to-seventeen-year-olds who smoke marijuana are eighty-five times more likely to use cocaine than those who do not."[4] You can just google "weed is a gateway drug" and see how many references pop up to validate this.

Guess what. If you're a teenager who is interested in trying illegal drugs, then you're going to try illegal drugs. If you can get your hands on weed or cocaine, you're going to try it. Most teenagers are curious, and I bet the Center on Addiction and Substance Abuse never thought to begin those studies where the data should truly begin: with alcohol and tobacco use. You know, the actual gateway drugs!

Think of it this way: Would you take a drug recreationally that has long term consequences of "peptic ulcers, liver failure, pancreatic cysts, high blood pressure, stroke, metabolic abnormalities, malnutrition, lung and urinary tract infections, brain damage, and cancers of the mouth, larynx, esophagus, pancreas, liver, stomach, colon, and breast"?[5]

Who in their right mind would use a drug like that? Well, those are the effects of alcohol, so that means the majority of Americans roll the dice every day when they drink. And I know those of you who drink are justifying to yourselves why you do it. Because this drug is familiar to us, we think that if we "control" how much of it we use on a recreational basis, then we'll be fine. We fool ourselves into thinking we're always in control when it comes to alcohol and we think these serious side effects are the worst consequences that occur only after heavy, prolonged use. Meanwhile, according to the National Highway Traffic Safety Administration, every two minutes, a person is injured in a drunk driving crash somewhere in America.[6] Sure, we're in control when it comes to alcohol. Absolutely.

And when it comes to teenagers and drug and alcohol use, there are a multitude of factors that these studies don't seem to go into like peer pressure and rebellion, but hey, let's just look at the facts: If marijuana were truly the number-one gateway drug that leads to heroin use, then why the hell isn't everyone a heroin addict? The federal government is in contradiction again! According to the government's own survey data, the number of Americans that have tried marijuana is twenty-four times greater the number of those who have tried heroin.[7] In what world does that make marijuana a gateway drug to heroin?

And let's be even more logical about this. A 2002 study by the RAND Corporation noted that prescription drugs and marijuana are more easily accessible for teenagers, so therefore, these drugs are tried before heroin: "Marijuana typically comes first because it is more available. Once we incorporated these facts into our mathematical model of adolescent drug use, we could explain all of the drug use associations that have been cited as evidence of marijuana's gateway effect."[8] So in essence, the "marijuana gateway effect" is total bs! How many people are in prison right now due to a bullshit law based on this bullshit science that has time and time again been debunked? According to the ACLU, marijuana arrests account for over half of all drug arrests in the United States. Between 2001 and 2010, there were 8.2 million marijuana arrests and 88 percent of those arrests were made for simply having marijuana![9] Again, not for attempting to sell it, not for getting caught smoking it, but hey, the cops pulled you over for speeding and found it in your car, so you're going to jail!

Let's just forget all the scientific evidence for a minute and pretend that I'm wrong and that the feds are right. Let's just say marijuana is the gateway drug. Here's how that makes any sense to me: once a teenager tries it, that kid will soon discover that the government has been lying about what it feels like to be high and what the "negatives" are. Let's just say that this particular teenager tried alcohol, got drunk, blacked out, and spent the next day praying to the toilet and hating his existence. Then that kid tries pot and thinks, *Not so bad. But wait a minute, isn't pot illegal? Wow, what other illegal drugs are out there that don't make me pass out, vomit and have a splitting headache? Well, maybe I'll give heroin a try next. After all, I just took out my iPhone and googled and that's in the same drug classification as weed, so the effects have to be similar, right?*

Now doesn't that sound like a government conspiracy to keep us all drugged up so we'll never know the true medical benefits of cannabis?

Some people in the medical community—and by medical, I mean pharmaceutical industry—think that marijuana isn't an effective medication because the effects aren't long term. Take glaucoma, for instance. Glaucoma is a qualifying condition for medical marijuana in every state that has legalized it. Smoking weed helps people with glaucoma see better, but scientists haven't found a way to make that effect last all day without the person smoking weed more than once a day.

The National Eye Institute, a division of the Federal National Institutes for Health, supported research that found that THC only helps glaucoma patients for three to four hours before the effects started to wear off.[10] Since glaucoma needs to be treated twenty-four hours a day, the development of THC eyedrops were recommended, so that a patient wasn't smoking weed six to eight times a day. Now, do you think Big Pharma was going to take up the torch to develop THC eyedrops, which are in direct competition with the eyedrops already on the market? They spent millions developing and marketing these products! Products, by the way—either in pill or eyedrop form—that can cause eye redness, itching, burning, stinging, tingling hands and feet, upset stomach, memory problems, depression, frequent urination, fatigue, headaches, dry mouth and nose, shortness of breath, low blood pressure, reduced pulse rate, blurred vision, and in the case of alpha agonists like Alphagan and iopidine, a great "likelihood of allergic reaction."[11]

Meanwhile, the American Glaucoma Society doesn't like to recommend smoking marijuana for glaucoma treatment, citing fears of lung problems (which we already know is bs), low blood pressure, memory issues, and potential problems from driving or operating heavy machinery when high.[12] But wait, how many Americans take opioid pills every day? The CDC stated that in 2012, health care providers wrote 259 million prescriptions for painkillers, which is enough for every American adult to have a bottle of pills.[13] And you can't operate heavy machinery or drive a car on those! So you're telling me all those people were responsible adults and took a taxi to work? Yeah, right! And isn't low blood pressure and memory loss already a side effect of Big Pharma's glaucoma medication? It doesn't sound like the doctors of American Glaucoma Society are on the side of their patients on this issue. And as for Big Pharma? In 2013, CBS News reported that nearly 70 percent of Americans are on at least one prescription drug.[14] Why on earth would the pharmaceutical industry even bother with weed, a nonaddictive substance with no harmful side effects, when creating addictive substances—or substances with adverse side effects that require another drug to balance the symptoms further—has worked out so well for them?

Now, I don't want to go into every drug Big Pharma has to offer and counter each with weed as a medical solution. That's another book for another time. But what I do want you to consider is Charlotte's Web and why no pharmaceutical industry had any intention of producing this CBD strain that cures children's epilepsy and seizures, even though the science was right in front of them.

Charlotte's Web is a special strain of cannabis that was invented by the Stanley Brothers in Colorado; the six brothers are legal marijuana growers and founding members of the Realm of Caring Foundation. They invented the strain, but then named it after Charlotte Figi, the strain's first customer. Since before she was even a year old, Charlotte experienced epileptic seizures brought on by Dravet syndrome.[15] She was experiencing up to three hundred seizures a week by the age of five, some lasting hours at a time, and she was unable to talk or even swallow. Her parents, Matt and Paige Figi, exhausted every option and were told nothing could be done for their wheelchair-bound daughter. After trying out medical marijuana for seven days, Charlotte went from three hundred seizures a week to not having a single seizure in those first seven days.[16] You've probably heard of Charlotte Figi because her story has been featured on many national news shows—from *Dateline* to CNN—and she's become the poster child for why medical marijuana is so important for severe health conditions, especially those considered incurable by Big Pharma.

But let me tell you what her parents went through first before they found this particular strain of marijuana. Charlotte went on a special ketogenic diet, used to treat Dravet syndrome; it's high in fat and low in carbohydrates. The diet helped her body produce extra ketones, which are natural chemicals that suppress seizures. The diet helped, but she suffered from side effects, including bone loss. Two years into the diet, the seizures came back, and there was nothing more that could be done. Her parents had to put her in a coma to stop the seizures, and then medical marijuana became legal in Colorado.

At that time, five-year-old Charlotte became the youngest person in Colorado to be issued a medical marijuana card. The Figis paid $800 for 2 oz. of cannabis oil from particular strain of marijuana called R4, which is low in THC and high in CBD.[17] It worked immediately, but they couldn't find any more of the supply. They then found out about the Stanley brothers, one of the state's largest marijuana growers and dispensaries, who were crossbreeding a strain of marijuana with industrial hemp, making a new strain high in CBD and low in THC. The brothers started the Realm of Caring Foundation soon after meeting Charlotte and after seeing the effects of this strain. This nonprofit organization now provides cannabis to those suffering from epilepsy, cancer, multiple sclerosis, and Parkinson's who cannot afford the cost of Charlotte's Web because it's not covered under medical insurance.

For every patient who takes Charlotte's Web or any medical marijuana product, the dosage is different depending on age, weight, severity of condition, and so on. Charlotte gets oil twice a day in her food; some others get 3 to 4 mg per day.[18] And what has her medication done for her? Charlotte is walking, riding a bicycle, feeding herself, and talking. As of 2013, Charlotte's parents reported that their daughter went from having about forty seizures per day to only about four seizures per month—something no other medication could provide for her.[19] They have not seen any negative side effects from Charlotte's use of medical marijuana.

Her father, Matt Figi, told CNN:

I literally see Charlotte's brain making connections that haven't been made in years. My thought now is, why were we the ones that had to go out and find this cure? This natural cure? How come a doctor didn't know about this? How come they didn't make me aware of this?[20]

Good questions. After all, when Charlotte's parents first discovered medical marijuana, it was largely an illegal product. The Figis also explained how difficult it was to find a doctor who would recommend cannabis to a five-year-old—probably most of them feared being sued—but I find this astounding because as I mentioned earlier, Israel has been conducting research on the medical benefits of CBD and THC for generations. In fact, Charlotte's Web exists in Israel. Over there, they call it "Rafael," after the healing angel called upon by Moses in the Bible, and it is mainly given orally to epileptic children.[21]

Here's just one of the more recent cannabis studies that was discovered in Israel last year: researchers reported that if rats with broken bones were given CBD for eight weeks, their bones were made stronger during the healing process, which could prevent future fractures.[22] That's right. In 2015, Tel Aviv University and Hebrew University published these findings in the *Journal of Bone and Mineral Research*, and Dr. Raphael Mechoulam—the patriarch of cannabis science—was one of the authors of the study. The scientists proved that CBD enhances the maturation of collagen, the protein in connective tissue that holds the body together. And in earlier research, the same team learned that the body's cannabinoid receptors "stimulate bone formation and inhibit bone loss."[23]

What do these two studies tell us? Well, aside from CBD possibly being better for strengthening bones than calcium, the findings open the doors to how marijuana could treat osteoporosis and other bone-related diseases. This is again bad news for the pharmaceutical industry, which has created many different types of osteoporosis medications, the kind that slow bone loss (antiresorptive medications) and those that increase the rate of bone formation (anabolic medications)[24]—and all of them have side effects. But what happened to the rats that were injected with CBD and now have stronger bones that are less susceptible to fractures? So far, there haven't been any side effects there because there are no known side effects from CBD. See what I mean about Big Pharma having a big beef with CBD?

Unfortunately, it's not just Big Pharma. Our federal government keeps saying more research is needed on CBD, but then it won't give any of our scientists grants for conducting the necessary studies because marijuana is a Schedule I narcotic and therefore illegal. Take the University of Florida, for example. As of 2014, the university received more than $300 million in federal dollars to conduct medical research. However, UF's College of Pharmacy won't be researching the efficacy of medical-grade marijuana any time soon. In fact, researchers were interested in researching Charlotte's Web, but they were too worried that it would risk their federal funding, so they couldn't participate in any studies. How do you like that hypocrisy?

But oh wait, the hypocrisy thickens. Since the feds aren't giving grants out to the universities that typically conduct these types of studies, those in the medical community who are backed by the pharmaceutical industry are stating that dabbling with Charlotte's Web is dangerous because there aren't any American studies to confirm that it isn't dangerous. Talk about a convenient catch-22!

However, a new study might just shut them up for good. Do you know what happened when marijuana was legalized in Colorado? State lawmakers said that the tax money collected from businesses and customers would be going to research and education. Do you know what one of the first things they decided to do with the revenue was? Start a study on Charlotte's Web at the University of Colorado Anschutz Medical Campus.[25] Researchers have been collecting data since 2014 to determine why some epilepsy patients see more positive results from this strain than others. Data will be collected until February 2016, and after that, researchers will be analyzing the data. Those in the epilepsy research community are calling this study the "Holy Grail" for determining the true value of Charlotte's Web.[26]

Now that Colorado is moving forward with footing the bill for the first major study on Charlotte's Web, Big Pharma must be getting worried. After all, about one percent of the US population has epilepsy, and about one third of that one percent has a form of epilepsy that can't be controlled with medication.[27] To put it another way, that's nearly three million Americans with epilepsy and one million Americans living with uncontrolled seizures, just like Charlotte Figi. So that means there's one million people living in the United States that the pharmaceutical industry has failed to sell a pill to. Well, not on Big Pharma's watch! GW Pharmaceuticals of London[28] proudly introduced Epidiolex in 2014—a pill derived from CBD.[29] The FDA approved a series of Epidiolex clinical trials in 2014 to test the drug on US patients with the median age of eleven years old. Side effects? Drowsiness, diarrhea, and a decrease in appetite. The drug was given to 213 patients for twelve weeks, and twelve people stopped taking the drug within those twelve weeks due to the side effects.[30] Results? On average, 137 patients found that their seizures decreased by 54 percent.[31] Conclusion? More trials are underway, but Dr. Shaun Haussain, who specializes in treating children with epilepsy at the University of California, stated the initial data is "certainly encouraging."[32] Meanwhile, the patriarch of cannabis science himself, Dr. Raphael Mechoulam, stated this of the initial study: "The side effects are disturbing. Pure cannabidiol is not known to cause drowsiness or tiredness."[33] Ha! I couldn't have said it better myself.

So again, why does Big Pharma have to reinvent the wheel here? Would I want my child seizure-free? Of course. Would I want my child to take a medication with no side effects or a medication with side effects? Seems like a pointless question to answer, yet here we are, with the FDA giving Big Pharma approval to conduct tests nationwide on our children for a drug with side effects. Charlotte's Web, on the other hand, receives no approval from the FDA. We already have a THC pill, it looks like we're going to have a CBD pill, but a team of brothers who invented a CBD oil with a small percentage of THC in it? They can't get the powers that be to validate that what they have works just fine.

Dr. Angus Wilfong, a pediatric neurologist leading the Epidiolex research at the Texas Children's Hospital, went so far as to say, "What's really astounding about medical marijuana is that there's no scientific proof that it even works."[34] Right. So Charlotte Figi is a figment of our imagination, right, Dr. Wilfong?

And Israel, the powerhouse of medical marijuana research, has yet to prove the benefits?

Dr. Wilfong also said it's too difficult to know exactly what's in a plant as opposed to a pharmaceutical-grade substance and had this to say about Charlotte's Web: "There's a great concern about exposing children to products where you're not really sure what they're getting."[35] Oh really? And the children in the Epidiolex studies were told exactly what they were taking and what it would do to them? Weren't they just guinea pigs for the pharmaceutical industry? Did the pharmaceutical industry have all the answers before the initial clinical trials? Or weren't those trials designed to determine the actual results and side effects of the drug? Even if you know exactly what is in a substance, you have no idea how it will interact with your body until you take it. Most people find out they have food allergies the hard way—they eat a peanut or a piece of shellfish and they blow up like a balloon. So why is it so difficult for a doctor to accept that clinical trials are also necessary when it comes to cannabis products that do help people, such as Charlotte's Web?

Though I'm not a scientist, I do have a theory as to why Charlotte's Web and even this Epidiolex pill don't work the same for everyone, and I'm curious if the research being conducted by the University of Colorado Anschutz Medical Campus team will prove my theory to be true. In September 2014, the Stanleys announced that they would ensure Charlotte's Web would consistently contain less than 0.3 percent of THC.[36] Now, some patients who take Charlotte's Web might not need THC, but some might actually require a larger dosage of THC to fully manage their seizures. Some people might need 0.3 percent THC, some people might need 1 percent THC.

Think of it this way: every pharmaceutical drug has different strengths for different people. Someone might need 10 mg of Lipitor to lower high cholesterol. Someone else might need 20 mg of Lipitor to get the same results. Yes, Lipitor lowers cholesterol, but there's no way to know for sure what the correct dosage is until after someone takes it for a few months to see the results. Sometimes after seeing the results, a doctor will prescribe a stronger dosage; sometimes a doctor will provide a weaker dosage.

Well, those who need medical marijuana are no different. There are different types of CBD oils and there are many different types of epilepsy. So it goes without saying that there are different dosages for different people. I understand why a parent might not want to give their five-year-old a medication with THC in it. THC gets people high, so why on earth would you want to make your five-year-old high? Well, remember our endocannabinoid system? THC and CBD both bind to our neurological system, which means that THC can also help those with seizures. Some people might not need THC at all to control their seizures, but some people might need a bit more than just CBD. Studies have also shown that too much THC can actually cause seizures, so again, it depends on the person. I agree that more needs to be done to determine the standard dosages for different types of seizures, and maybe the research being done by the University of Colorado's Anschutz Medical Campus is the first step.

And remember, there are medical values to THC—the pharmaceutical community just doesn't want you to know about them. *National Geographic* visited Manuel Guzmán in 2015 at the Complutense University of Madrid. Guzmán is a biochemist who has studied cannabis for about twenty years and he had something very interesting to show the Nat Geo reporter—four MRIs of a rat's brain. In the first two MRI images:

> The animal has a large mass lodged in the right hemisphere, caused by human brain tumor cells Guzmán's researchers injected.

> "This particular animal was treated with THC for one week," Guzmán continues. "And this is what happened afterward."

> The two images that now fill his screen are normal. The mass has not only shrunk—it's disappeared.

> "As you can see, no tumor at all."

> In this study Guzmán and his colleagues, who've been treating cancer-riddled animals with cannabis compounds for fifteen years, found that the tumors in a third of the rats were eradicated and in another third, reduced.

> Will cannabis help fight cancer? "I have a gut feeling," he says, "that this is real."[37]

National Geographic reports that a groundbreaking clinical trial based on Guzmán's research is going on right now at St. James's University Hospital in Leeds, England. Researchers are treating patients with aggressive brain tumors with Temozolmide (an oral chemotherapy drug) and Sativex, a THC-CBD oral spray developed by GW Pharmaceuticals.

So what exactly is this oral spray called Sativex? It's Big Pharma's version of liquid cannabis! It's a medication with a combination of THC and CBD and it's used to treat "spasticity" caused from multiple sclerosis and it is also used to combat cancer pain. It is used reduce spasms, improve sleep, lessen pain, and improve "normal functions."[38] It is currently approved for use in eleven countries, and the United States is not one of them. Each spray contains 2.7 mg of THC and 2.5 mg of CBD[39] and a patient can take up to eighteen sprays twice daily, depending on his or her condition. Some patients have used up to forty-eight sprays per day during clinical trials. You might want to reread what the American Glaucoma Society stated about why doctors shouldn't approve of cannabis use for glaucoma patients. The American Glaucoma Society didn't want people smoking pot or using THC eyedrops six to eight times a day, yet here comes Sativex, which contains THC and can be used up to forty-eight times per day! You know what's really astounding, Dr. Angus Wilfong? The hypocrisy of your pharmaceutical— oops, I meant medical—community!

Like I said before—cannabis itself is the cure. And here's your proof. Essentially, this Sativex is pharmaceutical-grade cannabis oil with THC and CBD in it and if it helps with multiple sclerosis spasms, maybe it could also help with epilepsy too. Who knows. Side effects? Due to the other chemicals that are in this spray, people get a lot of interesting side effects, among them: feeling drunk, "high" or euphoric, constipation, diarrhea, dry mouth, oral pain, vomiting, hypertension, abdominal pain, vertigo, blurred vision, anorexia, depression, hallucinations, balance disorder, and memory impairment. It is not recommended to drive a car or operate heavy machinery until you know how the drug will affect you.[40] But pure cannabis oil itself—a combination of THC and CBD—still isn't considered as a medication by many in the medical community because it wasn't invented in a lab.

Have you heard of Phoenix Tears and Rick Simpson Oil (RSO)? They're in the same boat as Charlotte's Web, only they're a high dosage of THC. These marijuana strains were invented by Rick Simpson, a Canadian man who had cancer and claimed he cured it through making an oil with an extremely high amount of THC. So if Guzmán is conducting studies on how THC can shrink or destroy tumors in rats, then who is to say Rick Simpson didn't already cure cancer, using the same method? But the pharmaceutical industry brushes Simpson aside. Like I said before—if Big Pharma can't invent it, they don't want to give it legitimacy, and Phoenix Tears and RSO were invented by someone who dropped out of school in ninth grade. So what could he possibly know?

Simpson's cannabis oil has THC levels in the ninety percent range and he claims it has been used by many to cure or control cancer, MS, pain, diabetes, arthritis, asthma, infections, inflammations, blood pressure, depression, and sleeping problems.[41] He refers to RSO and Phoenix Tears as "nature's answer for cancer" and he wrote a book with that same title to describe his personal experiences developing the oil through trial and error. Long story short, Simpson found out he had skin cancer back in the 1970s and he heard on the radio that THC could kill cancer cells and tumors. So instead of going the normal chemo route, he came up with his own strain of cannabis that had as much THC as the plant could produce.[42] Today, the man is cancer free. If you go to his website, PhoenixTears.ca, you'll see that Simpson explains how he produced the oil that saved his life and how the oil works. You can even buy the oil online or if you're able to get strains with high amounts of THC, Simpson explains how to break the buds down into oil. As a side note, I don't go into how to grow medical marijuana in this book, but if you live in a state that allows you to do so and you want to attempt to produce your own RSO from scratch, there are several books that can guide you through the process of growing your own marijuana at home, such as *Growing Marijuana: How to Plant, Cultivate, and Harvest Your Own Weed*, by Tommy McCarthy.

But wait a minute, as far back as the 1970s, there were studies that show THC kills cancer in lab animals? Yes, that's right. So what's taking scientists so long to cure cancer with THC?

Think about it this way: the problem is that since anyone can make this oil, then Big Pharma can't patent it, so therefore it doesn't want to invest any money into it. Have you ever seen the TV show *Shark Tank*? As Kevin O'Leary often says in his own unique way, there's no point in moving forward with a business opportunity if the product isn't patented. Someone else can come along and make the same product and that means there's too much competition. Competition is exactly what Big Pharma wants to avoid, so it will continue to create the Frankenstein's monster of cannabis in labs. That way, these pills and sprays can be patented, meaning they cannot be replicated like Charlotte's Web or RSO, and therefore Big Pharma can continue to make billions.

Again, the corporations win and we lose. Seeing a pattern yet? Like I said before, Hearst and DuPont and Anslinger still live on to this day. Even though we've legalized marijuana to some degree in twenty-three states and in Washington, DC, and the proof of marijuana's medical benefits is out there, people who claim cannabis is actual medicine are still considered a mockery thanks to the power of Big Pharma and our government. After all, since the DEA claims weed is the gateway drug, it can't possibly also be a medication. Now that would indicate a conspiracy.

10

The US Government's
Marijuana Patent Conspiracy

Remember when the federal government decided to patent cannabidiol through US Patent 6,630,507 (or Patent 507 for short)? Therefore patenting the cannabinoids that treat a wide range of neurological diseases such as Alzheimer's, Parkinson's, stroke and other conditions caused by oxidative stress such as Crohn's disease, diabetes, and arthritis? Well, what exactly does that mean, to patent cannabidiol?

For those of you who don't know, a patent is something proprietary—once you patent something, you hold the rights to it and no one else can produce it or use it without your permission by law until the patent expires. So for example, Marinol and Cesamet—the drug capsules containing synthetic THC—were patented and that patent expired in 2011.[1] Now that the patent expired, the chemical formula used to create the THC pill is available for other drug companies to use to create similar products. There's actually an American company right now working with Israel on developing a THC pill that releases the medication for ten to twelve hours. More on that later.

I can see how patents benefit a business—you have exclusive rights to something you invented for twenty years, and you can charge whatever you want for the product because no one can buy it anywhere else. And if another company wants to use your patented product, they have to either pay you a boatload of money or risk going to court for patent infringement. In essence, a business has a guaranteed monopoly for twenty years on a patented product.

That's all fine and good in the business world, but once you apply that to the healthcare industry, I'm against it. Big Pharma can charge whatever price it wants on a patented drug. It can also patent anything it wants to just so that a competitor doesn't use it to make a medication. What this means is there are hundreds if not thousands of patents out there on medical research that a particular pharmaceutical company owns. The company might at some point use to the patents develop a product, but they don't necessarily have to, and we're the ones who suffer.

That is essentially why there isn't a CBD medication to treat the neurological and oxidative diseases. The government's patent stopped anyone else from using those specific cannabinoids. That means Americans suffering from Alzheimer's, Parkinson's, strokes, diabetes, Chrohns disease, HIV dementia, arthritis, and other age-related, inflammatory, autoimmune diseases, and neurodegenerative diseases probably won't see a treatment or cure from CBD until the patent expires in 2021.[2] Meanwhile the government knows CBD can treat or cure these issues—that's why it patented cannabidiol in the first place. Our own government is allowing these people to suffer unnecessarily.

Under Patent 507, the government does not own the marijuana plant—products of nature aren't patentable. However, it does own the right to the methods of using certain cannabinoids for the purpose of treating a disease caused by oxidative stress or neurological disease (such as Crohn's disease and so on). What the government did is ensure that no other entity could use certain types of CBD for the purpose of treating a disease caused by oxidative stress or neurological reasons . . . unless the FDA decides to sell that right to someone . . . which it did!

Before I get into the details of what all that means for us as Americans who want to see marijuana legalized, I personally believe you cannot patent any form of nature, and I hope I see the day when the people rise up against the government and demand this patent be revoked. I can't patent an orange; therefore I cannot patent orange juice. It should be the same with marijuana. I cannot patent the plant; therefore I cannot patent the cannabinoids—THC or CBD—that come from the plant. How the government is getting around this is really astounding.

You see, the government is essentially claiming that its scientists invented a method of turning oranges into orange juice that hasn't ever been done before. The government is claiming they discovered how certain marijuana cannabinoids interact with our brains and they "invented" a method of extracting these specific cannabinoids from the plant to be used in treating certain diseases and conditions, and how to make synthetic versions of CBD. So if you wanted to extract CBD from the marijuana plant and then use it in a drug to treat certain diseases, you'd have to wait until the patent has expired.

Think of it this way: when Israeli Dr. Raphael Mechoulam used his knowledge of chemistry to extract THC from cannabis, he was the first to do this, and he was the first to study how it works in our brains. He named the endogenous cannabinoids that THC interacts with in our brains anandamine (which means "joy") because of how THC makes us feel. His research team was the first to determine the structure of CBD in 1963 and by 1964 he isolated and synthesized THC. If Mechoulam had patented how he synthesized THC, then Big Pharma would've had to pay him big bucks to create anything with THC in it. See, Mechoulam basically made the same discovery as the US government, only his was the psychoactive element, and the US patent deals with CBDs, the non-psychoactive cannabinoids. However, Mechoulam does hold over thirty patents, including how to treat or prevent diabetes with CBD.[3] Unless he decides to invest in a product or sell exclusive rights to that patent, no one else in the medical community can use those particular CBDs to help diabetes patients until that patent expires.

Meanwhile, in 1999, Aidan J. Hampson, Julius Axelrod, and Maurizio Grimaldi—all doctors who were employed by the US government—discovered how certain CBDs interact with our endocannabinoid system and they patented this so that no one but the federal government could have access to these particular CBDs.

These government researchers were no slouches either. Aidan J. Hampson is a neuropharmacologist at the National Institute for Mental Health. Julius Axelrod was a biochemist who won the Nobel Prize in Physiology or Medicine in 1970. Maurizio Grimaldi is a professor of neurology, neuropsychopharmacology and toxicology at the National Institute of Mental Health (NIMH). All three inventors of Patent 507 were National Institutes of Health (NIH) employees, and the patent was assigned to the US Department of Health and Human Services (HHS). Here's another fact you'll want to know: the FDA is housed under the

HHS. The FDA is what regulates clinical investigations of products assigned to the HHS.[4] Did you catch that? Only the FDA can approve a CBD study, and since the patent is a "product" of the HHS, the NIH would be in charge of CBD research and development.

Now, remember, in the pharmaceutical world, patents protect drugs from copycat versions for twenty years after the drug is invented.[5] And the drug's inventor can sell the drug in fifteen years after the drug is approved. Could this mean that the FDA is hoping to cash in big once Patent 507 comes close to expiring around 2021? Could this mean that certain people in our government are already working with Big Pharma to ensure the biggest payout imaginable? Or could this be a way for Big Pharma and the government to ensure that no research or development occurs on the patented cannabinoids for the next fifteen to twenty years? How about all of the above.

Our government already knows how much money can be made off of the medical marijuana industry and CBD in particular. Israel is the case in point. Israel is just one of three nations in the world with a government-sponsored cannabis program—with Canada and the Netherlands joining suit.[6] Israel first approved medical cannabis for a patient in 1992, for severe asthma. As of 2016, there are approximately thirty thousand medical marijuana patients[7] in a country of roughly 8.2 million people. In Israel, recreational marijuana is illegal, but the country remains the world leader in science on the medical uses of marijuana. How can that be? Because Israel understands that this plant can be used for more than just hippies getting high.

Look at it this way: a hammer is a tool that can be used to drive a nail into a wall to hang a picture frame. A hammer is also a tool that can be used to murder someone. A tool can be used for different purposes, but this basic understanding of marijuana—a valuable tool to the medical community—completely escapes the US government.

Meanwhile, the Israeli government will allow research on what is considered an illegal drug by Israeli law. However, the government will not allow any of the products resulting from the research to be exported. Israeli officials don't want their country to be known as the first country in the world to export what is largely considered an illegal and dangerous drug.[8] Could you imagine if they did though? The Israeli people would become more hated than Mexicans and Colombians due to our War on Drugs! They'd become the most dangerous people on the planet.

In Israel, researchers like Raphael Mechoulam are getting funding for all kinds of medical marijuana studies. This is why US scientists have been flocking to Israel—including Colorado doctor and Harvard-trained physician Alan Shackelford, who was the doctor that administered cannabis to Charlotte Figi and saved her life. That's right. Our best and brightest doctors and scientists are leaving the United States and going to Israel—a war zone country. They are essentially risking their lives to study pot. Isn't that incredible? And guess who benefits from all these medical studies? The Israeli people! They have complete access to the medical marijuana strains that their government will not export.

Through the development of different kinds of marijuana strains, Israeli doctors have figured out how to treat Crohn's diseases, basal cell carcinoma, psoriasis, Parkinson's, multiple sclerosis, and even PTSD in Israel military veterans. Did you catch that? The Israelis got around the US patent on CBD by using the plant only—which is not patentable. That's why dosages are available in cookies, caramels, chocolates, oils, and leaf form for smoking or vaporizing. The Israelis do not put CBD or THC in a pill form. They crossbred the plants to get the exact strengths they need for their studies. And I bet Israel is stockpiling and hording its marijuana medications. Wouldn't it be interesting to see the Israel become the healthiest nation on earth due to the development and use of medical marijuana?

Here's the strange thing: many governments, including the United States, Spain, Italy, Germany, the United Kingdom, and Brazil, are funding studies that Mechoulam conducts with his team. Even US-based institutions like the Kessler Foundation—an organization that helps Americans with disabilities—fund Mechoulan's research. Israel of course funds medical marijuana research as well, being that at the end of the day, the government sanctions medical marijuana research.

What's even stranger than our government funding Israel's marijuana research is what entity is funding it. As early as the 1960s, Mechoulam has been receiving funding from the NIH! That's right. The very organization that once upon a time filed Patent 507 is also funding marijuana research abroad, while the DEA tells everyone at home the drug has no medicinal value. According to Mechoulam:

> Although NIH does not generally fund foreign researchers, they made
> an exception in my case. They never interfered with my research and
> they never asked me (or suggested) to go into any specific direction.
> As a matter of fact I got a prize from NIDA, the National Institute of

Drug Abuse (NIDA) Lifetime Achievement Award, presented by the Director of NIDA, NIH, Bethesda, September 2011. [9]

Isn't that incredible? Our federal government puts us in jail for weed but gives a lifetime achievement award to a scientist who has dedicated his life to researching it!

Just one of the many studies being conducted in Israel right now is with researchers from Cannabics Pharmaceuticals—an American company. Scientists from Cannabics Pharmaceuticals are currently working on research in Israel to come up with a long-acting oil capsule, like Marinol, but an extended release version. The pill is being developed after an April 2015 Israeli study showed that cannabis kills or slows the development of some two hundred different types of cancer cells.[10] The main idea behind the new pill is to allow a steady ten to twelve hours of cannabis medication for cancer patients by simply taking one pill per day.[11] Now, remember, aside from getting people high and getting sick people to eat, THC is the main cannabinoid that attacks cancer cells, so Cannabics is creating another kind of THC medication derived from a Schedule I narcotic, and if its predecessor Marinol is any indication of what the FDA will do, you'll soon see a new THC pill on the market, listed as a Schedule III narcotic.

One issue I feel I have to address regarding cancer and cannabis is the conspiracy against it. I know there is a lot of back and forth in the medical community on whether or not cannabis kills cancer and I don't want to mislead anybody or give anybody false hope on the medical legitimacy of this plant. Let me just state that these cannabis cancer studies have been going on for generations, but the cancer cells are always in lab animals, such as rats, until recently.

Remember Dr. Manuel Guzmán from the Complutense University of Madrid, from chapter 9? His team has used human cancer cells in some of their research, such as a 2008 study on human breast cancer cells. Guzmán and his team used human breast cancer cells to prove that cannabinoids—or more specifically a strain of THC known as Delta(9)-tetrahydrocannabinol—can in fact reduce the growth rate of breast cancer cells.[12] But because none of these studies, including Guzmán's, have included human patients—just human cells—we keep hearing "there's no proof" that cannabis can actually cure cancer or shrink cancer tumors in humans.

Yes, to this day, no human has gone into a pot study with cancer and come out of the study cancer-free. You're welcome to form your own opinion on this, but I'm calling bs on "there's no proof." If cannabinoids shrink and eventually disintegrate human cancer cells, it's only a matter of time before a treatment and even a cure for cancer is derived from weed! Weed can cure cancer, Big Pharma just hasn't invented the product yet.

I do agree that it almost seems too good to be true. How can one plant provide so many solutions to so many different problems, including cancer? Well, remember the endocannabinoid system? The US National Institutes for Health (NIH) published a study in 2013 that proved the endocannabinoid system is involved in essentially every human disease,[13] so it goes to show you that a plant with cannabinoids that interact with our body's own cannabinoid receptors can practically cure or at least alleviate nearly every ailment in the human body. Again, that's a study that came from our scientists in the United States, yet we still have scientists in the United States stating there's no proof that cannabis has any medical value!

I could go into every single study that proves cannabis kills or shrinks cancer cells and cancer tumors in human cell tissue and animal cell tissue. But that's another book for another time. What I will do, if you're interested in researching this further, is direct you to a list of one hundred scientific studies published in medical journals that are approved by the NIH and on file at the US National Library of Medicine. I do refer to some of these studies in this book:

Cannabis kills tumor cells

http://www.ncbi.nlm.nih.gov/pmc/articles/PMC1576089

http://www.ncbi.nlm.nih.gov/pubmed/20090845

http://www.ncbi.nlm.nih.gov/pubmed/616322

http://www.ncbi.nlm.nih.gov/pubmed/14640910

http://www.ncbi.nlm.nih.gov/pubmed/19480992

http://www.ncbi.nlm.nih.gov/pubmed/15275820

http://www.ncbi.nlm.nih.gov/pubmed/15638794

http://www.ncbi.nlm.nih.gov/pubmed/16818650

http://www.ncbi.nlm.nih.gov/pubmed/17952650

http://www.ncbi.nlm.nih.gov/pubmed/20307616

http://www.ncbi.nlm.nih.gov/pubmed/16616335

http://www.ncbi.nlm.nih.gov/pubmed/16624285

http://www.ncbi.nlm.nih.gov/pubmed/10700234

http://www.ncbi.nlm.nih.gov/pubmed/17675107

http://www.ncbi.nlm.nih.gov/
pubmed/14617682
http://www.ncbi.nlm.nih.gov/
pubmed/17342320

http://www.ncbi.nlm.nih.gov/
pubmed/16893424
http://www.ncbi.nlm.nih.gov/
pubmed/15026328

Uterine, testicular, and pancreatic cancers

http://www.cancer.gov/cancertopics/pdq/cam/cannabis/healthprofessional/page4
http://www.ncbi.nlm.nih.gov/pubmed/20925645

Brain cancer

http://www.ncbi.nlm.nih.gov/pubmed/11479216

Mouth and throat cancer

http://www.ncbi.nlm.nih.gov/pubmed/20516734

Breast cancer

http://www.ncbi.nlm.nih.gov/pubmed/18454173
http://www.ncbi.nlm.nih.gov/pubmed/16728591
http://www.ncbi.nlm.nih.gov/pubmed/9653194

Lung cancer

http://www.ncbi.nlm.nih.gov/pubmed/25069049
http://www.ncbi.nlm.nih.gov/pubmed/22198381
http://www.ncbi.nlm.nih.gov/pubmed/21097714

Prostate cancer

http://www.ncbi.nlm.nih.gov/
pubmed/12746841
http://www.ncbi.nlm.nih.gov/pmc/
articles/PMC3339795/
http://www.ncbi.nlm.nih.gov/
pubmed/22594963

http://www.ncbi.nlm.nih.gov/
pubmed/15753356
http://www.ncbi.nlm.nih.gov/
pubmed/10570948
http://www.ncbi.nlm.nih.gov/
pubmed/19690545

Blood cancer

http://www.ncbi.nlm.nih.gov/pubmed/12091357

http://www.ncbi.nlm.nih.gov/pubmed/16908594

Skin cancer

http://www.ncbi.nlm.nih.gov/pubmed/12511587
http://www.ncbi.nlm.nih.gov/pubmed/19608284

Liver cancer

http://www.ncbi.nlm.nih.gov/pubmed/21475304

Cannabis cancer cures (general)

http://www.ncbi.nlm.nih.gov/pubmed/12514108

http://www.ncbi.nlm.nih.gov/pubmed/15313899

http://www.ncbi.nlm.nih.gov/pubmed/20053780

http://www.ncbi.nlm.nih.gov/pubmed/18199524

http://www.ncbi.nlm.nih.gov/pubmed/19589225

http://www.ncbi.nlm.nih.gov/pubmed/12182964

http://www.ncbi.nlm.nih.gov/pubmed/19442435

http://www.ncbi.nlm.nih.gov/pubmed/12723496

http://www.ncbi.nlm.nih.gov/pubmed/16250836

http://www.ncbi.nlm.nih.gov/pubmed/17237277

Cancers of the head and neck

http://www.ncbi.nlm.nih.gov/pmc/articles/PMC2277494

Cholangiocarcinoma cancer

http://www.ncbi.nlm.nih.gov/pubmed/19916793
http://www.ncbi.nlm.nih.gov/pubmed/21115947

Leukemia

http://www.ncbi.nlm.nih.gov/pubmed/15454482
http://www.ncbi.nlm.nih.gov/pubmed/16139274
http://www.ncbi.nlm.nih.gov/pubmed/14692532

Partial or full cannabis-induced cancer cell death

http://www.ncbi.nlm.nih.gov/pubmed/12130702

http://www.ncbi.nlm.nih.gov/pubmed/19457575

http://www.ncbi.nlm.nih.gov/
pubmed/18615640

http://www.ncbi.nlm.nih.gov/
pubmed/17931597

http://www.ncbi.nlm.nih.gov/
pubmed/18438336

http://www.ncbi.nlm.nih.gov/
pubmed/19916793

http://www.ncbi.nlm.nih.gov/
pubmed/18387516

http://www.ncbi.nlm.nih.gov/
pubmed/15453094

http://www.ncbi.nlm.nih.gov/
pubmed/19229996

http://www.ncbi.nlm.nih.gov/
pubmed/9771884

http://www.ncbi.nlm.nih.gov/
pubmed/18339876

http://www.ncbi.nlm.nih.gov/
pubmed/12133838

http://www.ncbi.nlm.nih.gov/
pubmed/16596790

http://www.ncbi.nlm.nih.gov/
pubmed/11269508

http://www.ncbi.nlm.nih.gov/
pubmed/15958274

http://www.ncbi.nlm.nih.gov/
pubmed/19425170

http://www.ncbi.nlm.nih.gov/
pubmed/17202146

http://www.ncbi.nlm.nih.gov/
pubmed/11903061

http://www.ncbi.nlm.nih.gov/
pubmed/15451022

http://www.ncbi.nlm.nih.gov/
pubmed/20336665

http://www.ncbi.nlm.nih.gov/
pubmed/19394652

http://www.ncbi.nlm.nih.gov/
pubmed/11106791

http://www.ncbi.nlm.nih.gov/
pubmed/19189659

http://www.ncbi.nlm.nih.gov/
pubmed/16500647

http://www.ncbi.nlm.nih.gov/
pubmed/19539619

http://www.ncbi.nlm.nih.gov/
pubmed/19059457

http://www.ncbi.nlm.nih.gov/
pubmed/16909207

http://www.ncbi.nlm.nih.gov/
pubmed/18088200

http://www.ncbi.nlm.nih.gov/
pubmed/10913156

http://www.ncbi.nlm.nih.gov/
pubmed/18354058

http://www.ncbi.nlm.nih.gov/
pubmed/19189054

http://www.ncbi.nlm.nih.gov/
pubmed/17934890

http://www.ncbi.nlm.nih.gov/
pubmed/16571653

http://www.ncbi.nlm.nih.gov/
pubmed/19889794

http://www.ncbi.nlm.nih.gov/
pubmed/15361550

Translocation-positive rhabdomyosarcoma

http://www.ncbi.nlm.nih.gov/pubmed/19509271

Lymphoma

http://www.ncbi.nlm.nih.gov/pubmed/18546271

http://www.ncbi.nlm.nih.gov/pubmed/16936228

http://www.ncbi.nlm.nih.gov/pubmed/16337199

http://www.ncbi.nlm.nih.gov/pubmed/19609004

Cannabis kills cancer cells

http://www.ncbi.nlm.nih.gov/pubmed/16818634

http://www.ncbi.nlm.nih.gov/pubmed/12648025

http://www.ncbi.nlm.nih.gov/pubmed/17952650

http://www.ncbi.nlm.nih.gov/pubmed/16835997

Melanoma

http://www.ncbi.nlm.nih.gov/pubmed/17065222

Thyroid carcinoma

http://www.ncbi.nlm.nih.gov/pubmed/18197164

Colon cancer

http://www.ncbi.nlm.nih.gov/pubmed/18938775
http://www.ncbi.nlm.nih.gov/pubmed/19047095

Intestinal inflammation and cancer

http://www.ncbi.nlm.nih.gov/pubmed/19442536

Cannabinoids in health and disease

http://www.ncbi.nlm.nih.gov/pubmed/18286801

Cannabis inhibits cancer cell invasion

http://www.ncbi.nlm.nih.gov/pubmed/19914218

If you go online and see who authored these studies, you'll notice that the majority of research is being done in Spain, England, Israel, Germany—few and far between were conducted on US soil. So at this point, it's obvious. Our country has decided to double down on the hypocrisy when it comes to marijuana. We'll fund research in other countries, our government will patent CBD, but we won't conduct any research in our backyard. And isn't it interesting that the research is being conducted by American researchers anyway? So the American government is fine with paying Americans to research weed—just so long as the research isn't being done in America.

Whatever our country's real underlying reasons are to stonewall cannabis research in the United States, they're certainly pathetic reasons, considering our stateside medical marijuana industry is only $3 billion[14] and that *Newsweek* estimates that if the feds legalized marijuana across the country, we'd gain the following:[15]

- New industry! Currently, the cultivation business makes $2.7 billion making heating and cooling systems for marijuana greenhouses.
- New jobs! Someone has to trim, manicure, and harvest hundreds of marijuana buds.
- More security guards! Someone will be needed to transport the weed, check IDs at marijuana dispensaries, and guard marijuana grow facilities.
- More entrepreneurs inventing paraphernalia! Just like the wine and alcohol industry has specialty glassware, the marijuana industry has everything from bongs to rolling papers. Electronic cigarette and vaporizer sales accounted for $3.5 billion in sales revenue in 2015.
- More tourism! People all over the world go to Amsterdam to smoke up can now travel to marijuana hot spots in the United States.
- More high tech development! From Eaze to Leafly to WeedMaps and Duby, there's plenty of smartphone apps popping up to cover nearly every aspect of the cannabis industry. There's even a dating website called *420 Singles*!
- A more stable economy! If marijuana is legalized in 2020, then state-licensed labs, which test marijuana for contaminants and THC levels, would become a $850-million industry.
- More in state tax revenue! We can expect a minimum of $2.91 billion in revenue when each state taxes cannabis like any other recreational drug.
- More in federal tax revenue! The federal tax revenue on recreational marijuana is estimated to be around $5.82 billion—how's that for putting a dent in the deficit?

But back to reality. Even though the National Institute on Drug Abuse (NIDA) admitted in 2015 that "marijuana extracts may help kill certain cancer cells and reduce the size of others,"[16] our government won't do a damn thing to change the drug laws. Right now, if you want to research cannabis in America and get FDA approval on your research, the only place to do it is at the NIDA's farm at the University of Mississippi. If you've ever watched Sanjay Gupta's documentary series *Weed*, then you'd know how much of a scam that program is.

Remember Robert Randall who received marijuana from the government for his glaucoma? Where do you think the weed came from? It was farmed at the University of Mississippi. That's right. Ole Miss has been the sole producer of federally legal marijuana since 1968.[17]

And get this: Remember how the government keeps saying we should do research on marijuana to find out what its true medical benefits are? Guess who decides how much marijuana can be grown at the University of Mississippi for research purposes? The good ole DEA!

From 2005 to 2009, the University of Mississippi had a DEA-established quota of producing and analyzing 9,920 lbs of marijuana. In 2010, that number went to 46.3 lbs and stayed there, and then it went back up again in 2014 to 1,433 lbs.[18] Again this is the world we live in, folks. A world where the Drug Enforcement Administration decides for our scientific community how much research can be done per year! The university has approximately twelve acres of land for growing weed. That's it. So our scientists and researchers are at the mercy of whatever can be grown on twelve acres and whatever the DEA tells them they can grow. Could you imagine how those researchers with PhDs in biochemistry, molecular biology, pharmacology, and toxicology must feel to be pushed around by a federal agency without any scientific knowledge or medical background? Leaving everyone you know to go to a war zone country to conduct cannabis research is starting to make a hell of a lot more sense now!

As of March 2015, the NIH gave $69 million to the University of Mississippi to grow up to thirty thousand marijuana plants. Why the sudden change of heart? Well, remember that FDA study that the DEA requested in 2014? (I mentioned it in chapter 7.) Where do you think the FDA is going to get their weed for this research? They're going to get it from Ole Miss! At least we know the scope of the FDA study is going to be significant. We should know once and for all if the FDA thinks marijuana should be downgraded from a Schedule I narcotic. (Or at least that's what they're trying to make us believe.)

Meanwhile, Ole Miss is really at the mercy of the FDA and NIH. Any cannabis-related research projects at Ole Miss are handed down from the FDA and the NIH. If researchers want to conduct a different study, they have to go through the FDA and NIH's approval first. Do you know how long it takes one federal agency to make a decision? Can you imagine how long a process like that takes? No wonder our top marijuana scientists are outsourcing their research to Israel!

And in the meantime, while everyone sits around and waits for approval to start a research project, scientists at Ole Miss told the *Los Angeles Times* that DEA agents guard whatever pot has been harvested "as if it were plutonium"![19] Isn't that incredible? The DEA won't let the researchers even touch the marijuana they harvested for studies without FDA and NIH approval!

What if a researcher wanted to compare the weed grown at Ole Miss to the weed sold at marijuana dispensaries in America? Not on the DEA's watch! That's illegal. I'm entirely serious. The DEA has told the researchers at Ole Miss that they "cannot receive materials from a non-DEA registrant."[20] So in other words, if Ole Miss can't grow it within twelve acres, it cannot be researched. And can you take a guess as to what kind of weed is grown at the University of Mississippi? Or what kind of cannabinoid research is being conducted? Our government didn't patent CBD for nothing! How much do you want to bet that cannabis research at Ole Miss has to do with the specific cannabinoil in the government's patent? How's that for government intervention and government-controlled scientific research!

But here's where the conspiracy really comes in. The US Department of Health and Human Services and the FDA have every right to grant another company the exclusive right to Patent 507. In fact, our government already has. Who do you think it gave the patent to? Big Pharma! Want to know the real reason why there will soon be a CBD pill for epilepsy? Because the FDA gave GW Pharmaceuticals the right to use the necessary CBD strains to create the pill—those same CBD strains in Patent 507. That's why the FDA approved the nationwide Epidiolex clinical trial to begin with! But don't take my word for it. You can go to GW Pharmaceutical's website and read all about it:

In November 2013, GW announced that the FDA had granted orphan drug designation for Epidiolex in the treatment of Dravet syndrome. . . . Under the Orphan Drug Act, the FDA may grant orphan drug designation to drugs intended to treat a rare disease or condition—generally a disease or condition that affects fewer than two hundred thousand individuals in the United States. The first NDA applicant to receive FDA approval for a particular active ingredient to treat a particular disease with FDA orphan drug designation is entitled to a seven-year exclusive marketing period in the United States for that product, for that indication.[21]

See how the FDA used the Orphan Drug Act to get around the fact that CBD comes from a Schedule I narcotic? GW Pharmaceuticals is based in England, so if the drug is created there, no US company breaks the law by creating a drug with cannabis. This benefits GW because Epidiolex is originally being marketed for Dravet syndrome, a rare seizure disorder, but GW knows this is a medication that can benefit all people who suffer from seizures. Which means they have much more money to make off of this deal than the initial two hundred thousand–patient customer base. All they have to do is change the Epidiolex formula slightly and they can cash in on all those who have epilepsy or any other seizure disorder. In fact, they're really upfront about this. You know that nationwide Epidiolex trial from 2014? That trial was for both Dravet syndrome and Lennox-Gastaut syndrome (LGS), so they're already using the Orphan Drug Act to their benefit. And did you catch that GW has exclusive rights to the product in the United States for seven years?

It is estimated that one in twenty to one in forty thousand people have Dravet syndrome[22] and approximately 14,000 to 18,500 people have LGS in the United States, and 23,000 to 31,000 people have LGS in Europe.[23] Even though this keeps GW Pharmaceuticals within the two hundred thousand range of eligible patients under the Orphan Drug Act, the company has another agenda: to get the FDA to approve its CBD and THC oral spray, Sativex. The company is currently in a "Phase 3" clinical development. Once the drug successfully passes Phase 3, GW can submit a new drug application for Sativex with the FDA.[24] And GW expects to get FDA approval for Epidiolex by the end of 2016.[25] When that happens, this will get really get interesting. No wonder the FDA is doing a study to determine if marijuana should be reclassified.

But that's not all GW Pharmaceuticals is up to, because the company is solely focused on discovering, developing, and commercializing medications from CBD. In December 2013, GW patented a method of treating brain cancer with

CBD and THC. Get this: GW Pharmaceuticals got the rights to use Patent 507 from the FDA under the Orphan Drug Act. So to develop this next drug, which is meant to treat brain cancer, Big Pharma is only focusing on treating glioma, a condition that causes brain cancer to form from the glial tissue of the brain, known as glioblastoma (GBM).

GBM patients have few treatment options and a life expectancy of a little over one year. The FDA considers GBM a rare disease because it affects 46 percent of the 22,500 people who are diagnosed with brain cancer each year. So that means, GW Pharmaceuticals can develop this new drug—with THC and CBD—under the Orphan Drug Act.[26] They can then tweak it and give it to everyone with brain cancer, a much larger patient pool.

You might find it interesting to know that GW Pharmaceuticals isn't the only company that the FDA and NIH gave the rights of Patent 507 to. In June 2013, KannaLife Sciences was able to acquire the exclusive license to the patent for only one disease: hepatic encephalopathy (HE).[27] KannaLife (its name is derived from the Greek word for cannabis[28]) is owned by Medical Marijuana, Inc.,[29] one of the largest companies in the medical marijuana and hemp field. GW Pharmaceuticals and KannaLife can't disclose how much they had to pay our government to use Patent 507, but Dean Petkanus, the CEO of KannaLife, said the product he is making to treat HE could be worth $1 billion to $2 billion and he's expecting a customer base of 1.5 million.[30] So whatever Big Pharma paid, it was well worth it!

But guess where KannaLife is doing their research? Unlike GW Pharmaceuticals, which is based in London, KannaLife is conducting their CBD research at the Pennsylvania Biotechnology Center of Bucks County in Doylestown, PA. But wait a minute—how is that legal? Isn't Ole Miss the only research facility in the United States that is sanctioned to do marijuana research? You might also be surprise to know that KannaLife doesn't get its weed from Ole Miss either.

Here's how they're getting around that loophole: according to a 2013 press release, KannaLife entered into a 50/50 joint-venture agreement with Biotech Inc., a Colorado firm and the creator of Cannatol and Haleigh's Hope, a CBD strain oil that is named after a four-year-old girl much like Charlotte Figi who suffered from severe epilepsy and has now gone from hundreds of seizures a day to just a few after taking the CBD oil.[31] Cannatol is a medical compound "derived from highly standardized, consistent and high-yielding cannabidiol phyto stock, free from pesticide and mold contaminants"[32] and it is what KannaLife is using to produce its orphan drug.

In other words, KannaLife is getting a quality strain from Colorado for its studies, and all production is going on in Colorado, where it's completely legal to grow weed. Cannatol is trademarked, it's organically grown, it's high in CBD and it does have some THC in it,[33] and KannaLife thinks this makes it perfect for a drug to treat neuronal injury, such as head trauma and neurological disorders.[34] How can a marijuana strain be trademarked? Because Cannatol didn't exist in nature prior to Biotech Inc. creating it. Cannatol is classified as a medical compound because it is artificially manufactured in a lab.

KannaLife hasn't actually come out with the drug yet, but it expects to before 2021, when the government's patent expires. And isn't it interesting that the company was given exclusive rights to the patent for one specific disease, but KannaLife's drug will be used as a form of "neuroprotection" to treat not only HE, but chronic traumatic encephalopathy (CTE)—which is the brain injury that NFL players suffer from when they get too many concussions. They also have Marvin Washington, a former NFL player, on the payroll to talk to the media on why a CBD-based drug is necessary for professional athletes.[35] If you've seen the movie *Concussion,* then you might remember Bennet Omalu, the doctor Will Smith played. Omalu is a real person, and he's on the board of KannaLife, so you can bet that the company has gotten some pretty favorable press lately.[36]

KannaLife CEO Dean Petkanus told CNBC that he's looking to "bring a product to market that can be a neuro-protectant and can prevent neuronal decay."[37] That sounds a hell of a lot more universal than one drug used to treat one specific illness known as hepatic encephalopathy.

And what is hepatic encephalopathy? Why, it falls under the Orphan Drug Act because it's an extremely rare condition. That's how KannaLife scooped the rights to the patent in the first place. HE is the loss of brain function brought on by disorders that affect the liver—such as alcoholism, cirrhosis, or hepatitis. If the liver is unable to remove toxins from the blood, a person can wind up with HE and experience unconsciousness, slurred speech, strange behavior or personality changes, disorientation, seizures, abnormal movements, drowsiness or confusion, or enter a coma. People with HE are often not able to care for themselves due to these symptoms.[38] There are fewer than twenty thousand US cases per year, which qualifies it for the Orphan Drug Act.

You know what I find to be the most astounding part about this? Under the Orphan Drug Act of 1983, if a company decides to dedicate research to developing an orphan drug—that is a drug for a rare disease such as Huntington's disease ALS, myoclonus, Tourette syndrome, muscular dystrophy, hepatic encephalopathy, or Dravet syndrome—then that company also qualifies for certain benefits from the federal government, such as reduced taxes! Ronald Reagan must be rolling over in his grave knowing that he signed the Orphan Drug Act into law and now the FDA is allowing companies the use of cannabis—the poster child of his wife's "Just Say No" campaign—and the federal government could also be giving reduced taxes to these companies! Oh, and the FDA also prioritizes orphan drugs and puts them on the fast track for FDA approval. Did you notice something else about all those rare diseases? Cannabis is able to treat them!

So what do you think GW Pharmaceuticals and KannaLife will do once they get their drugs approved by the FDA and get seven years exclusivity on them? Probably what KV Pharmaceutical Co. did when it made Makena. Makena is a drug to prevent premature births—it won FDA approval as an orphan drug in 2011. Guess how much the drug costs now? $1,500 per injection. A full treatment of fifteen to twenty shots runs the average patient $25,000.[39] Well guess what happened? Thousands of pregnant women couldn't afford the shots because their insurance providers wouldn't cover the cost![40]

So this is Big Pharma and the federal government's big endgame? We'll eventually get THC and CBD medication, but no one will be able to afford it. That's a hell of a way to "legalize" marijuana. Will everyone in America be at the mercy of Big Pharma when these new CBD and THC products get FDA approval?

I'm sure these medical breakthroughs that GW Pharmaceuticals and KannaLife are involved with right now will eventually do a lot of good for a lot of people, but the way we are going about this is ridiculous. The FDA is stonewalling this research in the United States, which means less jobs and less economic growth for America in general. Meanwhile, the FDA is picking and choosing who gets the monopoly on cannabis, but it won't disclose how much money it is making off of these deals. And we might never be able to actually afford these pills once they're FDA approved anyway.

All I can tell you is that the legalization of marijuana has benefited so many people in the United States, including children like Charlotte Figi, yet we still have a long way to go so that all can benefit equally. Isn't that what's most interesting about all this? We're all deemed equal under the US Constitution, but we sure as hell do not have equal access to life-saving medication. Depending on where you live, you could use marijuana to become seizure-free or you could go to jail for buying it.

You know what I think the government's patent on cannabis is really going to be used for? Before it expires in 2021, I would hope that the American people would stop being so ignorant and legalize marijuana nationwide. Even if we do it state by state, I would like to think that we'd see full legalization from sea to shining sea before that patent expires. And if that does happen, then that patent is essentially the government's insurance policy.

Think of it this way: since the government owns a patent on CBD, then that means it still has the capacity to make certain marijuana strains illegal for research and development. The government will be able to slap you with a lawsuit if you go anywhere near the specific CBDs in its patent. The FDA will sue you, bankrupt you, hell, probably even throw you in jail, all on the taxpayers' dime. And if marijuana is completely legalized before 2021, that means the government can still stop scientists and manufactures from creating synthetic CBD. All the FDA has to do is deny a company the rights to Patent 507!

11

Marijuana Invades Americana with Contradictions All Around

Even though I'm inclined to believe the federal government filed Patent 507 to control the American people's access to CBDs, I do have to say I was surprised to see the federal government side with Colorado to uphold its state marijuana laws.

In December 2015, Nebraska and Oklahoma (Colorado's neighboring states) brought a lawsuit to SCOTUS asking the Supreme Court to overturn the Colorado's marijuana laws, but the Supreme Court decided to let Colorado's right to pot stand.

In case you missed it, here's what happened:

- Shortly after Colorado legalized marijuana, Nebraska and Oklahoma sued Colorado and asked the Supreme Court to block the state's legal marijuana system.
- Nebraska and Oklahoma claim the legalization of marijuana created "a flood of modern bootleggers who are buying pot in Colorado and then illegally crossing state lines."[1]
- If Colorado's laws could be overturned, then the influx of marijuana in the states of Nebraska and Oklahoma would end, the lawmakers reasoned.
- Nebraska and Oklahoma lawmakers took this to the Supreme Court to argue that because marijuana remains completely illegal at the federal

level, then Colorado's marijuana laws actually violate federal law and should be overturned.

"If states are free to disregard federal laws they don't like, then our entire governmental structure is at risk," stated Zachary Bolitho, law professor and former federal prosecutor with the Department of Justice who is in favor of Nebraska and Oklahoma's suit. "What's next? Could a state that doesn't like the federal Clean Water Act pass a law authorizing the pollution of its waterways? Are congressional enactments simply suggestions that the states may accept or reject at their pleasure? That's not how our system is supposed to work."[2]

However, Colorado contended that marijuana is legal inside the state only, and anyone who chooses to leave the state with marijuana is conducting an illegal activity and should be prosecuted. Colorado lawmakers believe the state itself shouldn't be to blame for a private citizen's legal or illegal actions, as the state of Colorado has no bearing on an individual's decisions.

Colorado lawmakers asked the court to throw out the lawsuit, and in turn, the Supreme Court asked the federal government to weigh in, which it did. The Obama administration told the Supreme Court that Oklahoma and Nebraska shouldn't be allowed to sue Colorado over its marijuana legalization "because the state itself isn't causing a direct injury to its neighbors."[3]

This was the federal government's chance to state once and for all that Colorado legalizing marijuana under its state constitution goes against federal law. But here's what the Obama administration actually said:

> Nebraska and Oklahoma essentially contend that Colorado's authorization of licensed intrastate marijuana production and distribution increases the likelihood that third parties will commit criminal offenses in Nebraska and Oklahoma by bringing marijuana purchased from licensed entities in Colorado into those states. But they do not allege that Colorado had directed or authorized any individual to transport marijuana into their territories in violation of their laws. Nor would any such allegation be plausible.[4]

I would argue that unless law enforcement finds a receipt from a Colorado marijuana shop, where's the proof that a Nebraska or Oklahoma resident purchased weed there? It seems like a convenient way for Oklahoma and Nebraska to blame another state for what has been going on inside their borders all along.

In March 2016, the US Supreme Court took the Obama administration's advice and decided against hearing the case. SCOTUS didn't specify why it wouldn't hear the case, but Nebraska and Oklahoma now have the option of taking the matter to a federal district court. If the two states decide to continue the suit, the process could continue for many years. And in those years, many more states could legalize marijuana. In November 2016, some form of recreational marijuana legalization is on the ballot in states like California, Arizona, Massachusetts, Nevada, and Ohio.[5]

Here's another example of how the feds contradict their own marijuana laws: the government allows American companies to patent marijuana in some way.

A good friend of mine, Gary Johnson, the former governor of New Mexico who I endorsed for president in 2012, was the CEO of Cannabis Sativa, Inc.—a company that owns several patents on certain strains of marijuana. (He stepped down as CEO when he decided to run for president again in 2016 under the Libertarian ticket.)

How can Cannabis Sativa patent marijuana strains when they come from a plant? The company claims it produced these strains, and therefore they are proprietary because they did not exist in nature previously. Again, I find it disturbing that anyone can patent a plant, but here we are. And Cannabis Sativa isn't the only company doing this.

However, while we're on the topic of patenting marijuana, one conspiracy theory I have to debunk is Monsanto securing a patent for creating a GMO strain of cannabis. According to the company's website, this is actually a myth.[6] World News Daily Report, a fake news site, initially broke the story about Monsanto developing a GMO strain of marijuana, and the urban legend spread from there.[7] However, in 2011, the Chief Executive of Scotts Miracle-Gro Co.—the exclusive marketer of Monsanto's Roundup weed-killer in North America—told the *Wall Street Journal* that the company is interested in targeting the pot market.[8] Whether this means Miracle-Gro is going to come up with its own strain of weed or Miracle-Gro is going to come up with some kind of new pesticide for the pot industry is unclear. In 2015, the company did acquire General Hydroponics—which sells equipment that could be used to grow weed—and a soil company for a combined $130 million,[9] but that's hardly a toe in the water when it comes to being a leader in the pot industry. What I do know is that Monsanto's weed killer Kilo Max is used to destroy cannabis fields in South Africa.[10] I guess that's one way of "targeting" the pot market.

Monsanto claims that the Kilo Max herbicide, which contains glyphosate, is effective for killing plants, but it doesn't pose any health hazards. This is why the South African government decided to spray it aerially with helicopters to stop farmers who were growing pot. However, after the government did this, farmers who weren't growing marijuana noticed their food crops were killed in the process. Villagers of Bulawo in Port St. Johns found that their animals and water supply were poisoned and their overall health was adversely affected.[11] A 2015 study conducted by the World Health Organization concluded that glyphosate "probably" causes cancer,[12] so if you are in the pot business, I wouldn't recommend turning to Monsanto for any bug control products any time soon!

So why are companies patenting their own marijuana strains? Because whenever marijuana is legal nationwide, they'll be able to mass-produce certain kinds of weed. Look at it this way: if you buy a bottle of Pepsi or Mountain Dew, it tastes the same, no matter where you buy it. These pot companies want to do the same with their strains. So for instance, if you buy pot from the CTA strain (a Sativa strain from Ecuador that gives a "ceiling-less high"),[13] then it will be consistent wherever you buy it because it is patented.

I think the government will always approve products like these because it gives more validity to its CBD patent. And Big Pharma is also on the move to patent anything it can when it comes to cannabis too. Once marijuana is legalized nationwide, if a pharmaceutical company doesn't own the rights to cannabis, then someone else will. It's a race against time to patent whatever can be patented from a plant that is considered a Schedule I narcotic, something with no medical value whatsoever.

And did you know that the majority of these medical marijuana companies are publically traded on the stock market?[14] Even if medical marijuana isn't legal in your state, you can still invest in a pot company. So you might not be able to smoke up, but you can monetarily contribute to a company that allows others to.

Here are just a few examples of pot companies you can invest in:

- **GW Pharmaceuticals** (Ticker: GWPH; share price: $92.60; market value: $1.4 billion)
  Strategy: Developing cannabis-based pharmaceuticals.
- **Medbox** (MDBX; $17.75; $537 million)
  Strategy: Dispensary services. The company manufacturers self-service kiosks that dispense medicines including marijuana.

- **Cannavest** (CANV; $11.37; $381 million)
  Strategy: Makes and markets cannabis-related products, including hemp oil.
- **Advanced Cannabis Solutions** (CANN; $7.50; $101 million)
  Strategy: Leases growing space and related facilities to licensed marijuana business operators.
- **Medical Marijuana** (MJNA; $0.20; $105 million)
  Strategy: The first publicly held company vested in legal cannabis and industrial hemp markets is a holding company for a variety of industries and corporations including KannaLife.
- **GrowLife** (PHOT; $0.10; $81 million)
  Strategy: A marijuana equipment maker that sells hydroponic gardening gear.
- **Cannabis Sativa** (CBDS; $6.40; $75 million)
  Strategy: Produces cannabis-based oils, CBD water, edibles, and specialty strains of marijuana.

So now that marijuana has officially invaded Wall Street and twenty-three states plus DC, when will federal banks start taking hard earned cash from pot businesses? Isn't it interesting that pot companies are publically traded, but the banking industry as a whole won't give a loan to a pot business and won't allow a business owner to even open a bank account? The pot business is by and large a cash-only business because FDIC banks are worried that since marijuana is still illegal on the federal level, they could risk prosecution on the federal level. By taking money from an industry that's still illegal federally, a bank could technically be found guilty of violating money laundering statutes.[15] Credit card companies fall under the same jurisdiction, so in order for a marijuana shop to take credit cards, someone somewhere has to fudge the rules—such as a local bank without nationwide branches telling a pot shop to process a debit card transaction as an ATM withdrawal, so there's no proof the customer was at a marijuana dispensary.[16] Isn't that crazy?

In Colorado, the Fourth Corner Credit Union[17] is supposed to be a bank that caters to the marijuana industry; however, as of 2016, the credit union still isn't taking deposits[18] because it never officially opened. The credit union never received approval from the Federal Reserve and the National Credit Union Administration (NCUA) to begin offering financial services, even though it received a charter from the state of Colorado in 2014. The Fourth Corner Credit

Union sued both government entities because the NCUA denied it deposit insurance and the Federal Reserve denied it a master account (which is necessary to access the payments system used by banks).[19] Here's where it gets interesting: US District Court Judge R. Brooke Jackson dismissed the lawsuit because marijuana still remains illegal under the US Controlled Substances Act.[20] Isn't that some fancy footwork? The feds say Colorado's marijuana laws are sound, but they won't allow any pot business access to a bank! I'm with Senator Rand Paul on this one: it's time to audit and abolish the Federal Reserve!

Even though he hasn't gotten the chance to vote on the legislation yet, Senator Rand Paul is one of the politicians who has publically supported Colorado Representative Ed Perlmutter's bill: H. R. 2076—Marijuana Businesses Access to Banking Act of 2015. If H. R. 2076 passes, then that should put an end to the federal banking prohibition. Essentially, this bill ends the discrimination against pot businesses: a bank will have to allow a legitimate marijuana-related industry to operate like any other customer.

As of June 2015, H. R. 2076 was referred to the House Subcommittee on Crime, Terrorism, Homeland Security, and Investigations.[21] This committee has jurisdiction over the Federal Criminal Code, drug enforcement, sentencing, parole and pardons, internal and homeland security, Federal Rules of Criminal Procedure, prisons, and criminal law enforcement.[22] Notice how these guys don't deal with banking issues, or issues of commerce. Who knows how long it will take that committee to move the bill forward when the chairman is Republican Representative James Sensenbrenner of Wisconsin? He voted against medical marijuana in DC and NORML rates him as "hard-on-drugs" and anti-legalization.[23] Talk about an uphill battle.

Again, I don't understand what the issue is. How can certain pot companies be publically traded and then other pot companies be denied the use of a bank? Could you imagine being a business owner trying to figure out where to put all your cash? And then that business owner is paying his employees in cash. An entire industry is paying utility bills in cash, mortgages in cash, car payments in cash, taxes in cash, literally everything in cash. It's a domino effect.

The Native Americans are also trying to set up a banking system for the marijuana industry, since their casinos are basically smaller versions of banks—they receive large deposits from customers and the money is managed with commissioners and regulators.[24] For example, CannaNative working with Medical

Marijuana Inc. to get a legitimate bank operation up and running for pot companies nationwide.[25] CannaNative is also attempting to develop hemp-and cannabis-based products—including marijuana—on Native American reservations.[26] There are 566 sovereign American Indian nations, and they all fall outside of the federal government's restrictions. Some day in the near future, if you go to a Native American casino, you could purchase some weed that was grown on a reservation, light up a joint, and play blackjack—all of which would be completely legal!

Here's another strange contradiction within our government: the FDIC banks are afraid to touch money from the marijuana industry, yet the IRS is all too willing to collect taxes. Due to Internal Revenue Code Section 280E, the IRS does not allow pot growers and resellers to deduct expenses related to their businesses![27] If you're in the pot business, then everything from advertising costs to most employees' salaries is taxable—which means marijuana businesses are taxed on *gross* profits, not *net* profits (every other business in America pays taxes on net profits).[28]

Why are marijuana businesses being treated unfairly yet again? All because of a federal tax code amendment passed in 1982 called Section 280E. Section 280E denies tax credits or exemptions to businesses "trafficking" controlled substances.[29]

Do you want to know why pot businesses are bringing in so much tax revenue? Because they are overpaying! Due to Section 280E, their tax rates are anywhere from 40 percent to 70 percent—meanwhile the average corporate tax rate is around 35 percent[30] (that is, for the corporations that actually pay taxes). And some pot businesses in Colorado and Washington are forking over as much as 90 percent of their revenue to the IRS![31] Now do you see why the Obama administration sided with Colorado over Nebraska and Oklahoma? They want that tax money! And the IRS could very well put marijuana businesses out of business through this tax policy, so it's a win-win for the feds!

Some pot businesses such as the Vapor Room Herbal Center have actually tried to sue to get the same rights as any other business, but the courts held up the tax law due to the Controlled Substances Act that states marijuana is a controlled substance, illegal for sale, use, and distribution.[32] So it looks like the IRS is on the DEA's side when it comes to keeping marijuana classified as a Schedule I narcotic. In fact, the DEA and the IRS are thick as thieves when it comes to cannabis. If the IRS thinks a pot business isn't paying enough, it will send the DEA in to conduct a raid, citing money-laundering concerns. Since when does the IRS audit a business with a SWAT team? How is that even legal?

And just for argument's sake as to why that DEA classification is total hog-wash, let's go back to the fact that our country was founded on hemp, yet none of the Founding Fathers wound up as drug addicts. Flash forward to today, and you might find it interesting to know that since marijuana has been legalized, crime and hard drug use has gone down. Legalizing marijuana doesn't harm America, it helps America. Let's take a look at Colorado as case in point of this:

- Colorado collected almost $70 million in marijuana taxes in 2014, nearly double the $42 million collected from alcohol taxes.[33] The state even held a "tax holiday" on September 16, 2015 to celebrate— all marijuana products could be bought without the 10 percent sales tax that day.[34]

- Colorado schools earned $13.6 million in just the first five months of 2015, which is a huge increase from 2014—when the tax generated a total of $13.3 million for the entire year.[35] Tax revenue is being used to buy new roofs, boilers, and security upgrades in public schools.[36]

- Starting in 2017, marijuana taxes from Pueblo County, Colorado will be used to fund college scholarships and community projects, such as extending an Amtrak route to the county.[37]

- According to data released from the city of Denver, violent crime and property crime has been decreasing. Violent crime in Denver went down by 2.2 percent in the first eleven months of 2014, compared to the first eleven months of 2013. In the same period, burglaries decreased by 9.5 percent and overall property crime decreased by 8.9 percent.[38] I'm not saying legalizing weed was the sole factor that led to less crime in Denver, but clearly legalizing weed did not lead to more crime, as so many politicians thought it would.

- In 2010, there were 9,011 people arrested for marijuana possession and approximately 1,464 people arrested in 2014.[39] That means the state of Colorado is saving millions in costs associated with arresting and con-victing people for drug possession.

- According to the National Survey on Drug Use and Health, from 2010 to 2011, Colorado ranked second-worst among states for prescription drug abuse (Oregon beat out Colorado as the worst state by 0.37 percent).[40]

Since then, the state has improved. Colorado is now the twelfth-worst state in the nation. Again, I'm not saying legalizing marijuana was the sole factor that led to fewer people abusing prescription drugs, but I am saying that legalizing weed clearly did not contribute to more opioid addicts.

Weed has always been part of the American culture, no matter how much our federal government has tried to deny that fact. Currently, there are twenty-three states and the District of Columbia that have legalized marijuana and more and more states decriminalize it every day. As of 2016, 86 percent of Americans live in a state that allows some degree of legal cannabis use.[41]

So why are there still states that won't get with the program? Take South Dakota, for instance. When it comes to marijuana, it is illegal to ingest or possess it anywhere in the state. It is also illegal to have ingested it in another state, even if you legally ingested it weeks earlier. Yes, you read that correctly. Since marijuana can stay in a person's system for an estimated four to sixty-seven days,[42] South Dakota can punish someone to the full extent of the law for doing something that is one hundred percent legal in another state.

Here's a scenario to illustrate what this ridiculous law is implying: let's just say you ingested marijuana legally in Alaska, Colorado, Oregon, Washington state, or Washington, DC, and then you hop on a plane to South Dakota to visit family. You rent a car, and get pulled over for any number of reasons. If after peeing in a cup, police find marijuana is in your system, you're going to jail for up to 365 days and/or pay a $2,000 fine.[43] I guess that's one way for law enforcement to bring in revenue.

According to South Dakota's Codified Laws Chapter 22–42–15,[44] it is a Class 1 misdemeanor to ingest a "substance, except alcoholic beverages, for the purpose of becoming intoxicated," regardless of the "venue for violation." This is called "internal possession" of marijuana.

Going back to our scenario, under state law, if you are pulled over, police can't force you to pee in a cup. Police need "voluntary consent" or your urine test can be challenged in court. However, they do have strong methods of coercion, and they are not above threatening people to get a "voluntary consent."

South Dakota attorney Ron Volesky explains it further:

I defend a lot of drug cases and I've defended several of these urine sample cases, but I haven't yet seen an instance where we could challenge a court order because everyone has voluntarily consented. As a practical matter, when the police pick someone up they say, 'Look, we can do it the hard way or the easy way; you can voluntarily consent because we have probable cause, or we can wake up the judge, have him sign an order, and take you down and have you catheterized.' They basically threaten you.[45]

Essentially, if you're an out-of-state driver and you get pulled over by police in South Dakota, they may force you to "voluntarily" take a urine test for marijuana use. The only loophole in the "internal possession" law is if the marijuana in your system was "prescribed by a practitioner of the medical arts lawfully practicing within the scope of the practitioner's practice."[46] Therefore, medical marijuana users are off the hook in South Dakota if they travel with their state issued medical marijuana card and can prove they were prescribed the marijuana in their system.

Even in states that have legalized marijuana, the laws can be a bit strange. Washington, DC, legalized marijuana under Initiative 71, but the way in which the law is written, any public consumption of marijuana is still considered illegal:[47]

- The law is written for home growing and home use only.
- You cannot legally sell or purchase any form of recreational marijuana in DC.
- You cannot legally ingest any form of marijuana outside of your home.
- Residents can carry no more than 2 oz. of weed on them.

DC is considering opening marijuana dispensaries for recreational purposes, but right now, the only people who can purchase weed are those with medical marijuana cards. Isn't that the strangest thing? You can grow marijuana in your home legally for recreational purposes and you can legally consume it for recreational purposes, but you can't buy it or ingest it anywhere outside your home unless you need it for medical purposes. Name me any other product that is regulated in this way!

This kind of false legalization is holding our country back. According to *The State of Legal Marijuana Markets, Fourth Edition*:[48]

- America's homegrown marijuana industry is expected to grow by 25 percent in 2016, to bring in $6.7 billion in sales.

- In 2015, recreational and medical marijuana sales surpassed $5.4 billion in the states that legalized it.
- In 2014, those sales accounted for $4.6 billion, so you can see how this industry keeps growing exponentially each year.
- There are currently seven more states that could potentially legalize marijuana completely in 2016: Arizona, California, Massachusetts, Maine, Nevada, Rhode Island, and Vermont.
- And in 2016, Florida, Ohio, Missouri, and Pennsylvania will vote on passing medical marijuana laws.
- By 2020, nationwide sales could reach $21.8 billion

But think of how much more money could be made from marijuana if it were only legalized and taxed like cigarettes or alcohol!

Here's another contradictory thing: each state has different guidelines as to what conditions qualify for medical marijuana. For example, Delaware legalized medical marijuana in 2011 for debilitating pain, cancer, Lou Gehrig's disease, and Alzheimer's. Then in 2015, Delaware became the first state to add autism to the list. Now, autistic patents "who are prone to aggressive or self-injurious tendencies"[49] can apply for medical marijuana cards.

Now, just because Delaware is the first state to list autism as a qualifying condition for medical marijuana, that doesn't mean you're out of luck if you live elsewhere. Autism has a range of conditions, including intestinal disorders, seizures, and chronic pain. Many states will allow medical marijuana for one of those conditions. For instance, California residents who have autism have access to medical marijuana because doctors can prescribe it for any condition they see fit. Oregon residents with autism can also access medical marijuana because neurological disorders are a qualifying condition. But since Delaware is the first state to list autism as a qualifying condition, the state is planning to do some significant research studies in 2016—if it ever gets approval from the DEA and NIH, that is. You see, for any cannabis research study to be legitimate, it requires approval from these government organizations. The approval guarantees that the study is being conducted under certain universal standards. Without it, there isn't much chance that a product resulting from such a cannabis study can get FDA approval.

In 2015, Delaware passed Senate Bill 138 to allow for medical facilities that already meet FDA standards to conduct marijuana studies, particularly to help children with seizures or autism. I find Delaware's commitment to autism-cannabis studies interesting because according to the CDC, the official cause of autism is still unknown, and there are no medications that can cure autism or treat its core symptoms.[50] Currently, very little research has been done on medical marijuana and autism, even though one in every sixty-eight children is diagnosed with the disorder. However, Dr. Christian Bogner, the author of "The Endocannabinoid System as it Relates to Autism," has followed preliminary research in lab rats to determine that epilepsy treatments—such as an oil with high CBD content and low THC content—can also benefit those with autism.[51]

According to Dr. Christian Bogner, the endocannabinoid system plays a role in the progression of autism. He notes that certain genetic mutations—such as Fragile X syndrome, the most commonly known genetic cause of autism—"inhibit tonic secretion of endocannabinoids and disrupt their signaling."[52] Although Bogner admits more research must be done, he thinks that cannabinoids from marijuana might be able to provide treatment for autism because cytonkines (proteins that are secreted by CBD and THC) aid in the interactions and communications between cells in the endocannabinoid system.[53] So in theory, CBD and THC might be able to help autistic patents achieve more normal brain functions. Remember, the cannabinoid receptors in the brain play a direct role in virtually ever aspect of the human body, so it goes to reason that the cannabinoids in marijuana can help anyone with any condition that impacts the endocannabinoid system.

Now, if only we could get every state behind medical marijuana as a treatment for PTSD! Considering there already are studies that prove how much weed helps those with PTSD, it's alarming to see politicians and even the VA discredit marijuana as a treatment option.

12

Marijuana and Post-Traumatic Stress Disorder

The state of Colorado continues to make enemies with neighboring states—including Kansas. Medical marijuana is illegal in Kansas, and if you hear a story about Child Protective Services taking kids away from parents that smoke pot for medical purposes, there's a pretty strong likelihood that they live in Kansas. Kansas has a zero-tolerance policy when it comes to medical marijuana, so much so that a forty-year-old Gulf War veteran and his wife had their five youngest kids taken away while they were in the process of moving from Kansas to Colorado, where the veteran could get his PTSD medication legally.

Raymond Schwab, an honorably discharged Naval veteran, moved from Kansas to Colorado in 2015 so he could treat his PTSD and chronic pain with medical marijuana.[1] His chronic pain is so severe that he is currently on disability for it and cannabis remains the only effective treatment for both the pain and the PTSD symptoms. Schwab felt so strongly about how cannabis has helped his conditions that he started a business in Colorado to grow pot for veterans suffering from PTSD.

Prior to moving to Colorado, Schwab lived in Topeka, and the Department of Veteran Affairs (VA) prescribed him an assortment of pharmaceutical drugs to treat his PTSD and chronic pain—everything from pain pills to muscle relaxants to anti-anxiety drugs—but none of the medications helped. For years, his mental health issues went undiagnosed and he turned to alcoholism, and then he actually developed a heroin addiction due to the pain pills the VA prescribed. Eventually, he was able to overcome the addictions through cannabis therapy.[2]

When Schwab decided to move his family to Denver to gain legal access to his medication, his wife, Amelia, was supportive, but other members of his immediate family didn't seem to be thrilled with the idea. While Amelia and Raymond were preparing for the big move, they arranged for five of their six children to stay with relatives (the oldest was nineteen and did not need to stay with family).

One of the relatives caring for the children was Amelia's mother. Well, she must have really not approved of marijuana use under any circumstances because she took the children to the police station, claiming that their parents had abandoned them to go work on a pot farm in Colorado.[3] Included in this original police report is a screenshot of Raymond Schwab's Facebook post where he discussed moving to Colorado to start a marijuana business, so you can bet the cops took this grandmother's claim very seriously. So seriously in fact that the Kansas Department of Children and Families (DCF) placed the Schwab children in its custody, and the children are still in DCF's custody. Raymond has seen his children only three times since April 2015.

Amelia says her mother now regrets doing this to her family, but the damage is done. Kansas investigated the Schwabs and an official report was filed in July 2015 that says any allegations of emotional abuse and child endangerment were "dismissed as unsubstantiated."[4] Yet Kansas still won't return the children due to the stigma attached to medical marijuana. Even though authorities can't prove there was ever any harm being done to the children, they will not give them back knowing the father smokes pot . . . and does it legally with a Colorado state approved medical marijuana card!

Get this: If Raymond wants to visit his kids in Kansas, he has to submit a urine sample to the court first, to prove he's clean. Even though he now lives in Colorado, where he has a legal right to cannabis![5] And now, Kansas's courts state that if he wants his family restored, he has to pass drug tests for four consecutive months.[6] That means four months without cannabis. That means four months with his PTSD symptoms going untreated—symptoms that led him to alcoholism and heroin addiction in the past.

So the courts are telling Schwab that he'd be a fit father as a full-blown alcoholic and heroin addict with PTSD, but if he smokes pot, he's a danger to their well-being. How does that make any sense, given what we know about alcoholism, heroin addiction, and the effects of PTSD? How much do you want to bet that the people who made this horrendous decision for Schwab and his family weren't brave enough to serve our country like Schwab did?

"They're basically using my kids as a pawn to take away freedoms I fought for," Raymond Schwab told the *Denver Post*. "It's a horrible position to put me in."[7]

Yet Schwab is going to go through the agony of four months without cannabis to get his kids back. And he's planning on suing as soon as he gets them. He told *The Guardian* in February 2016:

> People who don't understand the medical value of cannabis are tearing my family apart. They're holding my kids hostage and threatening to terminate my rights if I don't seek cannabis-abuse therapy in a state that's legal. They're threatening other people with jail time or losing their kids if they speak out, but I will not submit. I'll take this to the supreme court if I have to.[8]

I wish my fellow Naval veteran all the luck in the world with that court case and in getting his constitutional rights restored. However, I would be shocked if SCOTUS actually sides with him over the state of Kansas, given that marijuana is illegal on the federal level. According to the US Department of Health and Human Services, cannabis use falls under parental drug use, and parental drug use is a form of child abuse:

> Exposing children to the manufacture, possession, or distribution of illegal drugs is considered child endangerment in eleven States [including Kansas] . . . the Federal Child Abuse Prevention and Treatment Act requires states to have policies and procedures in place to notify child protective services agencies of substance-exposed newborns.[9]

Raymond Schwab would have to prove what Robert Randall proved in federal court in the '70s: that marijuana is a medical necessity for his condition. Glaucoma is a "marijuana-responsive" condition and so is post-traumatic stress disorder. Cannabis helps with night terrors, flashbacks, and uncontrolled emotional processing associated with PTSD. Maybe Schwab will get FDA-approved access to government marijuana if he wins this case, just like Robert

Randall. One would only hope that history could repeat itself. But as Lenny Bruce once said, "In the Halls of Justice, the only justice is in the halls."[10]

Americans for Safe Access Chief Scientist Dr. Jahan Marcu states this about cannabis and veterans with PTSD:

> [Marijuana] works on the body's endocannabinoid system in five ways: It helps you to eat, sleep, relax, forget, and protect your body. In relation to PTSD, how cannabis is particularly useful is with the 'forgetting' part. If I remembered every face I saw today on the subway, my head would explode. Your body needs a system to get rid of information that is no longer useful, or harmful to you. In some situations, you cannot forget or adjust to painful circumstances. What we can say is that no study has conclusively shown any significant harm to vets with PTSD that are using cannabis. Studies looked for it—and what they found instead was better stress management.[11]

What the blockheads in the Kansas court system don't know is what it feels like to have PTSD and what people like Schwab have to deal with just to get through the day. If you have PTSD, you cannot get traumatic memories out of your head. Anything can trigger a flashback from war that you'd literally try anything to forget, and yet there isn't any way for our veterans get those memories out of their heads. That's the problem with the disorder. You get panic attacks, phobias, anxiety, emotional breakdowns, survivor's guilt, depression, nightmares, and thoughts of suicide as a result of experiencing combat trauma.[12] Most veterans with PTSD self-medicate, like Raymond Schwab did, with alcohol, prescription drugs, and harder drugs, like heroin.

And where does cannabis come in? Remember how memory loss is one of the effects of cannabis? Well, guess what it does for those with PTSD? It lets veterans let go of those horrible memories that haunt them day in and day out. Let me put it to you this way: The eighteen-year-olds of my generation who were drafted for the Vietnam War spent the majority of their time smoking pot in Vietnam when they weren't blowing things up.[13] At the time, commanding officers looked the other way. They knew smoking pot helped in compartmentalizing the horrors they were experiencing.

And let me tell you, I'm sick of chickenhawks sending our young men and women overseas to fight useless wars, and then denying cannabis as a medical solution. I'm sick of the VA stating there isn't enough medical data concerning PTSD and cannabis. These politicians who are all backed by Big Pharma seem to want our veterans to be alcoholics and heroin addicts. That way maybe we'll all be too wacked out to make it to the voting booth.

A 2012 study from the VA estimated that 20 percent of veterans returning from Iraq and Afghanistan suffer from PTSD.[14] Among these veterans, the suicide rate is 50 percent higher than the national average. The VA states that from 1999 to 2010, there were roughly eighteen veteran deaths per day in the United States.[15] Then that number increased to twenty-two deaths per day in 2013. Which means that every sixty-five minutes, a veteran commits suicide. In other words, there are more soldiers committing suicide every day at home compared to how many are being killed in action.

According to a report by the Cleveland Clinic Journal of Medicine:

> In military veterans, depression, posttraumatic stress disorder (PTSD), and suicidal thoughts are common and closely linked. Veterans are less likely to seek care and more likely to act successfully on suicidal thoughts.[16]

So what are the treatments for PTSD? Aside from therapy, anti-anxiety meds like Xanax or Ativan; antidepressants such as Prozac, Paxil, or Zoloft; and Adrenergic drugs like Propranolol and Clonadine.[17] And cannabis.

This may surprise you, but PTSD isn't a qualifying condition for medical marijuana in many states, including Colorado. Why? Because many states feel more research is necessary. Here are the states that have legalized medical marijuana but do not list PTSD as a qualifying condition for medical cannabis: Alaska, California, Colorado, Washington, DC, Illinois, Maine, Maryland, Massachusetts, Minnesota, Montana, New Hampshire, New Jersey, New York, Oregon, Rhode Island, Vermont, and Washington.[18]

Get this: If you live in one of those states and you have PTSD, you might still be able to get medical marijuana. If some of your PTSD symptoms fall under qualifying conditions for medical marijuana, then you can get a medical marijuana card. So for example, if chronic pain is one of your PTSD symptoms—or if a licensed physician can diagnose one of your PTSD symptoms as "debilitating"—you can most likely get medical marijuana for your PTSD in Colorado, Maryland, DC, California, Massachusetts, and many other states.[19] Don't you just love that loophole?

These are the only states that have officially approved PTSD for medical cannabis: Arizona, Connecticut, Delaware, Hawaii, Michigan, Nevada, New Mexico, and Maine. That's eight states out of twenty-three (or twenty-four if you include DC).[20]

As a side note, it's interesting that there are some conditions that are accepted in every state that has legalized medical marijuana—such as cancer, HIV/AIDS, glaucoma, seizures, multiple sclerosis, and Crohn's disease. For states that only allow CBD oil, such as Iowa and Florida, severe seizure conditions are the universal qualifying condition.[21] And for Louisiana, which just passed a medical marijuana law in 2015 but won't have legal access to it for at least two years, only three conditions are currently eligible: cancer, glaucoma, and spastic quadriplegia (a rare form of cerebral palsy).[22] Like I said earlier, state officials decide what conditions are qualifying and what conditions "need more research." No need to consult a doctor.

Okay, fine, so we need more studies on PTSD. Or do we? How is it that some states consider medical marijuana as a treatment for PTSD and some don't? Aren't our lawmakers looking at the same exact studies to determine what qualifies and what doesn't? How is it that Israel has approved cannabis for PTSD while weed is illegal throughout the country? Surely, there must have been some kind of significant study to allow that to happen. So why are we choosing to ignore its validity?

Israel has conducted medical marijuana studies for those who suffer from PTSD, and researchers are moving ahead with more. Don't get me wrong— cannabis isn't exactly flying off the shelves in the pharmacies over there. Medical marijuana is considered a last resort for people with serious illnesses; patients must exhaust all other medical options, and complete a long-winded bureaucratic process before they can receive medical cannabis.[23] To qualify for a cannabis permit in Israeli, a patient must have at least a 30 percent disability according to the National Insurance Institute criteria, must have tried at least two other medications for at least two months each, and must not have a history of psychosis or drug abuse.[24] Yet, even after jumping through all those hoops, the most common illnesses for cannabis therapy include cancer, Parkinson's, Tourette syndrome, and PTSD.[25]

In Israel, a country that considers marijuana an illegal drug, the medical marijuana industry is roughly producing $40 million per year[26] and PTSD is part of that thriving industry. As of December 2015, there were about 1,153

PTSD patients in Israel approved for medical cannabis.[27] If that seems like a low number, that's because the program for PTSD is extremely recent. In July 2014, the Israeli Health Ministry and the Israeli Psychiatric Association approved PTSD for the use of medical marijuana.[28] It is the only psychiatric condition currently approved for cannabis.

According to the patriarch of cannabis, Dr. Raphael Mechoulam, marijuana could very well be the answer for PTSD because of its role in "memory extinction."[29]

Memory extinction is normal for every human being, except for those with PTSD. The term "memory extinction" means that your brain is able to remove associations from stimuli—this is a normal process for a healthy brain, but it's something that someone suffering from PTSD is unable to do. Dr. Mechoulam tested his "memory extinction" theories on lab animals:

> An animal which has been administered an electric shock after a certain noise will eventually forget about the shock after the noise appears alone for a few days. Mice without cannabinoid systems simply never forget—they continue to cringe at the noise indefinitely. This has implications for patients with PTSD, who respond to stimuli that remind them of their initial trauma even when it is no longer appropriate. By aiding in memory extinction, marijuana could help patients reduce their association between stimuli (perhaps loud noises or stress) and the traumatic situations in their past.[30]

After conducting animal studies, Dr. Mechoulam tried a preliminary PTSD pilot study with ten people suffering from chronic PTSD in August 2014. The ten patients continued to take their PTSD medication while they received 5 mg of THC twice a day as an add-on treatment. Mechoulam determined that the dose of THC helped decrease the frequency of nightmares and "PTSD hyperarousal symptoms," thus allowing the patients to improve their sleep quality and overall quality of life.[31] These results also back up a PTSD study in New Mexico that was published in the Journal of Psychoactive Drugs in 2014.

New Mexico became the first state to list PTSD as a qualifying condition for medical cannabis, and researchers were eager to conduct a study to prove the healing power of weed. From 2009 to 2011, eighty psychiatric evaluations from PTSD medical marijuana patents were collected to determine that cannabis "significantly" reduces PTSD symptoms. The eighty patients reported "over 75 percent reduction in all three areas of PTSD symptoms while using cannabis."[32] But again, eighty patients is a small pool of people, which is why many in the medical community—including doctors in the VA—are continuing to doubt the effectiveness of medical marijuana.

Dr. Suzanne Sisley, a PTSD psychiatrist and researcher in the US, is in the process of conducting the first DEA-approved trial of medical marijuana as a treatment for PTSD in veterans. If you saw the CNN documentary series *Weed*, then you might remember her. She was doing medical research at the University of Arizona and received FDA approval to conduct the first study to determine the effects of smoking cannabis on veterans with PTSD. However, in June 2011, soon after receiving government funding and approval for the study, the university stripped her of all her existing contracts (which is a fancy way of firing someone who has done nothing wrong)[33]. Apparently, the University didn't want her conduct the marijuana study—even though the U.S. government had no issues with it, and even though Dr. Sisley had been working with veterans for *twenty* years.

After being booted from the University of Arizona, Dr. Sisley landed a $2.156 million-grant from Colorado's Department of Public Health and Environment to conduct the study,[34] but she had to wait to receive DEA approval so she could order the necessary medical grade marijuana from Ole Miss. On April 20, 2016—nearly seven years after sending in her application to the DEA—she finally received the go ahead, and today, she is making history. According to the *Military Times*: "this is the first randomized, controlled research in the U.S. for PTSD that will use the actual plant instead of oils or synthesized cannabis . . . advocates say the research will fill a much-needed gap in medical literature."[35] Dr. Sisley tells me that a study of this kind is necessary for her to achieve her long term goals: If the study proves marijuana helps PTSD, then she will work to get the whole plant approved by the FDA for medicinal use. Once she is successful in doing this, whole plant cannabis will be covered under medical insurance, just like any other drug.

This trial study is just phase 1 of this long-term plan. The US health department only accepts randomized, controlled testing when it comes to approving a drug, so it was completely necessary for Dr. Sisley to get the DEA on board before doing anything—including gathering participants. The trial focuses on on seventy-six veterans who are resistant to other forms of PTSD medication. Half of the veterans are being treated by Dr. Sisley in Phoenix, AZ and the other half are being treated by Ryan Vandrey, Ph.D, at Johns Hopkins University in Baltimore.[36] According to the press release announcing the DEA approval, the University of Colorado School of Medicine "will oversee the scientific integrity of the study," the University of Colorado will conduct blood analysis, and the Multidisciplinary Association for Psychedelic Studies (MAPS) "will work with the FDA to manage and monitor data, oversee drug accountability, and ensure the study follows Good Clinical Practice guidelines."[37]

The trial randomly divides the veterans equally into four groups: group 1 receives smoked cannabis with a high percentage of THC and a low percentage of CBD, group 2 receives smoked cannabis with a high percentage of CBD and a low percentage of THC, group 3 receives something more balanced, and the final group receives a placebo. Dr. Sisley's theory is that marijuana offers "a capacity not to forget bad memories but to not fixate on them."[38]

Again, I believe that a CBD strain with very little THC might help one person; a strain with more THC might help another. I don't believe this is an exact science where one dosage fits all.

Think about how many different kinds of antidepressant medications there are. Just because the term "depression" is a universal definition, that doesn't mean everyone's brain reacts the same to antidepressant drugs. Some people take Paxil. Some people take Prozac. And even those who take Prozac or Paxil don't take the same exact strength or dosage. It's the same with PTSD and marijuana. Everyone copes with trauma differently; no two people are exactly alike. Think about how many different drugs are being prescribed right now for those with PTSD. So shouldn't it go to reason that when treating PTSD with cannabis, each person should be monitored and the medication should be adjusted as needed? I'm curious to see if Dr. Sisley's study proves this to be true.

According to MAPS spokesperson Brad Burge, the study began in June 2016 at the Arizona and Baltimore testing sites.[39] MAPS has also conducted some fascinating studies in Israel and California that show how MDMA (the pure compound in Ecstasy) can help people with autism and PTSD.[40] Apparently, MDMA-assisted therapy can reduce "social anxiety symptoms" and increase "social adaptability" for autistic adults and those diagnosed with PTSD—and MDMA does not need to be used on an ongoing basis to achieve lasting results.[41] How's that for alternative medicine!

MAPS is responsible for purchasing the research-grade cannabis for this groundbreaking PTSD trial from the National Institute on Drug Abuse (NIDA) at Ole Miss. If the study goes as planned, the team will be able to develop "the marijuana plant in smoked form into an FDA-approved prescription medicine."[42] But the NIDA's Ole Miss pot supply ain't cheap. MAPS states that the NIDA once quoted the research-grade marijuana at $7 per gram. Meanwhile, Israeli pot producers offer research-grade marijuana to scientists at $1 per gram![43] That's the nice part about having a monopoly on something: The FDA can charge whatever the hell it wants.

Could Dr. Sisley get pot from Colorado for the study? Sure. But then the study wouldn't have gotten DEA approval. Isn't it interesting that companies like KannaLife and GW Pharmaceuticals aren't bound by those same rules? Big Pharma can bypass the NIDA and go with a privately-owned company to get their medical grade pot for research and development, yet Dr. Sisley has to do everything by the book—and the NIDA doesn't have to play by its own rules. Get this: Dr. Sisley said that she requested strains of marijuana with twelve percent THC or higher to conduct the study. By law, the NIDA must fulfill the requests of researchers, which means they must produce what she requests, but she doesn't know if they actually will. Ole Miss told her the strongest marijuana they had was with seven percent CBD and THC, so she's forced to take it—and she has no idea if this lower percentage will ultimately affect her results. She also has to test the marijuana to confirm its potency in a third party lab before giving it to the veterans, but the DEA specifies only labs with a DEA license can test DEA marijuana. She told me she requested a list of those labs, but the DEA won't disclose them to her!

Know what else I found interesting? Due to the fact that she's using whole plant cannabis, she can only order marijuana for a three-month supply, so that the quality doesn't degrade. The pot comes freeze dried and dehydrated from Ole Miss; she has to then thaw and rehydrate it before giving it to the vets. How is the weed shipped? Through FedEx! The government won't even ship its own weed through its own postal service.

Dr. Sisley and I are left wondering if the government will be able to keep up with the demands on a three-month supply basis. Again, Ole Miss is required by law to keep up with the demand, but will they actually grow enough? And will each batch be consistent when it comes to potency? Will the government sabotage the study on purpose? I wouldn't put it past them!

Dr. Sisley told me that she honestly doesn't know what the results will be, and she isn't going into the study with any bias. But she does feel that there is a "war on science." The government is concerned that American studies like hers will uncover the true benefits of cannabis. Up to this point, if you wanted to conduct a government-approved study on marijuana and do it on American soil, researchers had to focus on "safety studies," which can only explore what is wrong with marijuana. How's that for bias and researchers predetermining the results? This is why Sisley is also convinced that if the veteran community didn't stand with her to get national publicity about the project, the study would have been swept under the rug. She has no doubt that their immense public pressure granted her the DEA's approval (on 4/20, no less).

In any case, Dr. Sisley told me that results from the study might not be published until 2019 due to how much time it will take to collect and analyze data. She's estimating that she'll be spending the next two years just enrolling veterans in the trial. *The Denver Post* reports she is projecting that researchers will only be able to add four to five veterans per month due in part to how difficult it will be to track down the vets that meet the necessary criteria.[44] Her initial plan was to go to the VA and request volunteers—clearly those doctors would be able to recommend candidates for the study. However because of the recent VA scandals, administrators are "skittish" about working with her and aiding her "controversial" trial![45] But get this: She actually went to the VA to give a presentation about the study about three years ago, and the administration was eager to give her referrals. And now that she has the government's approval, the VA is only interested in the results, but they aren't interested in contributing. Or in other words, decision-makers at the VA yet again have no interest in actually helping veterans when they have the chance.

Meanwhile, the VA states on its website: "research has consistently demonstrated that the human endocannabinoid system plays a significant role in PTSD,"[46] but no VA doctor will prescribe medical marijuana—the one medication that is proven to interact positively with the endocannabinoid system—even in the states where cannabis is legal! The VA is basically saying, yes, we know that this could fix the problem but we won't give it to you.

If a veteran wants to get medical marijuana, then he has to go to a private doctor and get it prescribed and pay for everything out of pocket (or break the law by getting it from a drug dealer). And if a veteran does this, the VA will no longer provide medical services. Either the veteran takes *all* the VA's advice and medication and gets government healthcare, or the veteran forfeits all medical benefits by smoking pot.

Essentially, veterans with PTSD and chronic pain who rely on the VA for their healthcare are not able to access their state medical marijuana programs—and that's discrimination against our vets! Get this: if a veteran has medical marijuana on him and he's at a VA facility, he could be at risk for prosecution under the Controlled Substances Act![47] So even if medical marijuana is legal in your state, if you step on VA property with it, you are committing an illegal act and could be arrested for doing so.

Oregon House Representative Earl Blumenauer has been trying to change this for years. He introduced legislation such as the Veterans Equal Access Act to allow the VA to provide medical marijuana, but the bill was stalled *twice* in the Subcommittee on Health.[48] In April 2015, he tried to put a bipartisan amendment on the 2016 budget to allow for VA doctors to prescribe medical marijuana, and the measure failed narrowly by a vote of 210–213.[49] Then something interesting happened.

In November 2015, the Senate passed the Fiscal Year 2016 Military Construction and Veteran Affairs Appropriations Bill. In this bill was the H. R. 2029—Consolidated Appropriations Act, 2016 (sponsored by Pennsylvania Representative Charles W. Dent). Section 246 of this bill states that the VA is prohibited from interfering "with the ability of veterans to participate in a state-approved medicinal marijuana program," or denying services to veterans participating in a medical marijuana program, or interfering "with the ability of a VA health care provider care to comply with a program."[50] This House amendment passed unanimously with a vote of 93–0.[51] Victory at last? Unfortunately, no. The provision concerning medical marijuana was stripped from the final appropriations bill because the majority in the House of Representatives voted *against* it again![52]

On January 27, 2016 a group of twenty-one senators and *house* representatives sent a letter urging VA Secretary Robert McDonald to discuss and recommend marijuana as a treatment option for veterans in states where it's legal (because the law stating it is illegal for a VA doctor to even *discuss* the drug with patients was set to expire).

Vigilant US Senators Kirsten Gillibrand, Steve Daines, and Jeff Merkley and US Representatives Earl Blumenauer, Dina Titus, and Dana Rohrabacher led the charge in collecting the necessary signatures for the letter. The letter was also signed by US Senators Cory Booker, Barbara Boxer, Patty Murray, Brian Schatz, Tammy Baldwin, Michael Bennet, Ron Wyden, and Elizabeth Warren, and US Representatives Joe Heck, Sam Farr, Jared Polis, Chellie Pingree, Steve

Cohen, Justin Amash, and Mark Pocan. If you're passionate about this issue, you might want to check to see if any of those folks represent your home state and vote them back into office this coming election cycle. Politicians always say they support the troops, but actions like this speak louder than words. In April 2016, the Senate Appropriations Committee passed the same exact bipartisan amendment concerning medical marijuana again. The measure was sponsored by Senators Steve Daines and Senator Jeff Merkley. This time, they attached it to a must-pass military construction and veterans affairs spending bill, and they have high hopes that it will pass this time around in the House.[53] But who knows.

It's infuriating to see that the Department of Veteran Affairs—meant to help our vets in every way, shape, and form—has had a long history of actually doing the exact opposite. Since July 2002, over 300,000 veterans nationwide have been forced to wait over six months for a medical appointment. And if you recall in 2014 there was a huge nationwide VA scandal that started when at least forty veterans died while waiting for care at the Phoenix, Arizona, VA facilities. Veterans who went to the Phoenix VA waited an average of 115 days for an appointment,[54] and a federal investigation showed that VA facilities nationwide had similar problems. These facilities falsified records instead of hiring more doctors and nurses to keep up with the appointments. And these are the people who are telling our veterans that cannabis can't possibly help PTSD?!

When it comes to our veterans, they should receive the best care available in America. They should have the same benefits as Congress, plain and simple. Congress receives government-run healthcare, yet you never hear them complaining. Meanwhile, We the People are stuck with the Affordable Care Act and the VA. How did we get the short end of the stick when we're the ones who gave them their jobs in the first place? I say every Representative who votes in favor of going to war should have to send one of their own sons or daughters so they have some skin in the game. Maybe then we'll see some changes at the VA. Maybe then they'll vote a little differently on these bills.

If we as Americans really want to thank our vets for their service, then we have to stand up for veterans' rights. What happened to Raymond Schwab and his children should have never happened. Someone who fought for our country and took an oath to protect our Constitution and would have even died to uphold and defend our freedoms shouldn't ever have to worry about getting his kids taken away from him for using a legal medication. Veterans shouldn't ever have to make an "either/or" decision when it comes to their health and their family's well-being. They should never have to choose between either jeopardizing their mental and physical health by not taking their medical marijuana or losing their children because they're using medical marijuana. Mental and physical health is directly related to job performance and family life. So why on earth do we continue to deny our veterans the chance to treat PTSD with weed when it clearly helps their heath and well-being? The point is, we have no right to deny them access to this medication. I'm ashamed my country is doing this.

13

Jury Nullification—
How to Fight Back against
Marijuana Prohibition

To quote Martin Luther King Jr., "One has a moral responsibility to disobey unjust laws." I find it morally wrong for this country to deny a cancer patient the right to smoke pot. Why are we turning cancer patients into criminals? If you are in a state that won't be decriminalizing or legalizing marijuana in any way any time soon, you should know what jury nullification is. Jury nullification was used during the Civil Rights era and it can be used again to force the courts to stop prosecuting marijuana offenders.

As an American citizen, jury nullification is your last defense against unreasonable laws, but I bet the majority of Americans have no clue what it is and how it has been used in a court of law. After you are selected for jury duty, jury nullification is the one right you'll never be informed about when you're given juror instructions in court.

Jury nullification occurs when a jury returns a verdict of "not guilty" even though the defendant is clearly guilty of the violation. When the jury does this, they are deciding that whatever law the defendant disobeyed is either immoral or wrongly applied. So a jury can acquit a defendant—even if the defendant broke the law and did something illegal—because they believe the law is unjust and the person should not be charged or punished. It's the greatest tool available to a juror to restore balance between the law and justice.

Here's how jury nullification has been used throughout US history:

- Leading up to the American Revolutionary War, British prose-cutors gave up trying maritime cases and cases implicating free speech because colonial juries would never convict the person charged with the crime.[1]
- Prior to the Civil War, through the 1850s, juries refused to convict for violations of slavery laws, such as the Fugitive Slave Act, a law that stated if a slave ran away to the North to be free, that slave must be captured and returned to the slave owner.
- During Prohibition, juries nullified alcohol control laws approximately 60 percent of the time.[2] This resistance to Prohibition may have also contributed to its repeal.
- In the 1960s, during the Civil Rights era, jury nullification was prac-ticed to fight against segregation laws such as the Jim Crow laws.

So why aren't we taught about jury nullification in school? Because it's the best-kept secret in the legal system! In 1895, the Supreme Court decided in *Sparf and Hansen v. United States* that juries have the right to jury nullification, but the court is not legally bound to inform them about it![3] And the court takes that right of omission very seriously.

Get this: Just a few days before Thanksgiving in 2015, a former pastor by the name of Keith Eric Wood was arrested and charged with a felony for stand-ing on a sidewalk by a Michigan courthouse and handing out brochures that included information about jury nullification.[4] Bail was set at $150,000 and he was able to get out of jail twelve hours after being booked by putting $15,000 on a credit card. What a way to ruin a family's Thanksgiving!

Wood is now being prosecuted for a felony charge for obstruction of jus-tice. But wait a minute. What happened to the First Amendment? Isn't the state violating his freedom of speech? Wood was on a city sidewalk—a prime example of a public forum—where First Amendment rights are at their stron-gest.[5] Yet Michigan authorities are standing by the felony charge, stating he "knowingly and intentionally" gave the jurors a pamphlet encouraging them to "violate their oaths." Michigan viewed Wood's actions as "tainting the entire jury panel" and "willfully attempting to influence" jurors already assigned to a trial—even though the brochure he was handing out did not refer to any particular case![6]

In what world is informing someone of his rights as a juror violating anything? Apparently the world we live in. "Land of the Free" is officially an empty phrase as far as I'm concerned.

Folks, the First Amendment is there to protect unpopular speech. Popular speech does not need to be protected. The Founding Fathers felt the right to free speech—no matter how unpopular—was so profoundly important that they listed it first in the Bill of Rights. I truly hope that when the jury is picked for Wood's trial that they have done their homework on jury nullification. If there were ever a modern-day example of a case that required jury nullification, it should be this one.

Now don't get me wrong, jury nullification can be used inappropriately too. As much as jury nullification helped progress the civil rights movement, it also hindered it. White juries in the South would side with a white defendant, even if he obviously committed a heinous act against an African American. In 1991, the LA police officers that were videotaped beating Rodney King were acquitted. It was clearly obvious that the white officers beat an unarmed African American man nearly to death, but they faced no consequences for it.[7] Unfortunately, not much has changed in that department today. It's devastating to see how many people—even children—are gunned down by police in this country. It's infuriating to see the police get away with murder time and time again. It's astounding to see so few people in these police departments express any form of true remorse for these actions either. Yes, there are plenty of people in law enforcement who serve and protect their communities and put their lives on the line—but this nationwide problem of police brutality is more than a few bad apples. A vigilant cop is there to protect the public from the bad guys—and the bad guys include dangerous, violent, and corrupt cops. When was the last time you heard of a law enforcement whistleblower who exposed corruption within the police force? That's what a true public servant with integrity of the law is supposed to do.

There is no doubt in my mind that the laws concerning marijuana are unjust. There is no doubt that the laws concerning illegal drugs are also unjust. If someone is addicted to drugs, that person will not receive the treatment necessary inside of a jail cell. Addiction is a medical issue. Last I checked, medical issues were not within law enforcement's jurisdiction. The Baltimore police couldn't even transport Freddie Gray to Central Booking without killing him.

Do you really think they know what the hell they're doing when it comes to helping someone with a drug addiction? And what about all the people who are booked under the maximum minimum sentences for drugs. How are those laws helping anyone other than the people making money off of the prison system? By the way—you can thank President Bill Clinton for putting the majority of those laws on the books in the first place.

There are some states, however, that are moving toward informing juries of their right to nullify a case. In January 2016, West Virginia introduced a bill known as the Fair Trial Act, which would require judges in the state to inform juries of their right to nullify:

> The jury is the exclusive judge of the facts. The jury is bound to receive the law from the court and be governed thereby, except if a jury determines that a defendant is guilty according to the law and that the law is unjustly applied to the defendant, the jury may determine not to apply the law to the defendant and find the defendant not guilty or guilty of a lesser included offense.[8]

The bill hasn't been passed yet, but other states have also either adopted similar laws or are in the process of considering them—such as Georgia, Alaska, and New Hampshire.

Some drug policy reformers—including NORML and the ACLU—are also taking it upon themselves to educate people about how jury nullification can stop convicting people of drug charges. During Prohibition, juries refused to prosecute those who broke the law by drinking. In theory, we can all do our part to fight back against the government's War on Drugs by doing the same. NORML and the ACLU are holding town hall–style meetings about jury nullification in the states that have legalized marijuana. They're trying to level the playing field and fight back against the corruption of law enforcement.

Remember Hearst's war against marijuana and the racist propaganda he wrote in his newspapers about Mexicans and African Americans smoking pot and then raping white women? Well, as much as some people don't want to admit that today's War on Drugs has anything to do with racism, it absolutely does. The Centers for Disease Control and Prevention show that more whites are using illegal drugs and prescription pain pills and dying from overdoses than

African Americans. Yet our national incarceration figures would lead you to believe otherwise.

In 2016, the *New York Times* analyzed nearly sixty million death certificates collected by the CDC and determined the following:

- In 2014, the drug overdose death rate for whites aged twenty-five to thirty-four was five times what it was in 1999.
- The overdose rate for thirty-five-to-forty-four-year-old whites tripled during that same time period.
- Meanwhile, drug-related deaths for black and Hispanic adults have either been falling or have remained the same since 1999.[9]

So why are more white people dying from drug overdoses than African Americans? Could it be that black people just don't do as many drugs as white people do, as stereotypes that started with Randolph Hearst would suggest? And if African Americans aren't doing as many drugs, then why are there more black people in jail for drug-related crimes than whites?

For example, in California, where medical marijuana is legal, African Americans are four times more likely to be arrested for marijuana, twelve times more likely to be imprisoned for a marijuana felony arrest, and three times more likely to be imprisoned for that marijuana possession arrest than non-blacks. Overall, when you look at the odds, that means African Americans are ten times more likely to be imprisoned for marijuana than any other racial or ethnic group in California.[10]

Now I know some of you devil's advocates are saying, wait a minute, why do you have to make this all about race? What if there are more African Americans in California smoking pot than any other ethnicity? Wouldn't it then make sense that more African Americans are therefore getting arrested and going to jail for it? Well, get this: according to a 2010 study by the US Department of Health and Human Services, white people across the country between the ages of eighteen and twenty-five use marijuana at a higher rate than their black peers,[11] yet black people between the ages of eighteen to twenty-five have higher arrest and incarceration records than whites do—not only in California but nationwide. So the statistics from HHS and the CDC are in agreement: whites use more drugs and die from more overdoses than blacks, but whites are least likely to do the time for the crime.

What this means is that Nixon's War on Drugs has actually been successful. In *Harper's* magazine's April 2016 issue, (titled *Legalize It All*), journalist Dan

Baum referenced an interview he had with John Ehrlichman in 1994. Ehrlichman was a former Nixon staffer who went to jail for his involvement in Watergate— he was also Nixon's drug policy advisor. Ehrlichman admitted to Baum that Nixon launched the War on Drugs for one reason, "to decimate his perceived political enemies—the anti-war left, and black people." Here's the transcript of the interview:

> "You want to know what this was really all about?" he asked with the bluntness of a man who, after public disgrace and a stretch in federal prison, had little left to protect. "The Nixon campaign in 1968, and the Nixon White House after that, had two enemies: the antiwar left and black people. You understand what I'm saying? We knew we couldn't make it illegal to be either against the war or black, but by getting the public to associate the hippies with marijuana and blacks with heroin, and then criminalizing both heavily, we could disrupt those communities. We could arrest their leaders, raid their homes, break up their meetings, and vilify them night after night on the evening news. Did we know we were lying about the drugs? Of course we did."[13]

Doesn't that just make your blood boil? Well, jury nullification has the power to end the War on Drugs and all the racial bias that comes with it. If juries refuse to convict people for drug possession or nonviolent drug offenses, We the People can then police the police state. Together, we can reverse these statistics for good. We might not ever be able to weed out all the corrupt cops from law enforcement, but when those corrupt cops bring a defendant before us in the courtroom, We the People can reverse the charges. And what I'm suggesting isn't a radical idea because it is already happening.

In December 2010, national media outlets reported that there was a jury mutiny in Missoula, Montana over a case involving marijuana possession. Teuray Cornell, a thirty-seven-year-old African American man, was arrested and charged with selling marijuana—which is a felony in Montana—as well as marijuana possession (a misdemeanor) because he was arrested with a small amount of pot on him. While Judge Robert L. Deschamps III of Missoula County District Court was whittling down the jury pool, he quickly found that he could not find one person let alone twelve people to sit on the jury to hear this case.[14] Based on the charges, do you understand why? Cornell was charged with selling marijuana because the cops found two buds of weed on him.[15] Police did not actually catch Cornell in the act of dealing marijuana when they arrested him. So, those in Cornell's jury pool thought something didn't add up. Did the cops find weed on him and then proceed to build a case that he was a drug dealer? Two buds of weed is not a large enough quantity of marijuana to be considered intent to sell.

Montana voters legalized medical marijuana in 2004, so this case goes to show you that the average Montana resident finds a marijuana possession arrest to be completely unwarranted. One of the potential jurors even referenced a 2006 Missoula County initiative that advised local law enforcement "to treat marijuana crimes as their lowest priority"[16] as a way to voice concern and raise questions about Cornell's case.

Needless to say, Judge Deschamps ended up dismissing the case because of the initial reaction from the jury pool. This would have been the perfect example of jury nullification if Cornell hadn't accepted a plea agreement before the case was officially dismissed due to the felony drug-dealing charges. The plea agreement amounted to a twenty-year sentence, but the judge suspended nineteen of those years—meaning Cornell served a one-year sentence—so again who knows how substantial the evidence against him actually was.[17]

The moral of the story is that jurors have more power to define the outcome of a case than they are lead to believe. If the jury pool hadn't been vocal about their opinions on the laws surrounding marijuana possession, Cornell's trial would have proceeded and he would have most likely gotten at least a twenty-year sentence. But that's not what happened because of the way the potential jurors handled the situation.

Another example of vigilant jurors thinking for themselves are in cases involving driving under the influence (DUI) of marijuana. In Colorado, prosecutors are having a tough time getting convictions from juries for those who have been arrested for DUI marijuana charges. Apparently, completely sober jurors attempted to do the roadside sobriety tests for marijuana use and some actually failed. This led them to conclude that the drivers—although found guilty of driving under the influence of marijuana—aren't necessarily impaired or putting anyone at risk while driving.

Here's why: after the recreational use of cannabis was legalized in Colorado, authorities established a 5 ng/mL blood-THC limit for driving under the influence of marijuana (this is the same ratio in Washington state);[18] however, since

there isn't any study that proves there is a specific, universal number for marijuana impairment, law enforcement truly picked an arbitrary number for DUI
charges.

Think of it this way: a DUI for alcohol is .08 due to the many studies that
prove that a .08 blood alcohol ratio is where impairment begins for most people.
The first study to analyze the impact of marijuana on driving was conducted
in June 2015 by the University of Iowa. The National Highway Traffic Safety
Administration, National Institute of Drug Abuse, and the Office of National
Drug Control Policy sponsored the study. As expected, there was impairment in
all areas when alcohol and cannabis were mixed. However—and this is really
interesting—when cannabis alone was taken in moderate amounts, there was no
sign of significant driving impairment.

Here's what researchers at the University of Iowa determined:

> Once in the simulator—a 1996 Malibu sedan mounted in a twenty-four-
> foot diameter dome—the drivers were assessed on weaving within the
> lane, how often the car left the lane, and the speed of the weaving. Drivers
> with only alcohol in their systems showed impairment in all three areas
> while those strictly under the influence of vaporized cannabis only dem-
> onstrated problems weaving within the lane. *Drivers with blood concen-*
> *trations of 13.1 ug/L THC, or delta-9-tetrahydrocannabinol, the active*
> *ingredient in marijuana, showed increased weaving that was similar*
> *to those with a .08 breath alcohol concentration,* the legal limit in most
> states. The legal limit for THC in Washington and Colorado is 5 ug/L,
> the same amount other states have considered. (emphasis mine)[19]

The study also found that analyzing a driver's oral fluids can detect recent use
of marijuana but is not a reliable measure of impairment. Andrew Spurgin, a
postdoctoral research fellow with the UI College of Pharmacy, explained the
results further: "Everyone wants a Breathalyzer which works for alcohol because
alcohol is metabolized in the lungs. But for cannabis this isn't as simple due to
THC's metabolic and chemical properties."[20]

Essentially, these factors are contributing to a growing number of statewide
cases in Colorado where juries have acquitted marijuana users of driving under
the influence of marijuana—even when testing shows these people are over the
5 ng/mL limit. Jury nullification and common sense win again!

Here's another jury nullification scenario to consider: recreational and medical marijuana are legal in your state, but your employer can fire you for failing a drug test that indicates weed is in your system. How can an employer possibly deny you the right to access legal medical marijuana when your doctor has approved it? And in the case of recreational pot, what if you smoked pot over the weekend at a concert and failed the drug test on Monday. That doesn't mean you get high at work. How can you get fired for doing something off the clock that is completely legal? But that's exactly what happened in June 2010 to Brandon Coats, who used marijuana off the clock to deal with painful muscle spasms.[21]

Coats is a quadriplegic who legally used medical marijuana in Colorado. He worked at Dish Network and was fired in 2010 when he failed a drug test for marijuana use. He sued under wrongful termination because medical marijuana has been legal in Colorado since 2000. The case went all the way to the Colorado Supreme Court, and it was decided in 2015 that Coats was rightfully terminated. Remember, federal law still lists marijuana as a Schedule I narcotic. Since Dish Network's corporate policy is to abide by federal law, the company fired Coats because he was consuming an illegal substance.

In 2008, the California Supreme Court also sided with employers. Workers can be fired if they test positive for marijuana, even though medical marijuana is legal in the state of California.[22] Apparently state law protections don't extend to employment, and other states that have legalized marijuana are following suit with California and Colorado. Does that make any sense to you? Meanwhile, researchers from the University of Pennsylvania[23] found that from 1999 to 2010, there was a 25 percent drop in painkiller overdoses and opioid related deaths in states that legalized marijuana.[24] The hypocrisy is astounding.

Colorado and California are also employment-at-will states. This means that:

> Neither an employer nor an employee is required to give notice or advanced notice of termination or resignation. Additionally, neither an employer nor an employee is required to give a reason for the separation from employment.[25]

So you can be fired for any reason—and no reason has to be given—except for matters of discrimination. It is discriminatory to fire an employee based upon disability, race, creed, color, sex, age, religion, sexual orientation, national origin, and ancestry. It's also illegal to fire an employee for engaging in lawful off-duty activities.[26] See where Brandon Coats had a right to sue under state law? Jury nullification would have easily rectified his situation.

And as far as employers conducting drug tests to begin with? It's a total waste of time and money. If an employee is productive, keep the employee. Don't fire an employee for pot unless the employee isn't able to do his job because of it. And if your place of work conducts random drug tests, you can thank President Ronald Reagan for that. In the 1980s, he issued an executive order stating that "drugs will not be tolerated in the federal workplace," and then Congress passed a law to require companies that receive federal funding to adopt the same policies.[27] There hasn't been a single study that proves employees that smoke pot are more prone to more accidents or injuries on the job or that they take more sick and vacation time than any other employee.

I'll leave you with one last example of why Americans nationwide need to know about jury nullification: in states where pot isn't legal, some counties, towns, and cities are passing local laws so that residents will receive citations instead of jail time for marijuana possession. This is what is known as decriminalizing marijuana. So if local law enforcement is now not arresting people for marijuana—even though marijuana is completely illegal under any circumstances in that particular state—shouldn't juries also be able to not convict someone of the same crime? Because now this is getting ridiculous. We're just splitting hairs in the legal system.

Decriminalizing marijuana means that marijuana is still illegal, but the consequences of possessing it aren't as harsh. Small amounts of recreational marijuana are classified as a civil offense rather than a criminal offense. So you might pay a fine for an ounce of weed, but you don't wind up with a criminal record. Marijuana possession is reduced to a speeding ticket or a parking ticket. Larger amounts of weed, however, are still considered a criminal offense because it implies intent to sell. Here are some examples of recent decriminalization:

- Palm Beach County, West Palm Beach County, Miami-Dade County, and Broward County, FL: Possession of 20 g (about 0.7 of an ounce) or less of marijuana is punishable by a civil citation and a $100 fine or ten hours of community service.[28]
- Pittsburgh, PA: If you have less than 30 g (an ounce) of marijuana, police will seize the drug and issue a fine between $25 and $100, depending on the exact amount of weed. [29]

- Fourteen cities in Michigan have passed laws decriminalizing recreational marijuana possession and use, but each city has different rules on the maximum amount and the price of the fine: Berkley (2014), Huntington Woods (2014), Mount Pleasant (2014), Port Huron (2014), Saginaw (2014), Hazel Park (2014), Oak Park (2014), Jackson (2013), Ferndale (2013), Detroit (2012), Flint (2012), Grand Rapids (2012), Lansing (2013), and Ann Arbor (1972).[30]
- Harris County, TX: 2 oz. of cannabis or less means eight hours of community service or completing an eight-hour class.[31]

I'd like to think that cops who now give citations for marijuana possession are doing so without discrimination, but many years of drug war statistics state otherwise. When the system fails us, we have to stand up to the system and demand change. Marijuana should not be illegal. Marijuana should not be decriminalized. It's a plant and it should be legalized nationwide. If jury nullification worked during Prohibition, it could work again. So next time you get that little postcard in the mail for jury duty, remember your responsibility as a juror to exercise the right to nullify if you see fit.

14

Inside America's Prison Industrial Complex

So when juries fail to use nullification, which unfortunately they do the majority of the time, what happens to all those nonviolent drug offenders who are convicted?

Have you ever heard the Nazi death camp slogan "Work Shall Set You Free"? Our corporations aren't outsourcing labor to third world countries anymore. They aren't relying on global supply chains. They've found a cheaper form of labor inside the United States through a process known as "insourcing."

Instead of outsourcing work to sweatshops in China or Bangladesh, American corporations are insourcing work to the 2.4 million Americans behind bars and paying them literally pennies per day for eight hours of work.

Well, of course, these folks behind bars have nothing better to do, but if you're making between $0.23 and $1.15 per hour,[1] how the hell are you supposed to pay any bills or support your family while you're doing time for your crime? Do you think those 2.4 million people went to prison with zero debt to their names? They have mortgages, rent, credit card bills, student loans, car payments; you name it, just like everyone else. That means that aside from leaving prison with a criminal record, which makes it extremely difficult to find work, our prisoners are going back into society with massive amounts of debt. At what point will they ever be able to rebuild and reclaim their lives?

Now, don't get me wrong here. Prisoners should work and provide services to society, especially when the taxpayer is footing the bill. In most counties, residents can hire an inmate work crew from a local jail to paint walls or do carpentry for an extremely low rate. I'm sure we've all seen inmate work crews picking up trash on the side of the highway. At the end of the day, prisoners owe a debt to society for the crimes they committed, and our tax dollars pay for the cost of their food, healthcare, and so on while they're locked up. Having prisoners work for lower than minimum wage isn't necessarily a horrible idea, especially if picking up trash or painting public buildings is part of their sentences. However, next time you see something in the store with the label "Made in America," chances are, it was made in an American prison. That includes the American flag, by the way. And when it comes to insourcing, inmate work crews aren't typically working for the taxpayer's benefit, but they are working for the benefit of the corporations.

Before I go into which corporations are insourcing, I want to explain why I'm against it. Let's say you own a small business and you are paying your employees a decent living wage, plus healthcare. You're now at a disadvantage because you can't compete with the margins a corporation has when exploiting prison labor. Let's take that a step further. Let's say you own a small organic grocery store and you sell tilapia at the same price as Whole Foods. Whole Foods will always make more of a profit because they use prison labor to farm tilapia. Unless you start using prisoners to farm your tilapia, your profit margins will never come close to Whole Foods. You see, insourcing isn't helping a prisoner repay a debt to society. These prisoners aren't making the taxpayers' lives any better either—they're making the corporations richer and they don't have a choice in the matter.

So doesn't this then create a need to always have a certain amount of people in prison? If our corporations are relying on this cheap form of labor, what will happen if the prison work force fluctuates significantly? What if crime significantly goes down and everyone who was incarcerated due to marijuana-related offenses was released? Would major corporations and our entire economy be able to survive? All I know is that Whole Foods is one of many corporations that has a lot to lose if we ever end the war on drugs. Not just because of the cheap labor. Corporations that use prison work crews also receive added tax cuts and benefits from the government. Now do you see why it's so difficult for small businesses to survive in America?

The Federal Prison Industries, also known as UNICOR and FPI, is a corporation that was created by the US government in 1934 to use federal penal labor to produce goods and services. The idea was to have prisoners reenter society with relevant skills that can be used for the workforce, and in the meantime, they would produce products for society, for the taxpayer, such as license plates.

Under the Crime Control Act of 1990 (signed into law by George H. W. Bush), all inmates who are not a security risk or have a health exception are required to work for either UNICOR or some other prison job. There are 109 UNICOR factories in federal prisons that produce about 175 different types of products and services[2]—everything from clothing and textiles to electronics to prescription eyewear to office furniture to car parts to recycling activities to data entry and coding. Since 2011, UNICOR brings in at least $900 million per year in revenue[3] because its labor force is making $1 to $2 per hour at most. For example, according to the *New York Times*, in 2013 the federal government paid inmates $2 an hour to stitch more than $100 million worth of US military uniforms.[4] While this sounds like a great savings, keep in mind that an American-owed company probably lost the bid to make those uniforms.

Case in point: According to *CNNMoney*, UNICOR came close to putting Ashland Sales and Service, a Kentucky factory of one hundred employees located in Olive Hill, out of business. Ashland Sales and Service has been making windbreakers for the Air Force since 1998. The average employee makes $9 an hour, plus full medical insurance, 401(k) plans, and paid vacation.[5] In 2012, UNICOR tried to bid against Ashland Sales and Services by offering a work pool of thirteen thousand prison employees to make the windbreakers at $0.23 an hour.[6] If UNICOR got the Air Force bid, Ashland Sales and Service would have gone out of business, and that factory is the largest employer in Olive Hill. Michael Mansh, who runs the factory, had to contact Kentucky Senator Mitch McConnell, who was the Senate minority leader at the time, for help. McConnell then issued a public statement to UNICOR, urging it to back off. The next day, it did, and UNICOR did not place the bid,[7] and the people of Olive Hill continued to be employed.

To all those who support Donald Trump's idea of building a wall across the United States/Mexico border, stop worrying about immigrants taking your jobs. Worry about US corporations taking away your jobs and "giving" them to US prisoners. If you keep wondering when the unemployment rate is going to turn around, all I can say is don't hold your breath. UNICOR is not just in business for itself, but it is farming out the prison population to US corporations to make even more money for itself and for the corporations.

Get this: some prisoners even work for the corporations for free. According to *The Nation,* in states like Wisconsin, Virginia, Ohio, New Jersey, Florida, and Georgia, "inmates are not paid for their work, but receive time off their sentences."[8] Not even a migrant farm worker picking strawberries in California can compete with that rate of pay! And again, according to our nation's laws, the prisoners do not have a choice. They can't turn down the work because they are required by law to work. They can't negotiate their rate of pay because it is decided for them by UNICOR.

Again, I can't stress this enough: the United States has five percent of the world's population, yet we have 25 percent of the world's prison population.[9] Folks, that's a huge workforce. Who needs to rely on foreign sweatshops when there are 2.4 million people in the United States who will work for even less?

I keep saying the corporations have a vested interest in continuing the drug war, but let's look at just how much of a vested interest, in terms of money:

- In October 2015, ABC News reported that Whole Foods buys fish and cheese products from Quixotic Farming and Haystack Mountain Goat Dairy in Colorado. Inmates are hired by these companies to construct fish tanks to raise tilapia and to produce natural, organic cheese.[10] Colorado prison inmates are hired by Quixotic to construct fish tanks and raise tilapia in them. The inmates are paid anywhere between $0.74 to $4 a day. Meanwhile when Quixotic Farming sells tilapia to Whole Foods, Colorado's Department of Corrections (DOC) gets $0.85 per pound, and then Whole Foods turns around and sells the tilapia for $11.99 a pound.[11] Haystack Mountain Goat Dairy also pays the inmates the same rate. Four ounces of cheese sells for roughly $5.99 and eight ounces for $10. When this story initially broke, Whole Foods claimed it would stop using prison labor by April of 2016. However, at the time of completing this manuscript, we couldn't find a single source to verify that Whole Foods did in fact end the dependence on prison labor.[12]
- Walmart also relies on prison labor for its produce. Martori Farms in Arizona is Walmart's exclusive supplier for fresh fruits and vegetables,

for 2,470 stores.[13] The farm pays women from Arizona's Perryville unit $2 per hour (not including travel time to and from the farm) and expects them to work all day in the brutal sun—work without adequate sunscreen, water, or food.[14]

- In 1993, *Prison Legal News*[15] reported that prisoners in Colorado, Oregon, Arizona, New Mexico, Ohio, New Jersey, and Florida work a telemarketing call center called Unibase for $2 a day.[16] In 1993, AT&T increased profits by laying off thousands of telephone operators—all of which were union employees—and replacing them with prison inmates from Unibase call centers. Sprint and Verizon are also using inmates for their call centers.[17]

- Remember that huge BP oil spill in the Gulf of Mexico in 2010? When BP spilled 4.2 million barrels of oil and had to pay $18.9 billion in federal, state, and local fines?[18] Well, BP insulted coastal residents even further by paying inmate work crews to clean up the mess instead of hiring the people who were out of work due to the spill. And get this: Under the Work Opportunity Tax Credit (WOTC), BP received a tax credit of $2,400 for every work-release inmate used to clean up the spill! The tax credit is seen as a reward for hiring "risky target groups."[19]

Folks, BP is no exception when it comes to receiving a tax credit. All corporations receive a $2,400 tax credit for every inmate hired. That's why inmates are packaging everyday products in UNICOR factories—from Starbucks coffee beans to Eddie Bauer clothing.[20] That's why Wendy's and McDonald's use prison labor to produce frozen foods, such as processing beef for hamburger patties.[21] In the 1990s, a subcontractor called Third Generation hired twenty-five South Carolina inmates to stitch Victoria's Secret lingerie.[22] Two inmates were put in solitary confinement for telling journalists they were "hired" to replace "Made in Honduras" garment tags with "Made in USA" tags.[23] Subcontractors are why it's difficult to find out just how many corporations are using prison labor forces. A subcontractor works as a middleman or a shell corporation, and the corporation hires a subcontractor to "hire" prison workers so that all work goes through the subcontractor; in return, the subcontractor keeps the identity of the corporation private.

The Justice Department and the US Bureau of Prisons also won't disclose what corporations they do business with, but if you name a major corporation, chances are, that corporation has a stake in the expansion of the prison market: Microsoft, Dell, Hewlett-Packard, Intel, Nordstrom's, Revlon, Macy's, Target

stores, Costco, IBM, Boeing aircrafts, and Honda are no exception.[24] If a corporation is fed up with dealing with a union, they simply fire all union employees
and hire the prison labor force. For example, *Mother Jones* reported that in 1997,
Boeing's subcontractor MicroJet "had prisoners cutting airplane components,
paying $7 an hour" for work that union employees were paid $30 an hour.[25] And
when prisoners aren't busy making money for the corporations, they are busy
making products for the prison including uniforms, brooms, mattresses, and
toilets.[26]

In some cases, the UNICOR work program does help the taxpayer and provide inmates with skills they can use to support themselves after they're released.
Women at the Topeka Correctional Facility are taught how to use dental tools to
make dentures. As of 2014, the inmates accepted into this specialized program
earned $0.60 an hour.[27] Although that is a pathetically low wage for learning
a trade in the dental industry—an industry where American consumers spent
$119.1 billion in 2015[28]—the dentures the inmates produce aren't sold to a cor-
poration. Instead, they are given to the Kansas Association for the Medically
Undeserved and sold to patients at a reduced cost. So yes, in this case UNICOR
is helping the inmate learn a valuable skill that can benefit the taxpayer—both
behind bars and after being released.

However, this is not the case for the majority of the work done by prison
inmates. Even though the work is being done at a significantly reduced rate
of pay, the consumer does not receive any discount in price. The corporation
absorbs all the profits and takes the tax credits. Case in point: even though
AT&T, Verizon, and Sprint have saved millions by insourcing their call centers,
everyone's cell phone bill keeps goes up! The taxpayer is footing the bill to keep
these prisoners behind bars, and the corporations are making obscene profits in
the process of exploiting prisoners. Here's another problem: If you work at an
inmate call center, where do you expect to get a job when you get out of prison?
Customer call centers are either overseas or taken over by prison staff. Again, I
have to point out the fact that these corporations will lose their call centers if less
people are behind bars. This is why the corporations and the prison system have
a vested interest in keeping people locked up for as long as possible: they're both
making serious money off of the incarcerated!

And here's further proof of that: the measly $2 per day that the average
prisoner makes doesn't go directly to the prisoner. By law, at least half of that
money goes straight back to the justice system to pay off fines associated with the

crimes committed. In a 2007 Federal Prison Industries (FPI) report compiled for Congress, the FPI explained how UNICOR makes its money:

> In FY2006, FPI generated $718 million in sales. UNICOR uses the revenue it generates to purchase raw material and equipment; pay wages to inmates and staff; and invest in expansion of its facilities. Of the revenues generated by FPI's products and services, approximately 77 percent goes toward the purchase of raw material and equipment; 18 percent goes toward staff salaries; and 5 percent goes toward inmate salaries. Inmates earn from $0.23 per hour up to a maximum of $1.15 per hour, depending on their proficiency and educational level, among other things. Under [the Federal Bureau of Prison's] Inmate Financial Responsibility Program, all inmates who have court ordered financial obligations must use at least 50 percent of their FPI income to satisfy those debts, which accounted for $2.7 million in FY2005; the rest may be retained by the inmate.[29]

Did you get that? The inmate is slowly paying off fines and fees associated with the crime through UNICOR's program. Here's where I get concerned for the taxpayer: many states are also billing prisoners for the total cost of their incarceration once they have completed their sentences. Florida's state prisons can charge inmates $50 per day, plus the costs associated with other fees: hiring a public defender, police transport, medical care, DNA testing, probation, fingerprinting, you name it.[30] The ex-cons don't know the bill is coming until it shows up in the mailbox. But if the ex-cons are paying off these fees, where's the savings for the taxpayer when the costs associated with incarceration continue to go up every year?

To recap, prisoners earn less than minimum wage, they can then have more than half of that money taken away from them while they're in prison to pay legal fees, and then they still can't pay the outstanding bills they had prior to being incarcerated because they owe the state a big fat "room and board" check for being locked up in the big house.

Here's an example: Darlene Lorenz was released from the Mabel Bassett Correctional Center in McLoud, Oklahoma for nonviolent drug-related crimes in 2008. As of January 2015, she was sixty-five years old, and she owed $91,000 in court-imposed fines and other fees related to her case.[31] Meanwhile, while she was locked up, she earned $0.65 an hour as a darkroom technician developing camera film. That means she owed even more than $91,000 to the state of

Oklahoma because at least half of her earnings as a darkroom technician went to paying off her fines. And she's not alone. In Oklahoma, offenders literally pay for every aspect of their case:

- Those in court-ordered probation programs can pay up to $80 a month for supervision.
- Those required by the court to wear an electronic monitoring device can pay a monthly monitoring fee of up to $300.
- And if you're ordered by the court to go to Drug Court, those mandatory drug tests can cost you $80 to $100 a month in fees.[32]

Robin Wertz, another woman who did time in Oklahoma, was released from prison in 2007 and was slapped with $25,000 in fines. What did she do to get locked up in the first place? Just like Lorenz, she was convicted of several drug-related charges. When Wertz finished her sentence, she was having a tough time finding a job to pay off the fines, and she came close to selling drugs to pay off her debt. Do you see why there's a high rate of recidivism? Robin Wertz nearly became a statistic due to the financial burden handed down to her from our justice system.

Get this: from 2011 to 2014, the Oklahoma County District Court reaped nearly $28 million in fines and fees from offenders.[33] So these convicts might be freed in one sense, but now the state has made them prisoners of debt. They'll wear shackles for the rest of their lives, trying to pay off the debt. Again, I'm not opposed to prisoners paying an actual fee as part of their debt to society. What I'm against is how states come up with this fee. If a nonviolent drug offender is supposed to pay fines between $25,000 and $91,000 in the state of Oklahoma, what exactly is that person supposed to do to repay that debt? Win the lottery?

Many people in the media have referred to this whole system of insourcing as a form of modern day slavery. An opinion piece in *USA Today* by Jim Liske of Prison Fellowship stated the following:

Meaningful work can be part of a restorative corrections policy. Many prisoners need to learn skills that will make them employable after release. Prison jobs also help people maintain a sense of purpose and structure during long sentences. Society as a whole also benefits when prisoners' labor allows them to pay restitution. But slavery—labor that dehumanizes one person for the profit of another—has no place in prisons or in the Constitution.[34]

What he's saying is that today's prisoners are essentially slaves to the corporations and slaves to the justice system. Yes, prisoners are behind bars for a reason, but our justice system stopped giving them the same basic human rights as every other citizen. In some states, ex-cons lose their right to vote forever. In other states, ex-cons have to petition the state legislature to restore their right to vote. Yet they are all still expected to pay taxes just like everyone else. Folks, isn't that taxation without representation? Isn't that what our Founding Fathers fought against in the Revolutionary War?

And again, I'm not saying that people behind bars should have all the free time in the world to lift weights and work out as much as they want on the taxpayers' dime. They should be doing actual work as part of their punishment, but that work should be benefiting society in some way, and the corporations don't count. It's not like these businesses hire the inmates at a reasonable salary once they're released. That would be almost like an apprenticeship or an internship. But that's not what's happening.

Let me put it this way: How would it make you feel to know that you have over $91,000 in fines and you are working at least eight hours every day to pay that off while you're in prison, but you don't have a prayer of doing so because your rate of pay is literally pennies per hour. Then you're released back into society with a huge debt on your shoulders. How is that justice? Didn't you go to prison to pay off the debt to society? Shouldn't your debt be gone once you leave the prison walls? Apparently not. What you really did during your incarceration was provide free labor to corporations. And again, this directly relates to the War on Drugs because the vast majority of people in prison right now are there due to drug-related charges.

Believe it or not, nationwide, crime is at an all-time low—including violent crime. Even the FPI admitted this in their 2007 report to Congress:

> While the number of federal inmates incarcerated for violent offenses has consistently declined since 1980, the number of federal inmates incarcerated for a drug-related offense has consistently risen since 1980.[35]

This means that the growth rate of the War on Drugs and our prison population are closely linked. According to the Federal Bureau of Prisons, as of July 2015, there were a total of 207,847 people incarcerated in federal prisons and roughly half of those prisoners were there for drug offenses.[36]

You can bet that the corporations profiting from insourcing want the prison population to stay that way. Think about this: as the CEO of Boeing, do you want a sex offender, a murderer, or a nonviolent drug offender creating airplane parts? The nonviolent drug offender can't get high in prison, so essentially, "hiring" a prisoner with drug-related offenses is like hiring a typical employee that you know will always pass a drug test—except that employee basically works for free.

Here's a hint as to which corporations utilize the prison work force: UNICOR allows corporations to "hire" prisoners as long as that corporation abides by all federal laws. Federal law states that marijuana is illegal. Remember Brandon Coats from chapter 13? Under Colorado state law, he is legally able to smoke medical marijuana, but Dish Network fired him after he failed a drug test. What does that tell you? Here's my theory: Dish Network abides by federal law because if the company doesn't, then UNICOR will take away its prison labor force. So Dish Network had to fire Brandon Coats. Now, I can't prove this as the Justice Department and the US Bureau of Prisons feel they are above the Freedom of Information Act, and neither will ever disclose the American companies relying on prisoners, but you can bet if a corporation has a toll-free customer service line—and Dish Network has one—the "employees" taking your phone call are federal prisoners.

Here's where the taxpayer gets screwed again: with corporations making a huge savings by using prison labor, the price tag on goods and services should go down, right? But the price we pay on goods and services keep going up every year—even though corporations see bigger and bigger profit margins due to insourcing. This is case in point as to why there is no such thing as "Reaganomics" or the "trickle-down theory" of economics. American corporations do not pass on excess profits to the consumer—they keep it for themselves. They won't give their employees modest raises with that excess profit margin either.

Here's case in point: Walmart, the largest private employer in the United States, just announced in February 2016 that it would "boost" its minimum wage from $9 an hour to $10 an hour for store employees.[37] This is after the corporation shut down 154 stores in the United States, and with that savings, the company is still paying employees less than $15 an hour. According to the *Washington Post*, fifty years ago, the typical CEO made approximately $20 for every dollar a worker made, but today, the average CEO makes $300 for every dollar.[38] Care to guess how much Walmart's President and CEO makes? In 2015, C. Douglas McMillon earned a total of $19,070,249.[39] Remember that Walmart is one of the corporations that utilizes prison labor forces and gets a tax credit of $2,400 per inmate. Meanwhile Americans for Tax Fairness estimated that Walmart avoids paying at least $1 billion in federal taxes due to corporate loopholes.[40] Yet, the majority of the corporation's non-prison work force relies on food stamps to make ends meet. Excuse me? If you're saving $1 billion in taxes, why aren't your employees making enough money to eat? In one Wisconsin store of three hundred employees, taxpayers paid $5,815 per employee—or nearly $1.75 million per year—so Walmart employees could receive housing assistance and food stamps.[41] And nationwide? According to NPR, in 2013, Walmart saw approximately $13 billion dollars in revenue from food stamps,[42] mostly from its own employees!

Any way you look at it, the American people work for Walmart. If you're in prison, you're farming produce for Walmart. If you're a taxpayer, your money is going to Walmart employees so they can eat, and those Walmart employees are purchasing their food at Walmart. In return, Walmart tries like hell to get out of paying taxes, so taxpayers are stuck paying even more to the government to make up for the billions Walmart is supposed to pay.

Walmart's callous disregard for its employees starts at the bottom, with the prison labor force. America's largest employer is paying convicts pennies per hour to do manual farm labor, and the corporation has no problem paying the rest of its employees below the poverty line because in both instances the taxpayer is subsidizing the costs. We pay for prisoners to have food and shelter. We pay for Walmart employees to have food and shelter. How did we get stuck with all the bills?

I'll leave you with one last thought to consider: if our government suddenly reversed its marijuana laws today, every major corporation would go ballistic because our economy rests on the shoulders of insourcing. Remember: roughly half of the people in prison right now are there due to drug-related crimes. These corporations are profiting from the fact that as long as weed is a Schedule I narcotic, they will continue to have an abundance of cheap, prison labor. CEOs are only worried about their bottom line: how to make even more money by exploiting even more prisoners. When it comes to the prison industrial complex, there's one entity in particular that has found a way to do just that: private prisons.

15

Our Politicians Are Backed by For-Profit Prisons

By now, I hope you've noticed a running theme in this book. There is nothing wrong with consuming marijuana, and science has proven that CBD *and* THC are both medically beneficial. The only thing wrong with cannabis is that our government wants it to remain illegal.

There is no question that the United States has the largest prison system in the world, thanks to marijuana and drug related offenses. We have so many people behind bars that we've actually moved to a for-profit prison system without much hesitation from our hypocritical elected officials. Why is that? Because the for-profit prison system has some seriously scary lobbying power.

If you've read any of my previous books—in particular, *DemoCRIPS and ReBLOODlicans: No More Gangs in Government*—then you'd know the power that Big Oil, the Koch brothers, and Big Pharma have over our political system, especially after Citizens United. As long as our politicians are bought and paid for by special interest groups, then for-profit prison companies like GEO Group and Corrections Corporation of America (CAA) will do all they can to keep even more of the US population locked up for an even longer period of time.

The idea behind private prisons was for the government to save money. In theory, if a company in the private sector could house inmates for a lesser cost, then the government would save money. The problem with this concept is that the government isn't supposed to run like a business. The government is there to provide services for its people—that's why our elected officials are referred to as public servants. Somewhere we've gotten off track with this philosophy and we think that the private sector can run things like prisons more efficiently.

Any way you look at it, the prison system is supposed to be a service. In theory, it's where those harmful to society are kept for a period of time until they've learned from their mistakes. Once they've proven that they feel remorse for their actions, we allow them back into the general population so that they can go on with their lives. However, our current prison system couldn't be farther from that ideal.

Let me just say this: when you turn the prison system over to a private company, then the prison system becomes a business. A corporation is looking to make money off of the prison system, so corners are cut to save money. A corporation has no interest in helping drug addicts recover or providing actual services to inmates. Why? Because a corporation doesn't supply services. The government does. Corporations that own private prisons want those outpatient facilities like drug court, probation and halfway houses to disappear for good. Without those services, there's a greater likelihood for repeat offenders. When a prison is run like a business, it must make a profit, and to make a profit, it must be full at all times.

When a state grants a private company permission to run a for-profit prison, the state agrees to pay the private prison a day rate per prisoner (usually around $60 per day per inmate). There's also a special clause in every private prison contract: the state must work with the private prison to ensure it stays at least 90 percent full at all times. That way, the prison is profitable. If there are too many empty beds, the state will have to pay a penalty fee. The funny thing about this empty bed clause is that the 90 percent capacity rate doesn't fluctuate when crime rates rise or fall. In other words, We the People could have stopped doing illegal activities entirely, but that wouldn't matter to the private prison system. If there are beds to fill, the beds will be filled, or the state will pay a penalty fee with our taxpayer money.[1]

When I say we're living in a police state, you've got to follow the money to find out the serious reality of this situation. The revenue brought in from police quotas for traffic tickets and arrests are just one aspect of a police state—the corporations and our politicians are what drive our prison system. The average prison has at least one thousand beds. That means if the prison is 90 percent full, the state is paying these private companies around $55,000 to $59,000 per day. See how it's become profitable to keep us behind bars?

How did we get here? The War on Drugs! Under Reagan, prison populations soared, prisons became overcrowded, and the costs skyrocketed.[2] The
private sector stepped in to "help," and we've been stuck with them ever since
because with each new president came up with a new War on Drugs mandate
with harsher drug sentences and longer prison stays, which in turn has increased
our overall prison population.

President George H. W. Bush's 1989 "war on drugs" meant less money
was allocated to treatment facilities and more was given to the prison system to
account for how many people he locked up. The goal was to have a "drug-free
America." Meanwhile, it was no secret that his sons Jeb and George W. did drugs
with their friends:

- "I drank alcohol and I smoked marijuana when I was at [Philips
  Academy]. It was pretty common."[3]—Jeb Bush, former governor
  of Florida
- "I wouldn't answer the marijuana questions. You know why? Because
  I don't want some little kid doing what I tried."[4] —George W. Bush, in
  privately taped conversations with Doug Wead, a former aide to George
  H. W. Bush.

Here's what the forty-first president of the United States said in his address to the
nation when he announced his National Drug Control Strategy on September
5, 1989:

> I'm also proposing that we enlarge our criminal justice system across
> the board—at the local, state, and federal levels alike. We need more
> prisons, more jails, more courts, more prosecutors. . . . Our 1990 drug
> budget totals almost $8 billion, the largest increase in history. We need
> this program fully implemented—right away. . . . To start, Congress
> needs not only to act on this national drug strategy but also to act on
> our crime package announced last May, a package to toughen sentences,
> beef up law enforcement, and build new prison space for twenty-four
> thousand inmates.[5]

This is coming from a man who would not be alive today if it wasn't for hemp.
When H. W. Bush's plane was shot down in WWII over the Pacific, the cord
in the parachute that saved his life was made from cannabis, yet he made no

effort to differentiate industrial hemp from marijuana in his war on drugs.[6] Even more ironic is that Bush has repeatedly commemorated this experience—when American-grown hemp from the Hemp for Victory campaign saved his life—by parachute jumping from a plane on his seventy-fifth, eightieth, eighty-fifth, and ninetieth birthdays.[7]

In the early '90s under H. W. Bush, the annual bill for keeping one person in prison for drug-related offenses was anywhere from $25,000 to $50,000. As of 2010, the average cost of incarcerating one inmate was $31,307 per year. In states like Connecticut, Washington state, and New York it could cost anywhere from $50,000 to $60,000.[8] Why? Because of all the "tough on crime" and "three strikes, you're out" policies of the War on Drugs. After H. W. Bush and Bill Clinton's policies went into effect, they have been more mandatory sentences and longer sentences. In 2016, we're essentially paying a teacher's salary or a firefighter's salary to keep one person in jail. Overall, incarceration now costs taxpayers $63.4 billion a year![9]

As much as Nixon started this whole thing and Reagan and H. W. Bush continued it, the War on Drugs and our prison population really got out of control under President Bill Clinton. Clinton signed the North American Free Trade Agreement (NAFTA) treaty in 1993. NAFTA increased the amount of trade and traffic across the United States–Mexico border,[10] which made it more difficult for US Customs to find narcotics hidden within legitimate goods. This obviously benefited drug cartels and enabled more drug trafficking across the border.

So the following year, Clinton came up with mandatory minimum sentences in his 1994 Violent Crime Control and Law Enforcement Act, authored by then-Senator Joe Biden. The law offered states billions in funding for new prisons—but only if they adopted federal "truth in sentencing laws."[11] Nothing says justice prevails like a "truth in sentencing" law. Unless of course the law is designed to reduce prisoners' eligibility for parole. Which is what it actually did. The law also established Clinton's "three strikes" rule. Anyone convicted of a violent crime with two or more prior convictions—even if they were minor offenses, like marijuana possession—was given a life sentence.[12] The bill provided $10 billion to fund new prisons,[13] $8.9 billion for one hundred thousand new police officers, and $6.1 billion for crime prevention.

State legislatures really bought into the Violent Control and Law Enforcement Act, particularly due to the "more funding for prisons" incentive.

PolitiFact reports that within five years of enacting the Violent Control and Law Enforcement Act, twenty-nine states had truth-in-sentencing laws and twenty-four states had "three strikes" laws.[14] The phrase "school-to-prison" pipeline was born.

Guess what the Violent Control and Law Enforcement Act did to the prison population? The Brennan Center for Justice reports that by the end of the Clinton presidency, the number of people incarcerated in America's prisons rose by nearly 60 percent.[15] The Justice Policy Institute claims that:

> Under President Bill Clinton, the number of prisoners under federal jurisdiction doubled, and grew more than it did under the previous twelve years of Republican rule, combined.[16]

The Justice Policy Institute also states that during the Clinton administration, 63,448 people were put away in federal prison on drug charges—which means nearly 60 percent of the entire prison population sentenced under Clinton's reign was there due to drug related charges.[17] So you see, the War on Drugs and the US prison system are connected: they both just kept getting bigger and bigger.

And let me just say this about Joe Biden and his "tough on drugs" policies: he's a hypocrite. As a senator in the '80s, Biden was invaluable in creating the US Drug Czar's office. Under the 1986 Anti-Drug Abuse Act that Biden helped author, individuals caught with just 5 g of crack were subject to the same mandatory minimum sentence as those caught with 500 g of powder cocaine: a five year prison sentence.[18] Biden was also the main sponsor of the Illicit Drug Anti-Proliferation Act of 2003 (also known as the RAVE Act), which was passed under George W. Bush. The RAVE Act held club owners liable for selling their customers glowsticks and water and other legal goods the law classified as MDMA (or Ecstasy) "paraphernalia."[19] Then-Senator Hillary Clinton co-sponsored the bill.[20] To this day, Vice President Biden vocally opposes marijuana legalization, and he does not regret any of the bills he passed.[21] Yet, his own son Hunter Biden was discharged from the Navy Reserve in 2014 after testing positive for cocaine.[22] Forty-four-year-old Hunter Biden was in the Navy Reserve for two months before he was discharged for failing a drug test. So what's Hunter doing now? Well, he isn't sitting in prison. He's sitting on the Chairman's Advisory Board for the National Democratic Institute;[23] he's chairman of the Board of World

Food Program USA;[24] he's a director on the boards of the US Global Leadership Coalition,[25] the Truman National Security Project,[26] the Center for National Policy,[27] and the Ukrainian energy company Burisma Holdings (Ukraine's largest private gas firm).[28] He's also part of the president's Advisory Board for Catholic Charities in Washington, DC.[29]

If only all cokeheads had fathers in high places. Joe Biden is fine with putting our kids in prison for drug use, but he won't send his druggie son there. Unbelievable, isn't it?

Today, Bill Clinton says he regrets his 2014 Violent Control and Law Enforcement Act:

> The good news is, we had the biggest drop in crime in history. The bad news is we had a lot people who were locked up, who were minor actors, for way too long.[30]

But the damage is done, and thanks to a combined effort from Republicans and Democrats, private prisons are here to stay. In 2011, Arizona proved that privately operated prisons, such as the Saguaro Correctional Center in Eloy, Arizona, actually cost more to operate than state-run prisons. So when politicians say yes to a private prison system—a system that is supposed to save money—they are doing so when they know it will actually cost the taxpayer more. And get this: private prisons steer clear of the sickest, costliest inmates and they're still more expensive to operate![31] That's right. A private prison company can pick and choose what prisoners it wants. And guess which ones they take? The youngest ones with the longest sentences. Do you remember who the majority of those prisoners are? Nonviolent drug offenders! Do you really think they'll get a fair parole hearing or get out early for good behavior in a private prison when the goal is to keep a private prison 90 percent full?

Meanwhile, Arizona has a state law that stipulates private prisons must create clear "cost savings" for the state to justify paying the private company to run it. This is true for every state that has private prisons. And yet Arizona's Department of Corrections revealed that one inmate in a private prison costs as much as $1,600 more per year[32]—even though private prisons are allowed to cherry-pick the inmates so that only the healthiest and easiest are admitted. Arizona isn't alone in this either. In a 2007 cost analysis by the University of Utah, it was proven that cost savings from private prisons were "minimal at best"![33] Yet, private prisons are on the rise in Florida, Ohio, and just about every state due to lobbyists.

How we really got to be known as the country with the largest prison system in the world is due to the for-profit prison lobby. Take Florida as the case in point: In 2010, GEO Group and supporters of private prisons pumped $33,000 into SuperPACs benefiting Florida Republicans running for office. Remember, 2010 is the year Marco Rubio was elected to the US Senate. And how did this young Florida senator get there? Between 2009 and 2010, GEO Group gave $10,000 to Rubio's US Senate PAC.[34] George Zoley, GEO Group's co-founder and chief executor, also made personal donations to Rubio's senate campaign. From 2009 and 2010, Zoley gave $4,800 in personal contributions—then gave an additional $7,400 on September 13, 2010 to seal the deal for the Senate seat.[35] But that's not all GEO got with its money. The company used its money to ensure a GOP-controlled state legislature and a Republican governor in Florida. In fact, Corrections Corporation of America (CCA) and GEO Group have spent a combined $5.28 million on Republican races in Florida in the past twelve years,[36] so it goes to show you that the GOP/GEO Group/Corrections Corporation of America monopoly will continue in the Sunshine State.

Florida currently has seven private prisons,[37] none of which actually save the state any money. Just like the state of Arizona, the contracts Florida made with private prisons grantees a 90 percent occupancy rate, a day rate per inmate, and if extra services and programs are necessary, the state must then cough up extra money for those fees as well.[38] How can a prison rehabilitate people and get them back to being productive members of society when it must be 90 percent full at all times? That's part of the reason why the United States has half a million more people incarcerated when compared to China—a nation with a population five times greater than the United States.[39]

However, there was one thing and one thing only standing in the way of private prisons taking over state-run prisons in Florida after GEO Group and CCA bought their politicians. When Governor Rick Scott was elected in 2011 (yes, he was backed by the prison lobbyists) he tried to privatize twenty-seven state detention facilities to cut Florida's Department of Corrections budget.[40] In an interesting turn of events, he was unable to privatize due to the union representing prison employees. If Governor Scott turned state-run prisons over to a private company, all public employees would lose their jobs.[41] Roughly 3,800 state employees would be out of work once those twenty-seven state facilities became privately owned.[42] Their union, the Police Benevolent Association (PBA), took on the newly elected governor in several lawsuits, and even formed a nationwide coalition of union members to spread the word about Republicans being backed by private prison lobbyists to encourage union members not to vote Republican.[43]

Florida's Department of Corrections is the third largest in the nation, so it goes to figure that the PBA did not want to lose an overwhelming number of members and union dues. Even though the PBA did its job and ensured the twenty-seven facilities would not be privatized, the prison employees soon voted in a different union: the Teamsters. The difference between these two unions is quite interesting: the PBA doesn't seem to want private prisons under any circumstances. The Teamsters work with the PBA to oppose privatization, but if a facility is privatized, the union then works to unionize private prison staff.[44] Whether or not the Teamsters will negotiate with the private company so that the state prison staff can keep their jobs remains to be seen. So far, the unions are winning the fight. Governor Scott has been unsuccessful in overturning state-run prisons to his campaign contributors.

Remember all those 2016 presidential candidates before we were left with Hillary Clinton and Donald Trump (and Gary Johnson and Jill Stein, who I voted for in 2016)? Well, there were two from Florida for the taking. As of October 2015, Marco Rubio's PACs have received $133,450 from private prisons or groups that lobby for them. Jeb Bush, who dropped out of the race in February 2016, received $21,700 from groups affiliated with GEO Group and CCA. But before you get all up in arms about the Republicans, keep in mind that the GEO Group and CCA spread wealth around. Even though they give more to the GOP overall, the companies give to Democrats too. For example, the current governor of California—Democrat Governor Brown—was given $54,000[45] by GEO Group lobbyists. And Hillary Clinton is right up there with Marco Rubio. She's received $133,246 from prison lobbyists for her 2016 presidential campaign.[46] In fact, as of February 2016, Hillary received $274,891 in personal contributions from Richard Sullivan of Capitol Counsel, a federally registered lobbyist for GEO Group.[47]

Folks, I keep telling you that the Republicans and Democrats are owned by the same people! Hillary Clinton, Jeb Bush, and Marco Rubio all stand for the same thing: keeping the American people behind bars!

Here's what the Democrats and the Republicans don't want you to know, but the ACLU has vigilantly researched:[48]

- Today, six percent of state prisoners are in for-profit prisons and 16 percent of federal prisoners are in a for-profit prison.
- Nearly half of all immigrants detained by the federal government are in a for-profit prison.
- The Immigration and Customs Enforcement (ICE), a federal agency, locks up four hundred thousand immigrants each year and spends $1.9 billion on doing so. ICE is now looking for private companies to build massive immigration detention centers in New Jersey, Texas, Florida, California, and Illinois.
- In 2010, the two largest private prison companies—GEO Group and CCA—received nearly $3 billion in revenue.
- Geo Group rakes in $1.5 billion every year from ninety-eight prison facilities.[49]
- Between 2008 and 2013, Geo Group's CEO George Zoley earned $22 million, which is more than any other individual in the corrections industry.[50]
- Top executives in GEO Group and CAA received annual compensation packages over $3 million.
- CCA spent over $18 million on federal lobbying between 1999 and 2009.
- In 2010, CCA spent $970,000 on lobbying the federal government.
- Between 2003 and 2011, CCA hired 199 lobbyists in thiety-two states: Alabama, Alaska, Arizona, California, Colorado, Connecticut, Florida, Georgia, Hawaii, Idaho, Indiana, Kansas, Kentucky, Louisiana, Maine, Minnesota, Mississippi, Missouri, Montana, Nevada, New Hampshire, New Mexico, Oklahoma, Pennsylvania, Tennessee, Texas, Utah, Vermont, Virginia, Washington, West Virginia, and Wisconsin.
- During the same time period, GEO Group hired seventy-two lobbyists in seventeen states.
- Since 2000, CCA and GEO Group contributed over $6 million to candidates for state office and over $800,000 to candidates for federal office.
- In 2010, both companies contributed a combined $2 million to state political campaigns and state party committees on both sides of the aisle.
- If the private prisons in Arizona aren't 90 to 97 percent filled, the state must pay the company. In 2011, Arizona agreed to pay $3 million to Management & Training Corp. when the empty beds quota wasn't met.[51] Remember, this "empty bed quota" is a universal stipulation for any state that signs a contract with a private prison.

- GEO Group and CCA spent over $52,000 to get the current governor of Arizona, Republican Douglas Ducey, elected in 2014.[52] In return, CCA now has control over Red Rock Corrections in Eloy for the next twenty years.[53]

- In 2011, Ohio became the first state to sell its public-operated prison Lake Erie Correctional Facility to CCA for over $72 million.[54] I'll repeat that. The good people of Ohio who pay taxes? Over $72 million of their tax money went to CCA to run the state prison. Why? Because Ohio's corrections department head Gary Mohr, had served as a managing director of CCA and he made the deal happen. Mohr was appointed to his state position by Governor Kasich in January of 2011, and within that same month, Kasich's Congressional chief of staff, Donald Thibaut, became a lobbyist for CAA. Oh, and during the early 2000s, Kasich was an executive at Lehman Brothers, the financial firm that bailed out CCA when the company was going through financial problems. No crony capitalism to see here, right folks?

- How are the prisoners in CCA's Lake Erie Correctional Facility doing under CCA's care? They're being served meals that have maggots in them. Prisoners have access to as much heroin as they want from CCA employees who will sell it to them.[55] Inmates are triple-bunked, with some sleeping on cell floors, even though CCA rearranged the original 1,700-bed floor plan to add more beds.[56] Inmates requesting a nurse didn't see one within forty-eight hours, and staff didn't follow proper procedures for chronically ill inmates—including those with diabetes and AIDS. By the end of 2012, a full year after CCA took control of Lake Erie, the state docked the company nearly $500,000 in pay due to inmate conditions.[57] So I guess in this case, the state did save the taxpayer money at one hell of a moral expense.

- GEO Group also operates juvenile prisons. In 2007, a report of a West Texas facility found that children were segregated by race, disciplined for speaking Spanish, had not received church services in over two months, were not allowed to brush their teeth for days at a time, were forced to urinate or defecate in some container other than a toilet, and placed in cells with leaking pipes and vermin.[58]

More than one out of every one hundred American adults is behind bars and GEO Group, CCA, and our elected officials have a common interest to make that ratio even worse.[59] There are currently thirty states that have some form of private prison system, and seven states house more than a quarter of their prison populations privately.[60] What that means is that seven states currently outsource their prisoners to a private prison in another state. So if local facilities are overcrowded, prisoners can be selected and transported across state lines to a private prison to fill the empty bed quotas!

If a private prison is actually saving taxpayers money, rest assured it is doing so by treating the prisoners inhumanely. And the reality is, even if cost savings are 10 to 20 percent, like some private prisons claim, these companies enjoy government benefits—such as property tax exemptions and receiving water and sewer services for free or reduced rates.[61] If you wonder why the costs of your municipal services are going up, it could be because of the benefits a private prison is receiving. So any way you look at it, we're paying more for private prisons, and the corporations are winning again.

If you're thinking, well, at the end of the day—aside from those with minor, nonviolent drug offenses—these are dangerous federal criminals we are talking about. If they didn't do anything wrong in the first place, they wouldn't be in prison. Who cares about the horrible conditions and who cares if our elected officials are getting a little cash on the side? Wrong. These private prisons aren't above paying off our judges to get higher conviction rates with harsher sentences!

In February 2011, Judge Michael Conahan and Mark Ciavarella of Luzerene County, Pennsylvania were convicted of racketeering, money laundering, and conspiracy in accepting nearly one million dollars from the head of a private juvenile facility.[62] From 2007 to 2008, Judge Ciavarella and his supervisor Judge Conahan would get a kickback from Robert Powell and Robert Mericle for every child they incarcerated in Powell's PA Child Care youth detention center in Pittston. This "Kids for Cash" scandal tossed 2,500 kids in jail—many didn't even have a lawyer to represent them at their trials.[63]

I'm not talking about bad kids here either. Judge Ciavarella locked up a high school girl for three months because she mocked a school principal on Myspace.[64] This judge also jailed a twelve-year-old boy for two years because he tried to drive his mother's car and got into an accident. Today, the victims and the families of the "Kids for Cash" scandal have sued and won millions from Mericle and Powell's companies. All four conspirators are now behind bars—but that's not enough for me. The money awarded to these families and to these victims can't make up for unwarranted jail sentences.

Folks, just because you do something stupid as a teenager does not mean you should be incarcerated for it. As a society, we should be judged by the amount of children we keep out of jail, not by the amount of children we put in jail. The phrase "no child left behind" should really apply to the legal system. No kid should be put behind bars. There are other diversion programs like counseling and community service for that very reason. And these diversion programs actually work too.

For example, local law enforcement and the school board in Broward County, Florida, are using youth diversion programs to saving troubled youth from becoming part of the prison system. Broward County has a detention center for undocumented immigrants that GEO Group owns, and it earns the company $20 million a year. [65] But other than that, there are no other private prisons in the county. Since 2012, Broward County has been practicing school and law enforcement diversion programs like civil citations and the PROMISE program (PROMISE stands for Preventing Recidivism through Opportunities, Mentoring, Interventions, Support, and Education) to keep kids out of jail.

Between 2014 and 2016, over 90 percent of the juveniles in Broward County guilty of committing nonviolent crimes—everything from vandalism to drug possession—are not re-offending because they are being put through diversion programs instead of being sent to jail. The policies were put in place by Broward County Sheriff Scott Israel, who stated this about the "school to prison" pipeline in 2014:

> Zero-tolerance policies don't make our schools safer; they are disciplinary measures that are expensive to enforce. They push children off an academic track and on to a track to prison. Thus, students become the collateral damage of these policies. They lose sight of their future before they have the maturity to reflect on their career options.

> The Civil Citation Program and PROMISE intervene to discipline, educate, mentor, and ultimately provide a solution with a positive outcome, one that does not include an arrest record. Unfortunately, many youths who have entered the criminal justice system found it can haunt them for a lifetime.

> Whether you are applying for college, housing, or employment, there are countless applications that require a background check.

A criminal record can easily prevent a student from being admitted into a university, receiving a job offer, having a career in law enforcement, or even serving in the armed services.

After more than thirty years in law enforcement, I've witnessed countless youths re-offend, and I knew the zero-tolerance policy wasn't benefiting anyone.

Under this new agreement . . . eleven nonviolent misdemeanors will no longer result in arrests if the youth can be diverted through PROMISE or the Civil Citation Program. I am pleased to welcome this necessary change, which will eliminate lengthy suspensions, expulsions, and controversial arrests.

Programs that support education over incarceration will always have my support because they are effective. Since Broward's school district adopted PROMISE in August, schools have already seen arrests drop by about 40 percent and suspensions are down by 66 percent.[66]

Do you want to stop the progression of private prisons and the prison system? Get your local legislature to back juvenile diversion programs. In 2015, Florida TaxWatch found that when local law enforcement gives a minor a civil citation to avoid an arrest, that community saved $1,500 to $4,600.[67] That's per incident. So each civil citation saved up to $4,600 in taxpayer money. That's an estimated $44 million to $139 million annually. And guess what that would do to our prison population? Florida TaxWatch estimates that civil citations are reducing state prison populations by 10 percent a year—which is a savings of $72 million.[68] And civil citations can potentially decrease prison populations even further. The *Miami Herald* states that the counties in Florida that participate in civil citations, like Broward County, were seeing a greater reduction in repeat offenses when compared to youth who were sent to jail for the same crimes:

[Overall, state-wide] the number of youth who received civil citations who were caught a second time committing an offense was 4 percent, compared to a 42 percent recidivism rate for juveniles going to jail, 17 percent for those on probation and 13 percent for those in post-arrest diversion programs.[69]

What this means is that Florida's law enforcement is using civil citations to decrease arrest rates. If they keep jail and prison populations down—therefore decreasing the costs of jail and prisons—the governor can't justify the need for more private prisons. Governor Scott will continue to try though because GEO Group CEO George Zoley is already funding Scott's reelection campaign:

- In 2014, Zoley hosted a $10,000 per person fundraising dinner for Governor Scott.[70]
- Geo Group spent $1.3 million on the governor's reelection bid and other Florida GOP candidates in the 2014 election cycle. The company also gave $75,000 to the Republican Governors Association.[71]
- As of 2015, George Zoley gave $25,000 in contributions to the governor's mansion commission. This money will be used to build a park around the Tallahassee governor's mansion as Governor Scott's legacy.[72]
- Five out of seven private prisons in Florida are contracted to GEO Group, which accounts for 76 percent of all private beds in the state.[73]
- Florida has 101,000 inmates, which is the nation's third-largest prison population. Since crime rates have declined in Florida, more than two-thirds of all inmates are in prison for drug related offenses or some form of substance abuse problem. Seventeen percent are diagnosed with a serious mental illness.[74] Which means that the overwhelming majority of the folks in prison in Florida right now belong in rehab facilities or in counseling services—not behind bars!

When a politician is bought and paid for by the for-profit prison system, that politician will never have the people's best interests in mind. In just about every interview Senator Bernie Sanders gives on TV, he says he does not have a SuperPAC and he never will. Folks, this is why. When a major industry gives substantial money to a campaign, it's a conflict of interest. Every politician with a SuperPAC has been bribed. You can bet that the for-profit prison lobbyists have bribed the 2016 candidates, even though the majority of them should've had criminal record themselves for smoking pot.

16

Marijuana Lobbyists— The Good, the Bad, and the Ugly

When it comes to our elected leaders, politicians either deny ever using marijuana—which we know is a lie—or they willingly admit to trying it and then do nothing to change the laws.

President Barack Obama seems to want to go down in history as a marijuana enthusiast: "When I was a kid I inhaled frequently. That was the point."[1] Okay, Obama, you broke the law repeatedly. So what exactly did you do in eight years to stop today's generation from going to jail for using it?

In 2014, the president said marijuana laws were unfair because the government was "locking up kids or individual users for long stretches of jail time when some of the folks who are writing those laws have probably done the same thing."[2] But Obama hasn't actually done anything to stop that from happening— even though he has issued executive orders 227 times in his presidency.[3] If he really wanted to make marijuana legal, he could go around Congress to do it. When someone asks him if he thinks marijuana should be legalized, this is what he says:

> Middle-class kids don't get locked up for smoking pot, and poor kids do. And African American kids and Latino kids are more likely to be poor and less likely to have the resources and the support to avoid unduly harsh penalties. It's important [to move] forward [with legalization]

because it's important for society not to have a situation in which a large portion of people have at one time or another broken the law and only a select few get punished.[4]

Again, Obama was willing to issue thirty-three executive orders per year between January 20, 2009 and December 31, 2015. If he really felt that strongly about the unfair nature of marijuana laws, what's one more executive order? Fix the problem, Mr. President! You have the authority to do so. Instead, he has continued the drug war policies of his predecessors, and in some cases, he has even made it worse.

George W. Bush started the trend to militarize our police force, but Obama accelerated it.[5] Obama's administration has increased SWAT team raids and heavy-handed police tactics more than any other administration. Remember the *Avina v. United States* court case from chapter 4? In 2012, the DEA pointed their guns at an eleven-year-old and a fourteen-year-old during a drug raid on the wrong house and the family sued.[6] Obama stood by the DEA in this lawsuit, claiming the agents didn't do anything wrong. You see he's all talk when he claims he cares about how poor kids are being arrested and getting harsher penalties.

And here's why: under Obama, the tanks, armored personnel carriers, and M-16s that were used in Afghanistan and Iraq against our enemies were handed over to domestic police agencies to be used against us, the American people. In 2011, the Pentagon reported that "more than $500M, that is million with an M, worth of property" was "reutilized" to police forces around the country.[7] Under Obama, the Department of Homeland Security also gave out grants to police agencies so that they can purchase military-grade equipment to fight domestic terrorism. In 2011 alone, more than $2 billion was doled out to purchase bomb-disarming robots and Army tanks in states like Arizona and Idaho.[8] The Center for Investigative Reporting states that from September 11, 2001 to 2011, the Bush and Obama administrations give out a total of $34 billion in grants to arm local police as they would arm our soldiers overseas.[9] In his Fiscal Year 2016 budget proposal, Obama requested $27.6 billion to continue the war on drugs.[10] Where is he allocating most of that money? I'll give you a hint—it isn't for rehab facilities:[11]

- The Justice Department's drug war spending increased from $7.79 billion in 2015 to $8.14 billion in 2016 under the president's proposal.

- That includes nearly $3.7 billion for the Bureau of Prisons (up $187 million);
- A $2.46 billion increase for the DEA (up $90 million);
- A $519 million increase for the Organized Crime Drug Enforcement Task Force (up $12 million);
- A $293 million increase for the Office of Justice Programs (up $50 million).
- Drug Policy Alliance estimates that an additional $25 billion is spent at the state and local levels to fight the drug war every year, which is how we come to the total figure of at least $51 billion being spent to fight the War on Drugs.[12]

But let's not forget that my least favorite president, chickenhawk George W. Bush, is just as much of a hypocrite as Obama because he also smoked pot and used cocaine, particularly at Yale.[13] During Bush's presidency, he increased the drug war budget by $1.2 billion. And $23 million of that budget increase was used to drug test students in public schools![14] This may be difficult to believe, but Bush's War on Drugs gets even more hypocritical than that.

In December 2001, Bush's administration linked al-Qaeda groups in Afghanistan to heroin trafficking and he had the audacity to say to the American people, "If you quit drugs, you join the fight against terrorism."[15] Because quitting an addictive substance like heroin is really that simple, isn't it? This is coming from a man who had a severe alcohol problem in his thirties. Bush went so far as to illegally change the number on his driver's license in an attempt to hide a 1976 DUI arrest so he could run for office with a clean criminal record.[16]

What President Bush failed to mention about Afghanistan's heroin trafficking was that the Taliban actually banned opium entirely in Afghanistan because the terrorist group found the drug to be "anti-Islamic."[17] But after our troops went into Afghanistan in 2001 and destroyed the Taliban, local farmers started growing poppy crops again because they needed the source of income. Since the US occupation of Afghanistan, the United Nations has reported that the country now provides 90 percent of the world's supply of opium.[18] As of May 2015, the United States has spent $8.5 billion in counternarcotic programs in Afghanistan, but we might as well have put that money through the shredder. Afghanistan has roughly five hundred thousand acres devoted to growing poppy plants. That's larger than four hundred thousand US football fields put together. So yes, the War on Terror and the War on Drugs are related, but not in the way George W.

Bush would like you to believe. Think about it: if the US War on Terror and the occupation of Afghanistan never occurred, then Afghanistan wouldn't be the supplier of America's heroin epidemic. So doesn't that make George W. Bush somewhat liable for the national heroin epidemic? This cover up is coming from a president who was arrested for cocaine possession in 1972, but had his record expunged with help from his family's political connections.[19] Could you imagine where George W. would be today if his last name wasn't Bush?

And who could forget hypocrite President Bill Clinton—the champion of maximum minimum sentences, the guy who went nuclear with War on Drugs incarceration rates. He has also openly admitted his drug use: "I didn't say I was holier than thou, I said I tried. I never denied that I used marijuana."[20] Well, that's great. Thank you for your honesty, but what does that do for all those who were incarcerated for doing the same exact thing under your presidency?

Now I know some of you might be thinking—wait a minute, Governor. Didn't you also admit to smoking pot? Yes, I did. But I'm not a hypocrite like the last three presidents we've elected. In 2010, I talked about my history with marijuana on *Larry King Live*:[21]

I grew up in the '60s, in the days of Jimi Hendrix, the Rolling Stones, the Beatles and all of that . . . Marijuana was to rock 'n' roll what beer is to baseball . . . I'll tell you this, Larry, I've behaved far worse on alcohol than I ever have from marijuana.

When I was governor of Minnesota, I tried to introduce bills to change the marijuana laws and introduce hemp as a major agricultural solution. Unfortunately, I couldn't get anyone in the state legislature on board. They were only interested in continuing the War on Drugs, and I was powerless to stop them.

Bush, Clinton, and Obama are three of countless political leaders who admit to their past drug use, but who are all too willing to spend $51 billion of your tax dollars every year to eradicate plants that grow in the ground. And how are our hypocritical politicians spending that money? Not wisely.

In 2010, in anticipation of the fortieth anniversary of Nixon's War on Drugs, the *Associated Press* accessed archival records, federal budgets, and interviewed dozens of leaders to determine what exactly we spent $1 trillion on in the past forty years. Yes, that's right. The $1 trillion price tag on the War on Drugs is an outdated figure, calculated at least five years ago. Thanks to the Freedom of Information Act, reporters determined that in forty years, taxpayers spent over:[22]

- $20 billion to fight foreign drug gangs. For example, the United States spent more than $6 billion in Colombia, but coca cultivation increased and trafficking moved to Mexico—and the violence along with it.

- $33 billion in marketing "Just Say No"–style messages to America's youth and other prevention programs for nothing. In 2009, the CDC reported drug overdoses have "risen steadily" since the early 1970s to more than twenty thousand. In 2010, high school students reported the same rates of illegal drug use as they did in 1970.

- $49 billion for law enforcement along America's borders to cut off the flow of illegal drugs. In 2010, the AP estimated that "twenty-five million Americans will snort, swallow, inject, and smoke illicit drugs, about ten million more than in 1970, with the bulk of those drugs imported from Mexico."

- $121 billion to arrest more than thirty-seven million nonviolent drug offenders, about ten million of them for possession of marijuana. Yet, studies show that jail time typically increases drug abuse.

- $450 billion to lock those nonviolent drug offenders up in federal prisons. In 2009, half of all federal prisoners in the United States were serving sentences for drug offenses.

- At the same time, drug abuse is costing the nation in other ways. In 2010, the DOJ estimates the consequences of drug abuse—"an overburdened justice system, a strained health care system, lost productivity, and environmental destruction"—cost the United States $215 billion a year.

However, there are people within our government and within the lobbying community trying to change all this. Although this is an uphill battle, marijuana lobbyists are winning several fights against the War on Drugs. Marijuana lobbyists are armed with their own SuperPACs and they are taking on every issue from criminal justice to bank access to legalization.

The National Cannabis Industry Association (NCIA)

In chapter 11, we talked about how legal marijuana shops do not have access to any banking system and how the IRS tax code 280E denies tax credits to any marijuana business. There are lobbyists for Big Marijuana that are trying to change that.

In 2015, the National Cannabis Industry Association (or NCIA), a trade group for legal marijuana businesses, hired two lobbying firms—the first one has strong ties to Democrats (Heather Podesta + Partners) and the second with a proven track record with Republicans (Jochum Shore & Trossevin).[23] The two firms will partner with NCIA's in-house lobbyist, Michael Correia, who has been on staff since 2013.[24] Correia's main goal at the NCIA is to persuade lawmakers to do two things: change the tax code and give the marijuana industry access to banks.

Currently, the NCIA represents one thousand marijuana-related businesses, and the lobbying appears to be working. Democrats in Oregon and Colorado have introduced legislation in the House and the Senate to immunize banks from any federal prosecution for conducting business with legal pot shops.[25] Oregon lawmakers are also introducing state legislation to grant business tax deductions to marijuana companies.

The Marijuana Policy Project (MPP)

The national Marijuana Policy Project (MPP) is another lobbying group—it's actually the largest organization in the United States focused on ending marijuana prohibition. This group's objective is to educate people on the truth about marijuana, that it is safer than alcohol and therefore shouldn't be held to a higher standard of regulation or prosecution.[26] In 2015, MPP contributed $5,000 to the presidential bid of Republican Senator Rand Paul of Kentucky, as well as $9,500 to his senate reelection campaign.[27] He also received around $5,000 from the NCIA.[28] Paul was the only 2016 presidential hopeful to receive money from MPP, but MPP didn't put all its political eggs in one basket. Currently, the group is coordinating a ballot campaign in several states so that marijuana can be taxed and regulated like alcohol.

On Election Day in November 2016, if you live in Arizona, Maine, Massachusetts, California or Nevada, you can vote to make marijuana possession legal for adults aged twenty-one and older, and you can vote for it to be taxed and regulated like alcohol.[29] Yet, this isn't a revolutionary concept at the voting booth due to MPP.

MPP was able to get Ballot Measure 2 passed in Alaska on November 4, 2014. What is Ballot Measure 2? It's what made recreational marijuana legal in

Alaska—adults twenty-one and older are allowed to smoke weed legally *and* it is taxed like alcohol, thanks to the good people of Alaska who came out to vote for Ballot Measure 2.[30] In fact, MPP lobbyists have worked at the local level to change the majority of marijuana laws since 2000. The lobbyists were instrumental in getting Colorado's medical and recreational marijuana measures passed.

If you find MPP's work inspiring, the group has an open invitation for any vigilant citizen to join the movement. MPP's website lists ways to get involved in the legalization movement—including an easy form that allows you to send e-mails to your state senators and representatives: https://www.mpp.org/takeaction/

State Lobbying Groups

There are also local lobbying groups, such as Sensible Colorado, the Safer Alternative for Enjoyable Recreation, and the Marijuana Industry Group, that lobby for specific aspects of the marijuana industry. These groups tackle state issues that affect the existing marijuana industry. One such issue was in 2014 when Colorado's Department of Public Health and Environment tried to ban edibles— everything from candy, brownies, and drinks infused with cannabis.[31] This initiative went directly against Colorado's 2012 marijuana-legalization measure that stated, "retail pot is legal in all forms."[32] How can the Health Department then try to change the law two years later? Especially now that edibles account for 45 percent of marijuana sales in Colorado?[33]

The justification was that kids couldn't tell the difference between candy and edibles, and the Health Department was afraid that kids might eat a rice crispy treat without knowing it was actually an edible containing quantities of CBD or THC. However, I don't see how banning edibles from pot stores is going to solve that problem. Kids can't purchase edibles in a marijuana dispensary. By law, you have to be twenty-one years of age or older to even enter a marijuana dispensary. So if a kid gets to your box of THC cough drops, that's on you, not the marijuana dispensary.

What you do with your edibles when you get home is your business. If a parent leaves them within reach of children, then that's the parent's problem. The same with alcohol. If you leave a glass of wine on the table, it's your fault if your child drinks it and gets drunk. You can't sue the alcohol industry for your own stupidity. You can't blame a marijuana dispensary either. Plus, even if edibles were banned, what's to stop the same stupid person from baking pot brownies at home and leaving them somewhere that kids can access them? Colorado's marijuana lobbyists are out in full force on this issue because the new edible ruling will be coming in 2016.[34] If there is any kind of ban enforced, it would significantly affect the Colorado marijuana industry as a whole, and other states that have legalized marijuana might follow in the same footsteps.

The National Organization for Reform of Marijuana Laws (NORML)

By far, the most widely known and oldest marijuana-lobbying group is the National Organization for Reform of Marijuana Laws (NORML). NORML is dedicated to reforming marijuana laws and protecting marijuana consumers. Currently, it has 135 chapters and over 550 lawyers nationwide. It's also affiliated in other countries, such as New Zealand, Ireland, Canada, England, and France. Celebrities such as Willie Nelson, Tommy Chong, Woody Harrelson, and Bill Maher are on the NORML Advisory Board,[35] and they are often involved when NORML launches an advertising campaign or urges support for a particular piece of legislation.

The NORML Foundation is the nonprofit, tax-exempt unit that conducts educational and research reports on behalf of NORML. Many statistics about marijuana related arrests in America come from the foundation's reports. With all the new state marijuana laws, it can be tricky to know what is legal where. That's why NORML provides a breakdown of every state's laws on norml.org/states, including DUI, decriminalization, hemp, medical CBD, and specific regulations surrounding legalization. For example, it's illegal to grow your own weed in Washington state, but it's completely legal to do so in Washington, DC.

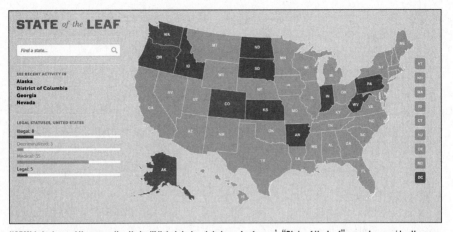

NORML is just one of the many sites that will list state-by-state laws. Leafy.com's "State of the Leaf" page also provides the same features. *(Photo courtesy of Leafy.com, 2016)*

These are just a few examples of the many lobbyists fighting to end the drug war. So how much money do these groups spend to push pro-marijuana legalization? In 2013, MPP spent more than $1 million on lobbying nationwide and Drug Policy Alliance spent $520,000.[36] Drug Policy Alliance (DrugPolicy. org) is the ultimate resource for facts surrounding the War on Drugs and incarceration. Since 2001, DPA has spent almost $4.2 million lobbying to end the War on Drugs.[37] The group advocates a wide range of issues including reversing zero-tolerance laws and abolishing the police state, the DEA, and asset forfeiture programs.

Since the 2012 election cycle, NORML has raised $109,900 for federal candidates, with contributions going mostly to Democrats. During the 2014 election cycle, NORML spent $28,000 in donations to House reps such as Earl Blumenauer (D-OR) and Dana Rohrabacher (R-CA) and to senators such as Cory Booker (D-NJ). However, the organization hasn't spent enough money on lobbying federal candidates to trigger reporting requirements. That's why NORML isn't listed as a special interest group.[38]

What has all that money contributed to? Aside from efforts to push state marijuana measures forward, you can thank Big Marijuana lobbyists for motivating Congress to do the following:

- In March 2015, Senators Cory Booker (D-NJ), Rand Paul (R-KY), and Kirsten Gillibrand (D-NY) introduced the Compassionate

Access Research Expansion and Respect States (CARERS) Act.[39] If passed, the bill would change marijuana's classification under the Controlled Substances Act from Schedule I to Schedule II. The change would allow more research on marijuana's potential benefits, plus doctors would be able to prescribe it nationwide. The CARERS Act would also forbid federal regulators from punishing or discouraging banks that work with marijuana-related businesses.

- Sen. Bernie Sanders (I-VT), introduced the Ending Federal Marijuana Prohibition Act in November 2015.[40] If passed, it would permit the states to determine their own marijuana laws, making the federal government's ability to punish those who possess or grow pot obsolete. Representative Barney Frank tried to pass the same bill in 2011, and Representative Jared Polis tried again in 2013.[41]

- In February 2015, Rep. Earl Blumenauer (D-OR) introduced the Veterans Equal Access Act,[42] which would allow healthcare providers at the Department of Veterans Affairs to prescribe medical marijuana. If you remember from chapter 12, a version of this bill was attached to the 2016 budget and it passed, but the VA has yet to take action.

- In April 2015, Rep. Dana Rohrabacher (R-CA) introduced the Respect State Marijuana Laws Act.[43] If passed, this legislation would amend the Controlled Substances Act so that anyone who legally produces, possesses, distributes, or delivers marijuana would not face federal prosecution.

- Rep. Jared Polis (D-CO) introduced the Regulate Marijuana Like Alcohol Act in February 2015,[44] which would remove marijuana from the federal drug schedule as well as give the FDA the same authority over marijuana it now has over alcohol.

- Blumenauer introduced another bill in February 2015 called the Marijuana Tax Revenue Act[45] to amend IRS codes for small businesses in the marijuana industry.

- In January 2015, Rep. Barbara Lee (D-CA) introduced the States' Medical Marijuana Property Rights Protection Act.[46] If passed, the law would stop the government from taking an individual's assets because of activity related to state-legal medical marijuana. This could be the beginning of the end of civil asset forfeiture.

- Oregon's House Representative Earl Blumenauer and Senator Ron Wyden introduced the Small Business Tax Equity Act in April 2015.[47] If passed, the legislation would allow marijuana-related businesses to take tax credits and deductions for their expenditures.

- Rep. Ed Perlmutter (D-CO) and Sen. Jeff Merkley (D-OR) introduced the Marijuana Business Access to Banking Act[48] in the House and Senate in April and July 2015. If passed, the bill would provide "safe harbor" to banks that serve legal marijuana-related businesses.

- In July 2015, Blumenauer introduced the Clean Slate for Marijuana Offenses Act.[49] If passed, we'd finally see amnesty for pot convicts. Those convicted of a federal marijuana-related offense in a state where marijuana was legal at the time, or those who were convicted of possessing an ounce of weed or less, could apply to have their records expunged.

I just listed fifteen pro-marijuana bills from 2015. Did you know about any of them? Did you notice how similar some of the bills are? This is because many of the same folks keep trying to pass the same legislation and it keeps failing. The wording of the bill changes slightly, or the name of the bill changes, or the person who introduces it changes, but each time the bill is reintroduced, it has another chance of passing. Rohrabacher-Farr's Medical Marijuana Amendment is case in point of this.

Do you remember in chapter 2 when I brought up how the DEA was going into legal marijuana dispensaries and trying to arrest people? The Rohrabacher-Farr Medical Marijuana Amendment, which was attached to the 2016 budget, was written to stop the DOJ from interfering with a state's medical cannabis program.[50] According to the Rohrabacher-Farr Medical Marijuana Amendment, if there is no violation of state law, the federal government cannot swoop in and raid a marijuana business or arrest anyone whom the state has approved for legal access to cannabis. This amendment was first introduced in 2003, but it got only 152 votes in the House. It took seven tries and eleven years to get this passed![51] Again, this is why it's important to pay attention to who is supporting pro-marijuana legislation. We need to vote these folks back into office if we want these bills to pass.

Did you know that you can contact your representatives to tell them to support these bills? Yes, the marijuana industry is starting to gain lobbying power, but keep in mind, these guys are going up against some of the oldest lobbying industries and all of these industries do not want marijuana to be legalized.

Case in point: private prison companies like GEO Group and Corrections Corporation of America do not want any of these bills passed. A 2010 report by CAA stated:

> Changes with respect to drugs and controlled substance or illegal immigration could affect the number of persons arrested, convicted and sentenced, thereby potentially reducing demand for correctional facilities to house them.[52]

So what does that tell you? The private prison lobbyists are going to be lobbying against those fifteen pro-marijuana bills!

Prison guard unions are also aware of what legalizing marijuana would do to the prison population. In 2008, the California Correctional Peace Officers Association spent a grand total of $1 million to defeat a bill designed to reduce sentences and parole times for nonviolent drug offenders by emphasizing drug treatment options over prison.[53] So if state and county prison guards aren't worried about losing their jobs to a private prison, then their union isn't going to lobby against private prison companies. Instead, the union and the private prison lobby will join together to keep prison populations on the rise.

Police unions are also major lobbying forces, and they want to see marijuana remain illegal for the same exact reason. Remember, the federal and state governments fund the drug war, which means police departments get additional funding based on their level of participation. Civil asset forfeiture has become a significant means of increasing a police force's budget because the police department can auction off any property seized during a drug raid. Since 2008, the National Fraternal Order of Police spends at least $220,000 per year lobbying. The National Association of Police Organizations is next with at least $160,000 a year. The International Union of Police Associations and the Internal Association of Chiefs of Police spend $80,000 each per year.[54] All together, that means the biggest players in police unions spend about $540,000 per year on federal lobbying.

But when it comes to lobbying, Big Pharma easily beats the police unions, private prisons, and the prison guard unions. This industry also does not want any pro-marijuana bills passed because that would end the monopoly on CBD and THC pharmaceutical pills. The Pharmaceutical Research and Manufacturers of America (PhRMA) spent $16.6 million on lobbying in 2014 alone. Get this: the entire drug manufacturing industry as a whole poured $14.7 million into the 2014 election cycle.[55] And in 2015, Pfizer spent more than $10 million in lobbying efforts.[56] Folks, 2015 was a non-presidential election year! This is an industry with millions to go around to everyone on Capitol Hill.

Guess which 2016 presidential candidate has collected the most donations from Big Pharma? Hillary Clinton! She collected a total of $336,416 in donations in 2015. Next up was Jeb Bush at $150,000—which is less than half of what Big Pharma gave Hillary![57] Want to know the difference between Hillary Clinton and Bernie Sanders? Vote for Hillary and Big Pharma will guarantee that marijuana is never legalized. Vote for Bernie and at least one of those fifteen pro-marijuana bills will be passed, since he went so far as to introduce one himself.

And let's not forget Big Booze and Big Tobacco. Since 2009, the beer, wine, and liquor industry has spent at least $20 million per year on lobbying issues concerning alcohol taxes and regulations. In 2014, the industry gave $17 million to federal candidates, their parties, and their committees.[58] Then in 2015, federal contributions went up to almost $25 million in the election cycle.[59] Both years, the majority of the money went to Republicans. As of February 2016, Big Tobacco has given $1.18 million in contributions to federal candidates on both sides of the aisle—but overall, the majority went to Republicans again.[60] Now do you see why the majority of Republicans are against marijuana legalization?

Again, what's most amazing about all these hypocrites is that statistically we know the majority of them have tried marijuana at some point in their lives. You're going to tell me that the folks at Big Booze and Big Tobacco and the legal drug dealers over at Big Pharma have never smoked a joint? Ha! When it comes to marijuana and the War on Drugs, it goes without saying that those who lobby, write, and enforce the law typically feel they are above it.

17

Why Ohio's Corporate
Marijuana Monopoly Failed

Now, as some of you probably already know, I am against lobbyists. When I was governor, I threw every last one of them out of the state capitol. During my administration, if the politicians of Minnesota wanted to participate in what I consider legalized bribery, then they had to do so off of state property.

Even when I ran for governor, I did not take any special interest money. I only took donations from the people of Minnesota and the average donation was under $30. I did not take any corporate money because I did not want to be in debt to anyone who had an agenda. I felt that if the people of Minnesota wanted to elect me, then it was my responsibility to do what was right for the people. And how could I do that if I had a list of corporate campaign donors to answer to first?

Well, if you know your history, then you know what happened: I raised less money than the Republican and the Democrat I ran against, but I won because I was able to debate them on TV. I proved that I wasn't bought and paid for by anyone but the Minnesotans who contributed to my campaign. And guess what. I had more personal donations than either of them! When people actually vote their conscience, the system works. I proved it. On November 3, 1998, not one Minnesotan threw his or her vote away on the third party candidate running for governor. The majority had the courage to vote for the candidate they wanted and I won, even though all the polls said I didn't have a chance.

Although I don't agree with everything he says, I was proud to see Senator Bernie Sanders running a very similar, anti-establishment campaign. He received more personal donations than any other Democrat or Republican candidate running for president. And his entire campaign was being funded by personal donations! So what does that tell you? That tells you he was not bought by any lobbyist or any special interest group. That tells you if the establishment ever allowed him to become president, on day one of his presidency, he would be going to work for the American people.

If you like that kind of politician, then I recommend you do some research on Jill Stein and Gary Johnson, the former governor of New Mexico and the Libertarian presidential nominee for 2016. He'll be on the ballot in all 50 states in November. And I know him well because we were both governors during the 90s. Even back then, he was advocating for the legalization of marijuana. And back then, he was part of the Republican party! Pretty obvious why he left and joined the Libertarians, isn't it? Anyway, back to lobbyists . . .

My problem with lobbyists is that any time a company trades money for power, that power can be abused. Even with the Big Marijuana lobbyists making a dent in the system and working toward legalization, corporate interests can override the good deeds NORML and MPP are trying to accomplish. When corporations see the profitability of the marijuana industry, they send in their lobbyists to see about getting a monopoly on a plant. In 2015, this almost happened in Ohio.

A measure known as Issue 3 would have legalized medical and recreational marijuana in the state of Ohio if the people voted for it. As much as that sounds like a good deal on the surface, Issue 3 would have also created the first marijuana monopoly and one of the worst examples of false legalization to date.

Issue 3 was designed to give ten facilities exclusive commercial rights to grow marijuana, and those ten facilities were already predetermined by the very people who put Issue 3 on the ballot in 2015.[1] Get this: the people involved in ResponsibleOhio, the SuperPAC that supported Issue 3 and petitioned to get it on the ballot in 2015, were the property owners of the ten marijuana growth, cultivation, and extraction (MGCE) facilities. Each property owner had at least one investor and each investor contributed $2 million to get Issue 3 on the ballot.[2] So essentially, this bill would have made anyone involved in those ten facilities super rich. Meanwhile, Ohio's farming community wouldn't see a penny from the legalization.

Keep in mind that agriculture is Ohio's number one industry. It supports one in six jobs and almost 50 percent of the land in Ohio is classified as "prime farmland" by the US Department of Agriculture, which means 50 percent of Ohio's land is fertile and productive. The state grows more than two hundred crops and 91 percent of Ohio farms are family farms.[3] So if Issue 3 passed, Ohio farmers—who obviously know what they're doing when it comes to agriculture—would not benefit at all from marijuana legalization. Why wouldn't Ohio want its farmers to make money off of marijuana legalization, especially when the majority of American farms are struggling to make ends meet? And besides, couldn't Ohio's farming community also then take on the hemp industry? Could you imagine what industrialized hemp could do for Ohio farmers!

The justification behind this Issue 3 monopoly was quality control. These ten facilities would grow and cultivate the marijuana with the same standards, and then sell it to marijuana dispensaries. Under Issue 3, those who owned and operated the ten growing facilities could not own any marijuana dispensaries, but they did have total control of the wholesale price of cannabis and could therefore sell it to marijuana dispensaries at any price, giving them direct control over the market. In other words, Issue 3 was designed to outlaw homegrown pot and create the OPEC of marijuana in Ohio.

In 2015, Issue 3 lobbyists went out in full force to try to cover up the corporate take over of marijuana. They knew that as many as nine out of ten Ohioans supported legalizing medical marijuana and the majority of Ohio voters approved of legalizing recreational pot.[4] So that's what they told everyone they were doing. Issue 3 would legalize marijuana, yes, but at what cost to the consumer? ResponsibleOhio even had a marijuana mascot named Buddie at college campuses, trying to get young people to vote yes on Issue 3.

What Buddie didn't tell anyone was that the wealthy investors of the ten grow facilities spent nearly $25 million just to get Issue 3 on the ballot.[5] They were then planning on spending over $40 million to build the facilities if Issue 3 passed. Folks, if these guys are willing to spend around $65 million, can you imagine what kind of profits they intend to make off of marijuana? Ohio's Issue 3 would have created legal drug kingpins!

Ohio's marijuana legalization also divided pro-pot lobbyists. On one hand, they wanted marijuana to be legalized. This was the first time in American history that there was a measure to legalize both medical and recreational marijuana at the same time. In every other state, marijuana legalization was a two-part battle: medical marijuana is passed first and then recreational marijuana might or might not eventually be passed. Issue 3 would certainly fast-track the legalization process. And other states might follow Ohio's lead.

On the other hand, pro-pot lobbyists really didn't want weed to be legalized in this way. According to the *New York Times,* Drug Policy Alliance and the Marijuana Policy Project stayed neutral rather than endorsing Issue 3 "because of the problematic oligopoly provision," and NORML gave it an "uneasy endorsement."[6] They all saw the measure for what it truly was: corporations having complete control over the quality of the product. And if Issue 3 did pass, wouldn't that mean corporate interests in other states might then try to do the same thing? Before you know it, corporations in America could be running all aspects of the marijuana industry, keeping all the cash, and paying very little, if any, taxes. Keep in mind that it's not like any of the investors or property owners of the ten MGCE facilities had any prior experience in growing marijuana. But if your investors have unlimited funds of money, doesn't that then trump experience? That's what ResponsibleOhio was banking on. They also laid out a lot of promises to the people of Ohio if they passed Issue 3.

ResponsibleOhio claimed that by 2020, the sale of pot would generate $554 million a year in tax revenue for Ohio, and 85 percent of that revenue would go to safety services and infrastructure repair.[7] However, the majority of Ohio voters didn't buy into that as a reason to legalize marijuana for a corporate conglomerate. In November 2015, over 63 percent of voters said no to Issue 3 and it did not pass.

People, this is why I keep saying it is so important to vote! ResponsibleOhio had the propaganda campaign out in full force for Issue 3—the SuperPAC spent millions—yet the measure did not pass because the majority of Ohio residents saw it for what it was. In this instance, every vote counted. Issue 3 could have very well reversed all the progress we've made with limited forms of marijuana legalization. Sure, it would have created more jobs, it would have created more tax revenue, it would have given people access to marijuana, but at what cost? Folks, if a state law is telling you it is illegal to grow a plant in your backyard but ten properties can grow acres of that same plant and profit off of it, that is not marijuana legalization. If a law states it is illegal to grow a plant in your backyard, but you can go to work for $10 an hour and grow that plant for someone else, that is not marijuana legalization. That's false legalization. I don't care what *Citizens United* states. Corporations are not people. People are people. And people deserve the right to grow marijuana in their backyards. I commend Ohio for being vigilant. Again, the majority of people wanted marijuana to be legalized. They realized this was their chance to do so, but they voted their conscience, and they did the right thing. And now one year later, MPP is doing what it can to give the farmers of Ohio the opportunity to grow marijuana and hemp.

Since Issue 3 was defeated, Rob Kampia, the executive director of MPP, has been on a mission with the Ohioans for Medical Marijuana to collect the 305,591 necessary signatures to get a new marijuana measure on the November 2016 ballot.[8] If Kampia is successful, there will be a new amendment in the Ohio Constitution called the Cannabis Control Amendment (CCA) that legalizes medical marijuana *and* recreational marijuana *and* industrial hemp throughout the state. The Cannabis Control Amendment will do the following:[9]

- Remove the state of Ohio's laws that prohibit producing, processing, and selling of cannabis.
- Create the Division of Marijuana Control, which will license and regulate all forms of cannabis.
- Establish a list of qualifying medical conditions for marijuana including chronic pain, seizures, and PTSD.
- Allow patients and caregivers to possess and grown personal-use amounts of medical marijuana at home. A patient can grow up to twelve mature marijuana plants at one time, but if two or more patients live in the same home, they are limited to twenty-four mature marijuana plants combined.
- Require the state government to issue licenses to businesses to grow, process, test, distribute, and sell medical marijuana.
- Impose a standard sales tax similar to what is imposed on "paper towels or juice at the retail level." This means there is no excise tax or special sales tax like in Colorado or Oregon, which should make medical marijuana much more affordable to the consumer.
- Approve hemp! Ohio Department of Agriculture Ohio will allow farmers to grow industrial crop, just like any other crop.
- Allow adults twenty-one years of age and older access to recreational marijuana on January 1, 2017. Adults can grow up to six mature marijuana plants at home, or if two or more adults live in the same home, they can grow up to twelve plants. The state doesn't require a license to grow recreational marijuana and there are no additional fees for doing so.

- Legally, residents will be able to possess up to 100 g of marijuana, 500 g of marijuana infused solids, 2 L of marijuana infused liquids, and 25 g of marijuana concentrates. However, there is no limit to the amount of marijuana or marijuana products a person possesses at home.

In this new Cannabis Control Amendment, Rob Kampia explains "the deck won't be stacked against anyone" because it "will embrace a healthy, free market approach to the production of medical marijuana, which will drive down the cost as compared to, say, an oligopoly" such as the 2015 Issue 3 measure.[9] If the new amendment passes, then the Ohio Department of Health would begin issuing patient identification cards on March 1, 2017.

In the meantime, the Ohio legislature passed House Bill 523 on May 26, 2016, which will legalize medical marijuana, but lawmakers estimate it can take anywhere between sixteen months to two years to set up and implement all the asinine rules associated with this bill. Honestly, I don't know how House Bill 523 is considered "legalization" of medical marijuana. The lawmakers have decided once again that they know better than anyone else when it comes to which patients can access marijuana for medical reasons. Twenty conditions are approved. And even then, lawmakers decided to only legalize non-smokeable marijuana. So in other words, you can't smoke your medicine (vaping the oil is permitted) and the law doesn't allow you to grow any marijuana either. According to the *Columbus Dispatch*, as a patient, you're limited to "a 90-day supply of marijuana edibles, patches, oils and plant material."[11]

When it comes to drug tests at work, medical marijuana patients have no protection. They can be fired for violating a "drug-free workplace policy" if marijuana is found in their systems, which also would make them ineligible for unemployment benefits![12] Okay, folks, in the real world, how does this help someone with epilepsy or a seizure disorder, exactly? How does this law help someone with crohn's disease, PTSD, parkinson's, sickle cell anemia, alzheimer's, fibromyalgia, or the rest of Ohio's qualifying conditions?

So hypothetically, as a medical marijuana patient in Ohio, I can take a medication that can help my condition and then lose my job, or I can go on suffering and keep my job and therefore be able to support my family. See how House Bill 523 doesn't actually legalize anything?

Here's something interesting about this new Cannabis Control amendment that MPP and the Ohioans for Medical Marijuana are trying to get on the ballot in November 2016: employers *won't* be able to fire those with a medical marijuana card if they test positive for marijuana. However, if you consume marijuana recreationally, there is no protection from a failed drug test—even though the CCA would make recreational marijuana legal. So the CCA might be the most common sense and comprehensive cannabis law to date, but we're still seeing false legalization. In Ohio, CCA would make it legal to consume marijuana recreationally, but a corporation could still fire employees for doing so. That still doesn't sit well with me, but that's the way it is in every state that has "legalized" marijuana.

If it passes, the CCA will save Ohio millions of taxpayer dollars within a year. The state spends over $200 million per year just to prosecute marijuana-related crimes.[10] Could you imagine what the state could do with an extra $200 million in the budget? This amendment will also allow the Ohio Department of Health to establish the Ohio Medical Marijuana Research Lab to conduct research and provide public and private medical marijuana research grants.[11] I'm sure the DEA will not be pleased with this! I'm also curious to see if the investors for Issue 3 and the ResponsibleOhio SuperPAC supporters will idly stand by while MPP gets the support necessary needs to pass CCA. Will their lobbyists try to intervene to stop CCA? We'll see what happens in November 2016.

While most pro-pot lobbyists are focused on the medical and recreational aspects of marijuana, and that's all fine and good, I'd like to see more of a push for the agricultural aspect of cannabis, as we're seeing in the CCA. Hemp is multibillion-dollar industry that could rejuvenate our pathetic economy. Again, we don't have to elect someone who promises to fix the economy when we can fix it ourselves.

Every 2016 presidential candidate swears fixing the economy is priority number one. Or maybe priority number two for those who want to turn our country into East Berlin by building a wall across the United States/Mexico border. But when it comes to the economy, we don't need a president to fix the problem. The private sector could create an entirely new industry from hemp if it is legalized. Besides, name me one president who has actually fixed our crumbling infrastructure or added more jobs in the private sector after promising to do so! Expanding the federal government with political hires doesn't count as growing the economy. If hemp were legalized nationwide, we'd see a whole new industry and a whole new future for our country in a very short period of time. This is why I hope the CCA passes. I want Ohio farmers to show the rest of the country how much money there is to be made from farming industrial hemp.

18

Hemp for Victory!

Did you know that we import American flags? Other countries manufacture our flag, and we pay them for it. We pay nearly $4 million per year on imported American flags, to be exact.[1] Guess where the majority of American flags are produced. China! China makes $3.6 million per year selling our flag to us. I don't know about you, but that just doesn't sit right with me. It doesn't sit right with our military either. The US military will not purchase or use flags that aren't made in the USA. Folks, if anything should be manufactured in the United States and only in the United States, it should be our Stars and Stripes. Think about it: When you stand to solute the flag, the symbol of our country, aren't you also saluting something that is made in China? Therefore, aren't you in some way paying homage to China? I'm sure the Chinese could see it that way.

On November 11, 2015—also known as Veterans Day—something momentous and historic happened at the US Capitol: a new American flag made entirely in the United States by US veterans flew proudly.

On Veterans Day, the federal government flew an American flag made entirely out of industrial hemp that was grown in Kentucky by US veterans.[2] Dozens of veterans from the Growing Warriors Project got together to spin and dye hemp yarn to make the three-foot-by-five-foot, handwoven American flag for the Capitol.

But wait a minute—doesn't the federal government classify hemp as a schedule 1 narcotic? Why yes, it does. Hemp has been classified as a dangerously addictive drug since 1971. So on Veterans Day in 2015, our federal government proudly raised the emblem of our country up on the Capitol's flag poll, and it was made entirely out of a Schedule I narcotic. Blasphemy? Not necessarily. Remember: there is no humanly possible way to get high off of hemp. But again, the government has known the difference between hemp and the "mother" cannabis plant since the Founding Fathers because American flags used to be made from hemp. The only blasphemy here is that hemp was the commodity that built our economy and that now it's illegal for American farmers to grow it.

During the early 1900s, when Wisconsin was profiting from its booming hemp farms, Wisconsin Agriculture Experiment Station researcher Andrew Wright characterized "three fairly distinct types" of cannabis: "that grown for fiber, that for birdseed and oil, and that for drugs."[3] Still, as of 2016, the federal government won't differentiate hemp from marijuana—it's all viewed as public enemy number one.

Do you remember how we're importing our own flag and losing at least $4 million in revenue for doing so? Well, get this: in 2015, US consumers bought between $500 million and $600 million in *imported* hemp products like food, cosmetics, fabrics, paper, construction material, insulation, and plastics.[4] We're buying these products from other countries because it is illegal for farmers in America to grow and cultivate hemp. In fact, the United States is the world's largest consumer of hemp-related products.[5] Yet, the United States is the only industrialized nation where hemp production is illegal. Do you see the problem here? When it comes to demanding hemp products, our country is number one. When it comes to making money off of hemp products by manufacturing them? Sadly, not one person vying to be president in 2016 has addressed legalizing hemp production as a solution to fixing the economy.

To coincide with the 2015 historic hemp flag made by veterans, the National Hemp Association (NHA), a Boulder-based nonprofit representing the entire US hemp industry, launched a federal campaign to pass the Industrial Hemp Farming Act of 2015. If this bill passes, then hemp will be removed from the Controlled Substances Act, and it will be legal under federal law to grow and manufacture it. NHA Communications Director Neshama Abraham had this to say about the importance of the bill:

> That single bill is the most important thing we can do, essentially removing the bottleneck to allow farmers to get seeds. If they can get

seeds, then they can start cultivating a domestic crop of hemp. In that way, this is the most important jobs bill to come in front of Congress this year. Right now, all the hemp products that are made in the U.S. are made from imported hemp. Why not cultivate it domestically and create jobs for rural farmers, here, in our own country?[6]

The bill also has the support of Vote Hemp, another grassroots hemp advocacy organization, as well as the Growing Warriors Project, which employs disabled veterans to make flags from hemp—they are planning to produce two hundred hemp flags in 2016 by hand.[7] I have to commend the Growing Warriors Project. These vets were injured in battle, but they continue to serve our country by being on the frontline of one of the greatest American battles of all time: a battle against an agricultural crop.

The Industrial Hemp Farming Act was introduced to Congress in January 2015 with support from Democrats and Republicans, including Senators Ron Wyden (D-OR), Mitch McConnell (R-KY), Jeff Merkley (D-OR), and Rand Paul (R-KY), and House Representatives Thomas Massie (R-KY) and Jared Polis (D-CO).[8] Isn't that an interesting mix of support? Colorado and Oregon have both legalized marijuana, but Kentucky is still debating if CBD oil should be legalized for kids suffering from seizures. If you remember, Kentucky does have a strong history with growing hemp, so this legislation might help educate the good people of Kentucky on what cannabis really is and how it can benefit them.

However, 2015 marks the *fifth* time our representatives are trying to pass this freaking bill! It was first introduced in 2005 by Ron Paul, Pete Stark, Jim McDermott, and Raul Grijalva. It was reintroduced in 2007, again in 2009, and then again in 2013, but each time the bill was stalled in one of those wonderful subcommittees—such as the Subcommittee on Crime, Terrorism, Homeland Security, and Investigations.[9] Now, again, we're talking about an agricultural crop. Why, exactly, is a crop considered a terrorism concern?

The most astounding thing about this law is that it is redundant. On February 7, 2014, President Obama signed the Farm Bill of 2013 into law (what is commonly known as the 2014 Farm Bill, because it didn't go into effect until 2014). Section 7606 of the Farm Bill is called Legitimacy of Industrial Hemp Research and defines industrial hemp "as distinct" from medical and recreational marijuana.[10] The Farm Bill allowed universities to conduct studies with hemp, and it allowed states to develop cultivation programs for farms that are state regulated under the state's department of agriculture. Therefore, the federal government has already classified industrial hemp as separate from what is sold in medical and recreational pot shops. But now we need to have another bill, Industrial Hemp Farming Act of 2015, to further clarify to the DEA what the 2014 Farm Bill actually means.

Get this: Kentucky tobacco farmers have already found the 2014 Farm Bill to be a blessing. Due to the decline of cigarette sales, tobacco farmers have been struggling, and they were looking for another crop that could supplement their income and eventually replace their dependence on farming tobacco. Kentucky farmers filled out the proper paperwork to be enrolled in the cultivation and research projects available to farmers under the Farm Bill. Then the DEA had to get involved. The agency unlawfully seized all the hemp seeds that Kentucky's Department of Agriculture had legally purchased under the Farm Bill. Why? Because the seeds are a Schedule I narcotic and an illegal substance.

In May 2014, Kentucky's Department of Agriculture had to go so far as to sue the DEA to stop them from interfering with six Kentucky hemp research projects—all of which were approved under section 7606 of the Farm Bill. Kentucky brought forward the lawsuit after the DEA confiscated 250 lbs of certified industrial hemp seed from Italy that was bound for the state's agricultural department.[11] In other words, the shipment wasn't going to some random farmers. The seeds were going directly to the state of Kentucky, where they would be distributed to those who were already approved to receive it. After a weeklong standoff, the DEA got off with a warning, and the seed was returned to Kentucky. But that didn't stop the federal agency from continuing to do this. The DEA also seized hemp seed going to Colorado farmers from Canada, and the agency had to be told again to respect the 2014 Farm Bill that POTUS signed into law.[12]

Because of the 2014 Farm Bill, there are currently twenty-seven states[13] that have defined industrial hemp as agriculture, which means twenty-seven states have legalized hemp and are either growing it or intending to grow it for commercial, research, or pilot programs, but the DEA could swoop in at any time to seize the seeds. So Congress introduced the Industrial Hemp Farming Act of 2015 in an attempt to stop the DEA from ignoring (and essentially breaking) the 2014 Farm Bill, which is federal law. But because hemp is included under the federal drug classifications, the Industrial Hemp Farming Act can't be passed without going through the DEA. Isn't that something?

Hemp was once considered America's most important cash crop, but today's hemp legalization is pathetic. Hemp farmers cannot transport seeds across state lines, obtain bank accounts, or get crop insurance.[14] The DEA and local law enforcement can come inspect the crops at any time and even seize and burn crop fields if they claim to find one mother cannabis plant growing among the industrial hemp. Farmers could go to prison or have their property confiscated under civil asset forfeiture.[15] Remember, under civil asset forfeiture laws, you don't have to be charged with a drug crime or even be found guilty of a drug crime for the cops to take everything you own and sell it at auction to increase their budgets. People, we're down to about one percent of the American population who choose to make a living as farmers.[16] And what about our neighbors to the north? Canadian farmers have built a fifteen-year hemp seed oil business that made $1 billion in 2014.[17] They make $300 per acre, per season, farming industrial hemp. Let me put that into perspective: $300 per acre is as much as ten times what our farms in Missouri, Wisconsin, Illinois, North Dakota, and Kentucky are currently making for growing GMO wheat, corn, and soy.[18] Are you embarrassed by your country's hemp laws yet?

Industrial hemp could really be the next big industry. Think of it this way: Who makes more money, beer companies like Coors and Budweiser or oil and gas companies like Exxon Mobile? Fully legalizing medical and recreational marijuana

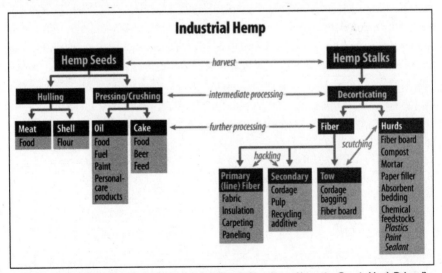

Source: CRS, adapted from D. G. Kraenzel et al., "Industrial Hemp as an Alternative Crop in North Dakota," AER-402, North Dakota State University, July 23, 1998.

will bring in a ton of money, no doubt about it. But when compared to the revenue that industrial hemp can bring in, you're looking at Coors versus Exxon Mobile.

So what makes hemp more lucrative than pot? It comes down to hemp seeds, hemp oilseed, and the hemp stalk fibers—which are all are used for different purposes. As George Washington said in 1794, "make the most of the hempseed . . . sow it everywhere."[19] And he said that for good reason.

Hemp Seed and Hemp Oil

Remember the difference between the father and mother cannabis plants? The father plant does not flower like the mother plant, but it does produce seeds. The hemp-seed is actually a tiny nut, with a hull and a meaty inner core. As Andrew Wright mentioned back in 1918, the hemp seed makes great birdseed. Today's farmers also use it for animal feed for horses, cows, and chickens. Recent studies in Kentucky have shown that "hemp-fed cattle require less feed and digest it more efficiently."[20]

However, there's also a surprising amount of nutrition in hemp seed, and its oil can be used for cooking—just like grape-seed oil. Hemp seeds are used in protein powders and health foods such as energy bars. The seeds can even be turned into nut butter for sandwiches (more on that in chapter 19). In addition, hemp seed oil is used for cosmetics like body lotion, and it's actually a preferred ingredient in many all-natural, organic cosmetics. This is why you can find hemp-based products in the personal care aisle of major US retailers including Whole Foods, Trader Joe's, and Kroger's. Hemp-seed oil is also used in Europe for household products such as laundry detergent and home-cleaning products. Like I said earlier, there is great demand for hemp products, so we are importing them. Could you imagine how much cheaper the products could be if we could grow, cultivate, and manufacture hemp right here in the USA?

Again, hemp seed, and hemp oil produced from the seed is just one aspect of industrial hemp. Next up is the stalk of the hemp plant. The stalk contains two types of fiber: the outer "bast fiber" that is processed into long strands, and the inner woody core known as "hurds" that are processed into a material resembling wood chips.

Bast: The Outer Fiber of the Hemp Stalk

The bast fiber is what the American textile and apparel industry is sadly lacking. Practically anything you buy in the store can be made out of bast fiber: footwear, luggage, rugs, clothing, rope, paper, plastic, you name it. Hemp blends well with other fibers like cotton, silk, rayon, linen, and wool, but if an American manufacturer wants to use hemp fiber in 2016, raw materials can only be imported due to our asinine hemp laws. Since the mid-1990s, manufacturers have seen the durability of hemp and have used it in their products and designs: Adidas created a hemp fabric for sneakers, Armani designed a tuxedo from hemp, and Calvin Klein has somewhat secretly used hemp for years by listing it as a "vegetable fiber," which it technically is.[21]

Here's the interesting thing about using hemp bast fiber for paper: it's more environmentally conscious to use hemp fibers, *and* hemp makes stronger paper. The process involved in taking wood and turning it into pulp for paper is a chemical-intensive process. Manufacturers use fewer chemicals and the process is done in far less time when they use hemp fiber, so it's better for the environment and more paper can be made at a faster rate.[22] Do you see why William Randolph Hearst needed hemp to go away for good? Who the hell would buy paper made from wood if hemp was an alternative?

Henry Ford discovered how to use bast fibers in the 1940s to construct cars, and in 1941, he constructed what people refer to as the first plastic car, or the first soybean car, or the first hemp car—all of which are accurate ways to describe the car.[23] This car was lighter than steel, yet it could handle ten times the impact without breaking or even denting. The car weighed 2,000 lbs, which was 1,000 lbs lighter than a steel car. Henry Ford developed a plastic comprised of "green" ingredients including soybeans, wheat, hemp, and flax to make the car's exterior.[24] The formula for producing the plastic has unfortunately been lost over time, and sadly very few people today would consider Henry Ford an environmentalist, but that's what he was. He wanted his products to come from the earth and be returned to the earth without leaving what is referred to today as a carbon footprint. But don't take my word for it—here's what Henry Ford told the *New York Times* in 1925:

> The fuel of the future is going to come from fruit like that sumach out by the road, or from apples, weeds, sawdust—almost anything. There is fuel in every bit of vegetable matter that can be fermented. There's enough alcohol in one year's yield of an acre of potatoes to drive the machinery necessary to cultivate the fields for a hundred years.[25]

Rudolf Diesel, inventor of the diesel engine, also warned that since fossil fuels were not a renewable resource, it was not wise to rely on it to power machines. Here's what he had to say about renewable resources in 1912:

> The fact that fat oils from vegetable sources can be used may seem insignificant today, but such oils may perhaps become in course of time of the same importance as some natural mineral oils and the tar products now. In any case, they make it certain that motor power can still be produced from the heat of the sun, which is always available for agricultural purposes, even when all our natural stores of solid and liquid fuels are exhausted.[26]

Get this: Rudolf Diesel felt so strongly about this when he displayed his first diesel engine at the 1900 Paris World's Fair that the fuel it ran on was petroleum based. To this day, certain diesel engines can run on cooking oil or vegetable oil. Today, we do add ethanol to some of our fuel sources, such as bioethanol (also known as Flex Fuel), which is an alcohol made by fermenting the sugar components of plant materials. But are American car companies really following in Diesel's and Ford's footsteps? I don't see Dodge or Chevy lobbying Congress to get hemp production underway, do you? And it might interest you to know that in 1932, Nazi Germany invented the Scholler process to create a form of fuel out of wood waste and sawdust to power their cars, tanks, and airplanes because the Allies cut off their supply chains to oil.[27] The United States briefly entertained this concept in the 1940s, but, long story short, Big Oil won that fight, and we've been at their mercy ever since.

How does all this relate to hemp? I would go so far as to classify hemp as a vegetable, since 12 tbsp of hemp seeds contain 40 g of protein, which is the same amount of protein found in a single-serving fillet of salmon. And speaking of using vegetables for a fuel source, did you know that you can break down the entire hemp plant and produce biofuel fuel from it? Willie Nelson does. His tour buses run entirely on biofuel produced from vegetable fats and seed oil crops, such as hemp.[28] His dream was to get American farmers to produce biofuel for American trucking companies through a company called BioWillie, but he couldn't come up with enough revenue to do so and had to abandon the project in 2008.[29] This is unfortunate because several studies in Sweden have proven just how valuable hemp can be if it is reduced to oil and used as biofuel:

Biodiesel production from hemp seed oil has been reported to have a much lower overall environmental impact than fossil diesel, even in case where the stalks and leaves were not used for energy purposes. Industrial hemp has a high-energy yield per hectare for both solid bio-fuel and biogas production that is similar or superior to that of most energy crops common in northern Europe. Hemp as a biogas substrate surpasses crops used for first-generation biofuel production (e.g., wheat, rapeseed) and with pretreatment might even compete with maize and sugar beet for biogas production. Industrial hemp is a high-yielding crop for biofuel production. Fuel properties of hemp are similar to those of wood and willow and superior to those of straw, miscanthus, and reed canary grass.[30]

Did you catch that? The Nazis were able to power an entire country *and* their war efforts from breaking wood down into fuel, and hemp is proven to be a better fuel source than wood.

Out of all the car manufacturers out there, the British car company Lotus seems to share the most in Ford's and Diesel's holistic approaches to green technology. Eco Elise is a concept car that is made of hemp and other renewable resources, water-based paint, and biodegradable parts. The entire process of manufacturing and building the car, driving the car, and even the inevitable end of the car's "life" are all taken under consideration to reduce global emissions and waste. You'll never guess who came up with the water-based paint system, which is being used to lower the emissions of solvents and other toxic chemicals during the manufacturing process. One of hemp's greatest enemies of all time: Henry DuPont![31] Isn't that incredible? DuPont would be rolling over in his grave if he knew the company is creating paint specifically for a company that uses bast fibers from hemp to construct cars!

Hurds: The Inner Fiber of the Hemp Stalk

Again, using the bast fibers in the outer layer of the hemp stalk is just one way we could cultivate hemp to create endless possibilities for economic growth, and the inner core of the hemp stalk, known as "hurds," has something incredible to offer as well. Hurds have a low density and a high absorbency. It can be mixed with plaster and concrete for building materials. It is also used in thermal insulation. Currently, hemp hurds manufactured in the European Union are sold for bedding for horses and other animals. Hemp hurd bedding absorbs much more than cereal straw or hay, which means there is less dust, fungal spores, and odors. Get this: the queen of England actually uses hemp bedding for her horses. Plus, there's less maintenance with hemp hurd due to its high absorbency. Could you imagine how much the pet supply industry could make off of a cat litter made out of hemp hurd?

Aside from the pet and animal industry, hemp hurd can be used for organic fertilizer. It cleans up biohazards and toxins in the soil. So the next time BP has an oil spill, bring in the hemp hurd! We currently "clean" oil spills with clay and polypropylene-based products, which, of course, impacts the delicate environment even further.

I want you to understand exactly what I mean when I say hemp hurd is so absorbent it can clean up an entire oil spill. This is not an exaggeration. On April 26, 1986, there was an explosion at a nuclear reactor in Chernobyl, a power plant in Pripyat, Ukraine. Until an earthquake caused Japan's nuclear facility in Fukushima to fail, Chernobyl was the world's worst nuclear disaster, and many experts still consider it to be, given the rage of the damage. The explosion at Chernobyl contaminated agriculture and water in a 30 km radius.[32] According to ABC News, the disaster "affected 3 million people and forced the evacuation of over 300,000."[33] Toxins accumulated in the meat and milk products as well as any vegetation—new children near Chernobyl were born with massive birth defects. This was not only a monumental disaster for Ukraine but for the world as well. How the hell do you get rid of nuclear contaminants in a population's food and drinking water supply? Well, hemp.

Hemp: The Phytoremediation Miracle Plant

Now, I must preface this next section by saying that when I discovered the full extent of how useful hemp is for restoring the environment, I had to shake my head in shame and embarrassment for my country. Due to the fact that hemp is widely illegal, there are so few studies that prove how the plant actually removes toxins from the soil and water better than any other naturally growing plant. But we soon found out exactly how useful this illegal plant could be after the tragedy at Chernobyl.

In 2015, a research book called *Soil Remediation and Plants: Prospects and Challenges* was compiled by scientists who study soil, plant biology, forestry, and agriculture in universities around the globe, in places like Turkey, Malaysia,

Canada, Turkey, and Pakistan. In the book, the authors explain the hemp case study that took place at Chernobyl. Phytotech Inc., a Princeton, New Jersey–based research company, was involved in the study. Phytotech is no longer in existence, but the company studied phytoremediation, or how certain plants can clean up polluted sites simply by being grown in the contaminated soil.

In February 1996, Phytotech developed transgenic strains of sunflowers called helianthus "that could remove as much as 95 percent of toxic contaminants in as little as twenty-four hours." [34] The company took the special sunflowers to Chernobyl and planted them in Styrofoam rafts at an edge of a contaminated pond. Within twelve days, the roots of the sunflowers had absorbed a significant amount of radiation. When compared to the radioactive concentration in the water, the roots of the sunflowers were between 2,000 and 8,000 percent *more* radioactive. If you don't know anything about radiation, then I'll explain further: the cesium concentrations within the plants' roots were 8,000 times greater than the water, and the strontium concentrations were 2,000 times greater than the water. [35] This means the helianthus was successful in removing a significant amount of toxins within those twelve days.

Now, I'm sure sunflowers created in a lab aren't cheap, so in 1998, Phytotech, Consolidated Growers and Processors, and the Ukraine Institute of Bast Crops planted something else near Chernobyl. The fact that the Ukraine-based company has "bast" in its title should give away what was planted, but yes, they planted Ukrainian hemp to remove contaminants in the water and soil. What they found was that the regular, good old industrial hemp extracted the radioactive elements just as efficiently as the special strain of sunflower that Phytotech invented.

Unfortunately, for unknown reasons, this hemp research project wasn't implemented in all the contaminated areas to completely minimize or even reverse the effects of the radiation, and today we have no way of knowing how successful the project could have been if it were conducted on a grand scale. But, folks, the Chernobyl disaster happened thirty years ago, and only a handful of studies on hemp's phytoremediation abilities have been published since that time. That tells you exactly how dangerous this plant is to corporate America. These companies would rather invent a new plant in a lab than use hemp! Why? Because then they'd get obscene amounts of money. If hemp were legal, then anyone could plant it to clean up polluted soil. Since hemp isn't legal, we're forced to rely on corporations to concoct new ways to clean up radiation leaks and oil spills, and their stocks will continue to soar with every natural and every man-made disaster. Imagine what hemp could do for Fukushima if the crop wasn't illegal in Japan. Hell, imagine what hemp could do for any soil or water contaminated with lead in Flint, Michigan!

People: hemp has been proven to absorb heavy metals from soil—and lead is a heavy metal.[36] Let me repeat that: hemp has been proven to take out toxic heavy metals from the soil, including zinc, cadmium, lead, and arsenic. Here's why heavy metals like lead are so toxic: they cannot be destroyed biologically. Lead does not degrade over time. If you drink water with lead in it, the lead not only permanently damages you but the effects are so severe that they can be passed onto your children. Studies have shown that lead not only diminishes fertility, but when it is ingested or inhaled by girls, the toxin will accumulate in their bones. Years later, the accumulated lead can leave the bones, just like calcium does, and enter the womb "during pregnancy, affecting the fetus," causing all kinds of severe abnormalities.[37]

An article published in 2004 in the *Reviews in Environmental Science and Biotechnology* proved that through the process of phytoremediation, hemp can actually remove these toxic heavy metals from the soil—and if you float hemp on a body of water, like they did with the sunflowers at Chernobyl, hemp can probably remove toxins from drinking water too.[38] Of course, this study was done in Spain because we live in the Fascist States of America, where corporations have taken over every aspect of our government, and no corporation would ever let the American people know that after hemp absorbs the toxins, the crop "leaves a clean, balanced, and nutrient-rich soil, which can then be safely used for agriculture or improving conservation habitats."[39]

Another study from 2003 published in *Industrial Crops and Products* studied how fibre crops (or fiber, as we spell it in the United States) absorb heavy metal deposits from industrially polluted areas in Bulgaria. The researchers exposed flax, hemp, and cotton plants to soil contaminated with heavy metals. Let me just quote their findings:

> Flax and hemp are . . . suitable for growing in industrially polluted regions—they remove considerable quantities of heavy metals from the soil with their root system and can be used as potential crops for cleaning the soil from heavy metals.[40]

Get this: according to *Hemp Diseases and Pests: Management and Biological Control*, the phenomenally researched and all-encompassing book that tells you everything you need to know about how to grow cannabis, hemp has also been known to absorb lithium, uranium, thorium, and even gold from the soil. In Silesia, a country in Eastern Europe with large deposits of minerals, hemp is "deliberately cultivated in wastelands contaminated with cadmium and copper."[41] In every instance:

> The crop efficiently extracts the toxic metals from soil and accumulates the metals in seeds. The crop is harvested, and the metals are recovered by leaching seeds with hydrochloric acid.[42]

Need I say anything further? Well, what the hell, I'll add another study to the list for good measure. The University of Hawaii (UH) used to have a research program to study industrial hemp. The DEA issued a permit for an experimental, quarter-acre plot at the university known as the Hawaii Industrial Hemp Research Program from 1999 to 2003.[43] Much of the research was focused on the phytoremediation properties of hemp and Phytotech was included in part of that research—that is, before UH lost the funding for hemp research in 2003. [44] However, UH conducted a study in 2002 that was published in 2006 in the *International Journal of Phytoremediation* that showed that when hemp was grown in polluted silty clay soil over a brief, twenty-eight-day period, the contaminant levels of the two pollutants—benzo[a]pyrene and chrysene—"were consistently lower."[45] This study was particularly important to Hawaii because it used Hawaiian soil. The study proved how effective growing hemp could be for restoring Hawaii's polluted land so that it can be farmable again.

As of 2016, UH is scheduled to get its funding back for hemp research projects. Under the 2014 Farm Act, the state agreed to allow the university to continue its research uses of hemp, such as biofuel and toxin removal. Local businesses are getting into hemp production too. Alexander and Baldwin Inc. is an agricultural corporation that grows sugar in Maui. In January 2016, the company announced it would start growing hemp on its 36,000-acre plantation and phase out sugar operations by the end of the year.[46] The corporation sees hemp as the economic future for Maui. In fact, Maui is the prefect place to grow hemp. According to Hawaii House Representative Cynthia Thielen, Hawaii "can grow three crops a year, and no other state can" due to its tropical climate.[47] This is why she's been actively pushing for industrial hemp for Hawaii for the past twenty years: she wants her state to lead the nation in producing industrial hemp, and it very well could when we won't even use hemp to restore hazardous waste sites in the United States.

Don't Plant a Tree, Don't Grow Cotton, Plant Hemp

Folks, the EPA estimates that one in four Americans lives within three miles of a hazardous waste site.[48] Why are we not utilizing hemp to restore our homeland? It's a natural resource that grows to full maturity in a four-month growing cycle! It takes twelve to fourteen weeks for hemp to reach maturity, yet it takes twenty years for a tree to do the same! People, forget about planting a tree. Plant hemp! Hemp breathes in four times the carbon dioxide of trees, and one acre of hemp produces as much cellulose fiber pulp as 4.1 acres of trees.[49] It should be illegal *not* to grow hemp! Every American should be contributing to everyone's heath and well-being by growing hemp in the backyard. We have water filtration systems, so why don't we use the best soil filtration system known to mankind, hemp?

Plus, when you consider growing hemp as a crop, it takes less water and leaves less of an environmental impact than cotton (or really any other crop). But since cotton and hemp have been competitors for generations, let's just do a simple comparison between the two crops:

- Cotton plantations need 50 percent more water per season than hemp. That amounts to around 1,400 gal. of water for every pound of cotton you intend to produce.[50]
- Hemp can be grown with little irrigation or little intervention—it's no secret why it's referred to as a *weed.51* In fact, a British study noted that all the water necessary for hemp to grow in the United Kingdom "is met entirely by rainfall."[52]
- On an annual basis, 1 acre of hemp will produce as much fiber as 2 to 3 acres of cotton.[53]
- Hemp fiber is stronger than cotton, it lasts twice as long, and it doesn't mildew.[54] By the way, all those reasons explain why hemp was so valuable for the rigging for ships and parachute chords.
- Then when it comes to processing cotton, the plant uses more than four times the quantity of water that hemp requires to process.
- Hemp doesn't require pesticides or chemicals to grow, but cotton sure does. Some resources state that cotton takes up about 25 percent of the

world's pesticide use.[55] This is why cotton leaves a huge ecological footprint when compared to hemp.

When the Industrial Hemp Farming Act was introduced for the fourth time in 2013, *Forbes* magazine called industrial hemp "a win-win for the economy and the environment."[56] California can grow hemp in a drought. And those wildfires in California that burn acres of forests? Hemp can restore the natural balance of a forest within weeks.[57] People, no further research needs to be done here. To paraphrase *Forbes*, hemp is invaluable to the economy and to the environment. It is an agricultural crop. It is a vegetable. It is *not* a Schedule I narcotic.

But do you want to know something that's truly embarrassing about our government's ban on hemp? It is something worse than paying China for American flags. Even though America's first cash crop was hemp, there is not one original American hemp seed that exists today. We have completely eradicated our hemp seeds.

When the Marijuana Tax Act went into effect, hemp farmers were completely caught off guard. They were under the impression that the Marijuana Tax Act applied to marijuana, not hemp. Everyone knew the difference between the two, or so they thought. Then the federal government showed up and torched the hemp fields in Kentucky and Wisconsin. Only to ask the same farming community to regrow the crop in World War II. And now, here we go again, for the *third* time, trying to make this renewable resource legal again.

To start over with industrial hemp production, we have to import hemp seeds from one of the thirty countries that grow it legally. In 2003, France produced 70 to 80 percent of the hemp used in Europe, with the majority going to pulp for cigarette papers and technical applications,[58] so maybe we'll turn to France for not only seeds but also for advice on how to grow it and how to build necessary machinery. That's why hemp faces so much criticism today: to start up the industry again, we literally have to build it from scratch, and that takes time, money, and commitment, three values our politicians historically don't have the patience for. You can see the lack of patience in the USDA/Bureau of Plant Industry's 1913 *Yearbook of the Department of Agriculture*, when the future of hemp cultivation was so offhandedly dismissed:

Hemp is one of the oldest fiber-producing crops and was formerly the most important. The cultivation of hemp is declining in the United States because of the (1) increasing difficulty in securing sufficient labor for handing the crop with present methods, (2) lack of labor-saving machinery as compared with machinery for handling other crops, (3) increasing profits in other crops, (4) competition of other fibers, especially jute, and (5) lack of knowledge of the crop outside of a limited area in Kentucky.[59]

Yet in the early 1940s, the federal government was encouraging hemp production for WWII and even went so far as to instruct farmers how to grow it (as anyone who had grown it back in the early 1900s was now most likely dead and gone). The USDA's 1935 *Farmers' Bulletin* stated this about hemp:

Hemp is not a hard crop to grow . . . It produces twice as much fiber per acre as flax, and [hemp fiber strength and durability] is known to be suitable for culture and preparation on machinery in this country. . . . Hemp is recommended as a good crop for the Corn Belt States, because of their favorable climate and soil conditions. . . . Although hemp requires a rich soil, it does not remove from the farm an excess of plant-food material . . . [Hemp] returns to the land a large part of the plant nutrients that it removes during its growth. . . . Hemp has been recommended as a weed-control crop. Its dense, tall growth helps to kill out many common weeds. . . . In Wisconsin and Kentucky, where only experienced farmers have grown the crop in recent years, the yields have not varied a great deal. The crop has been reasonably dependable and has not often been injured by storms or droughts."[60]

And when the federal government really needed to convince farmers to grow hemp for the war—this is after the American public was traumatized with the 1937 propaganda film *Reefer Madness*—the USDA had this to say in the 1942 *Hemp for Victory* film:

Hemp is not hard on the soil. In Kentucky it has been grown for several years on the same ground. . . . A dense and shady crop, hemp tends to choke out weeds. Here's a Canada thistle that couldn't stand the competition, dead as a dodo. Thus hemp leaves the ground in good condition for the following crop. . . . This is Kentucky hemp going into the dryer over mill at Versailles. In the old days breaking was done by hand. One of the hardest jobs known to man. Now the power breaker makes quick work of it. . . . All [manufacturing plants] will presently be turning out products spun from American-grown hemp: twine of various kinds for tying and upholsters work; rope for marine rigging and towing; for hay forks, derricks, and heavy duty tackle; light duty fire hose; thread for shoes for millions of American soldiers; and parachute webbing for our paratroopers. . . . American hemp will go on duty again: hemp for mooring ships; hemp for tow lines; hemp for tackle and gear; hemp for countless naval uses both on ship and shore. Just as in the days when Old Ironsides sailed the seas victorious with her hempen shrouds and hempen sails. Hemp for victory![61]

Twenty-nine years later, those five reasons the USDA gave to justify the end of industrial hemp have disappeared due to a world war. Please do not tell me it will take another world war for our country to legalize hemp for good. Knowing our track record, I do fear that will be the case.

Notice that in the 1940s, the bast fiber was primarily utilized for all production purposes. Thanks to technological advances, we now know so much more about what this plant can do. Even though we don't know if or when the Industrial Hemp Act of 2015 will be passed, we do have the 2014 Farm Bill. If you want to see hemp make a comeback without another world war becoming the rational for it, you can check with your state's agricultural department to see how to apply to grow hemp.

Even if our government continues to be willingly ignorant, you can be a hempreneur and grow it for yourself. Remember, hemp benefits the crops grown after it. Hemp is a natural fertilizer; it adds nitrogen to the soil, so it can benefit anyone's backyard vegetable, herb, or flower garden. Hemp also kills weeds naturally, so you don't need to use any herbicides or GMO-modified seeds to keep weeds out of your garden. As the USDA pointed out in 1942, hemp even kills thistle! So in honor of the Hemp for Victory campaign of WWII, here's how to plant hemp as a crop, according to the US government.

The following seven photos were presumably taken during the "Hemp for Victory" campaign. These are the only photographs in the US National Archives that pertain to government-endorsed hemp production in the 1940s. (After the Archives photos, I've included the entire Hemp for Victory brochure.)

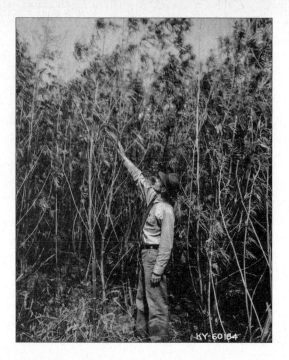

Hemp grown for seed, not fiber, on the farm of Patterson Moore, Georgetown, KY. During the growing season, after pollination, the male stalks are cut out, leaving only the female, or seed-bearing stalks standing. This is the 1940s process of gathering nutritious hemp seed, or most likely, this is the process used to gather hemp seed for more industrial hemp production.
(Credit: Courtesy of the National Archives, photo taken Sept. 1942)

Step one of harvesting hemp for seed on the farm of Patterson Moore. The hemp on this farm has been harvested by an old fashioned reaper that leaves the hemp in bunches on the ground. These bunches are then spread by hand so the hemp can dry before being placed into stacks.
(Credit: Courtesy of the National Archives)

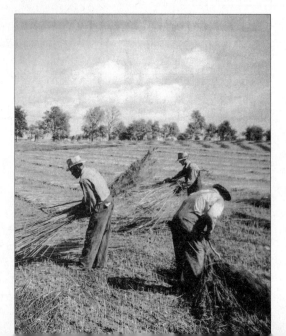

Next 3 photos: On another farm in Lexington, KY, the hemp stalks are cut by hand, then placed in bunches on a canvas sheet. The seed is then threshed out of the plant by hand with flails. (Credit: Courtesy of the National Archives, photos taken October, 1942)

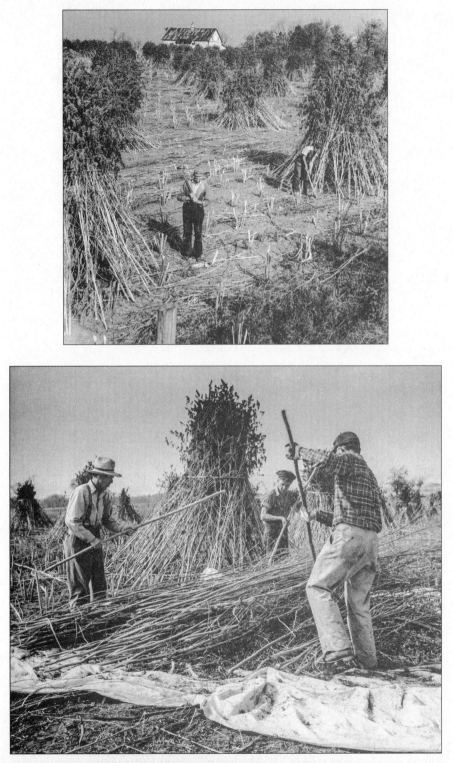

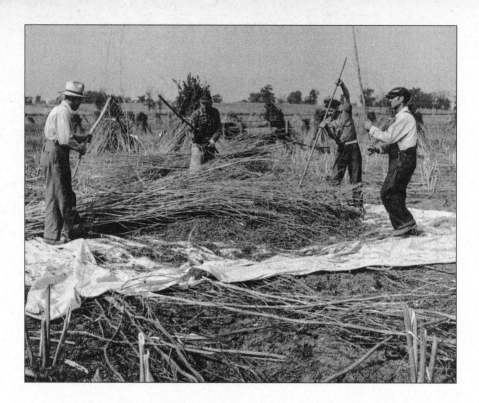

Hemp grown for fiber production. Hemp is seeded with a common grain drill. If a drill especially designed for seeding hemp is not available, many fiber growers double drill to obtain a better distribution of seed.
(Courtesy of the National Archives, taken April, 1942.)

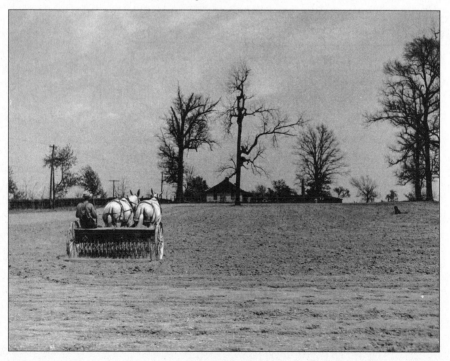

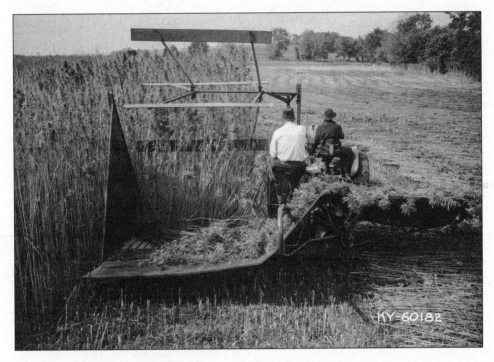

Harvesting hemp on the farm of Brooks Barnes, Winchester, KY with a hemp harvester that cuts and automatically spreads the stalks on the ground. This is the standard type of harvester used in the northern part of the Corn Belt. It is not adapted for use in most Kentucky farms because Kentucky hemp grows tall, and if it is spread immediately, it may sun scald (weakening the fiber) due to Kentucky's climate.
(Credit: Courtesy of the National Archives, taken Sept. 1942.)

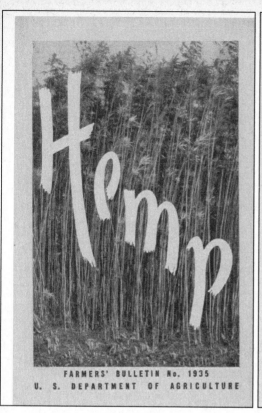

FARMERS' BULLETIN No. 1935
U. S. DEPARTMENT OF AGRICULTURE

Caution

THE HEMP PLANT contains the drug marihuana. Any farmer planning to grow hemp must comply with certain regulations of the Marihuana Tax Act of 1937. This involves registration with the farmer's nearest Internal Revenue Collector and the payment of a fee of $1. Although the fee is small, the registration is mandatory and should not be neglected, as the penalty provisions for not complying with the regulations are very severe. The registration must be renewed each year beginning July 1. This so-called "license" permits a farmer to obtain viable hemp seed from a registered firm dealing in hemp, to plant and grow the crop, and to deliver mature, retted hemp stalks to a hemp mill.

Washington, D. C.

Issued January 1943
Slightly Revised April 1952

HEMP

By B. B. ROBINSON, Senior Agronomist

*Division of Cotton and Other Fiber Crops and Diseases
Bureau of Plant Industry, Soils, and Agricultural Engineering
Agricultural Research Administration*

HEMP is a fiber used in making twines and light cordage. It is also used as an extender for imported cordage fibers, particularly abaca, sisal, and henequen, when supplies of these are not adequate to meet domestic demands. The size of the hemp industry, therefore, is greatly influenced by the availability of imported cordage fibers.

Hemp is not a hard crop to grow. It should be planted on the most productive land on the farm—land that would make 50 to 70 bushels of corn per acre.

The crop is planted with a grain drill and harvested with special machinery rented from hemp mills.

It is allowed to lie on the ground until the outer part of the stalks has rotted, freeing the fibers. This process is called dew retting.

The most important step in hemp farming is to stop the retting process at the proper time. (See pp. 12 and 13.)

This bulletin tells how to grow and harvest hemp. For more information write to the Bureau of Plant Industry, Soils, and Agricultural Engineering, United States Department of Agriculture, or to your State experiment station, or consult your county agent.

What it is

Hemp is an annual plant that grows from seed each year, and therefore it can be brought readily into production. It produces twice as much fiber per acre as flax, the only other fiber that is its equal in strength and durability and that is known to be suitable for culture and preparation on machinery in this country.

When hemp seed is sown thickly for fiber production, the plants usually grow from 5 to 8 feet tall. However, when the plants are thinly spaced in rows for seed production, they may, under favorable conditions, reach a height of 12 to 16 feet. If the plants are not crowded, they become much branched and are bushy. Uniform stems approximately ⅛ inch in diameter and 5 to 8 feet long are especially desired for fiber production, because they can be handled well by the harvesting and processing machinery available in this country.

Hemp is a dioecious plant, that is, the staminate (male) and pis-

---

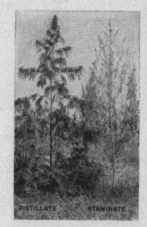

tillate (female) flowers are borne on separate plants, rather than both on one plant. The flowers of the two types of plants are different, but the male plant is easily distinguished from the female, as the anthers are about the size of a wheat kernel. The male plants die soon after discharging their pollen; this is usually about 3 to 5 weeks before the female plants mature seed and die.

The fiber of commerce ranges from 4 to 8 feet in length and has the appearance of a flat, fine ribbon. It lies very close to the epidermis or skin of the plant. Spinners desire the fiber ribbon 1/16 inch or less in width. The long strands of fiber are called "line" fiber to distinguish them from "tow" fiber, which consists of shorter, broken, tangled pieces.

It grows well in the Corn Belt

Hemp is recommended as a good crop for the Corn Belt States, because of their favorable climatic and soil conditions.

Most fiber-producing varieties of hemp require a frost-free growing season of 5 months or longer to produce seed and approximately 4 months for fiber production. Hemp will endure light frosts in the spring and survive frosts in the fall better than corn. It grows best when well supplied with moisture throughout its growing season and especially in its early stages of growth. Drought conditions, if accompanied by high temperatures, appear to hasten maturity before the plants are fully grown.

The vegetative growth of hemp should be uniform. This growth is noticeably affected if the soil is flooded or saturated with moisture for too long a period. The leaves turn yellow, and the plants die. Rainfall, well distributed during the growing season, is, therefore, desirable for uniform vegetative growth. Hemp should be planted only on well-drained soils and not on flat, heavy, impervious soils.

Climate is important not only in the growth of the plant but also in the preparation of the crop after harvest. It influences the method used in handling the crop and the labor requirements, which determine the cost of production. In the United States the common practice (known as dew retting) is to cut the crop and let it lie on the ground. Exposure to the weather causes the fiber in the outer part of the stem to separate. Light snows and alternate freezing and thawing seem to improve or make the retting more uniform.

How to grow it

Soils and Fertilizers

Hemp should not be grown on poor soils. To obtain good yields and fiber of high quality, it is necessary to have a growth of uniform stalks 6 to 8 feet long. Short stalks, from poor nonfertile soils, seldom produce a high-quality fiber.

Fiber hemp grows successfully on soils of the Clarion, Tama, Carrington, Marion, Hagerstown, and Miami series, which, in general, are deep, medium-heavy loams, well-drained, and high in organic matter. Artificially drained areas of the Webster, Brookston, and Maumee series also give satisfactory yields. These soils are among the most productive soils of the Corn Belt. They produce average yields of 50 to 70 bushels or more of corn per acre. If land will not produce from 50 to 70 bushels of corn per acre, it should not be planted to hemp for fiber production.

Muck or peat soils are not recommended for the production of high-quality hemp fiber. The quantity of fiber produced per acre on these soils may be very high, but experience has demonstrated that the fiber lacks strength, which is the first requirement of hemp fiber for good cordage.

The inexperienced farmer usually gets advice from an experienced hemp-mill superintendent in the selection of the right soil. In fact, the farmer's contract to grow hemp usually specifies the exact field that it has been mutually agreed should be used for the hemp crop. This type of supervision by the company contracting for hemp has helped to prevent many crop failures.

Hemp should not be grown continuously on the same soil, for the same reasons that many other crops are not adapted to such practices. In Wisconsin, fields previously used for a cultivated crop are selected for hemp planting in preference to ones upon which small grains have been grown. In Kentucky, bluegrass sod, if obtainable, is selected. Old pastures plowed up are well suited for hemp culture. Fields previously cropped to soybeans, alfalfa, and clover are excellent for hemp. A good rotation is to follow corn with hemp, and in Kentucky a fall cereal may follow the hemp.

Although hemp requires a rich soil, it does not remove from the farm an excess of plant-food material. Nearly all the leaves on the hemp plants, containing much of the plant nutrients removed from the soil, fall off during the growth and maturing of the plant. The remaining leaves may drop off in the field during the process of retting. Further, the plant stems lose about 90 percent in weight of soluble and decomposed materials, which leach out upon the fields, and the stubble may be plowed under. The plant in this manner returns to the land a large part of the plant nutrients that it removes during its growth.

Commercial fertilizers may be used to advantage on soils that are not well supplied with organic matter. Ordinarily, the best ferti-

5

---

lizer for hemp is barnyard manure, but commercial fertilizer can be used to advantage to supplement manure. Lime applications may be supplied on acid soils to advantage. Consult your county agent for recommendations as to amounts of fertilizer and lime to apply.

Seed

The period of flowering of the hemp plant may extend over several weeks, and as a result the seed does not all mature at one time. Hemp seed for sowing frequently contains some immature green to yellowish-green seeds that may not germinate well. Good hemp seed for sowing should be relatively free of such seeds and should germinate 90 percent or better. As the oil content of hemp seed usually ranges between 29 and 34 percent, the seed should be kept cool and dry, as it spoils rapidly under warm and damp conditions. Hemp seed seldom retains its germinating power well enough to be used for seed after 2-years' storage.

When to Plant

Hemp should be planted in the spring just before corn. In a program calling for small spring grains and corn, the farmer should plan to plant his hemp between the time he plants his small grains and the corn.

Seeding

Hemp grown for seed production should be sown in rows or hills. The hills are commonly spaced 5 by 5 feet, with 6 to 10 seeds to the hill, planted not more than ½ inch deep. The plants are thinned to 3 to 5 to a hill. If care is taken to save seed, about 1½ pounds will sow an acre. Most farmers use more seed, and frequently the crop is replanted because of late floods or failure to obtain good stands.

Hemp grown for fiber should be sown with a broadcast seeder or with a grain drill. A drill with 4 inches between drill tubes is preferred to one with 6 inches or more. The seed should not be planted deeper than 1 inch, and a depth of ½ inch is preferred. If the seed is planted deep, the hemp seedling is not capable of pushing its way to the surface of the ground. A slight crust on the ground frequently results in a poor stand. If the seedbed is loose, disks on a seed drill may cut too deep into the soil and the seed will be sown more than 1 inch deep. In such cases, to make certain that the disks do not cut too deep into the seedbed, they should be tied to the seed box.

A standard bushel of hempseed weighs 44 pounds. The rate of seeding hemp for fiber production ranges between 3 and 5 pecks of seed per acre. In Kentucky, where hemp is hand-broken, it has been the practice to sow 3 pecks (33 pounds) per acre. However, when the hemp is to go to the mill, 1 bushel per acre gives a product that is better suited to milling. Wisconsin and other Corn Belt farmers have commonly sown 4 pecks per acre. The lighter rate of seeding in Kentucky produces larger stalks. These stalks are easily broken, and the fiber is easily prepared by the hand-breaking methods that have been used there since colonial days. Machine methods of breaking and scutching to prepare the fiber are used in Wisconsin, and

6

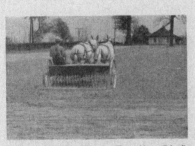

recently to some extent in Kentucky. The machines will handle finer stems, and the sowing of 5 pecks is advisable where hemp is to be prepared by machine.

A good practice in planting hemp for fiber production is to sow around the edge of the field next to the fence a 16- to 18-foot width of small grains, which may be harvested before the hemp. Space is thus provided for the harvester to enter the field and begin cutting without injuring the hemp. It also prevents hemp plants at the edge from growing too rank. Uniform plants are necessary for uniform fiber quality.

Culture

Fall plowing in Wisconsin gives better results with hemp than spring plowing.

Hemp for fiber production requires little or no cultivation or care after planting until the harvest; but if, after seeding and before the seedlings emerge, the ground crusts badly it may be advisable to roll the field to break the crust. Hemp for seed production should be cultivated the same as corn; that is, sufficiently to keep back the weeds. Spudding out Canada thistles where they appear in dense stands in hemp fields should be done when the hemp is only a few inches high. In most cases hemp will compete well with weeds, if the hemp gets off to a good start.

Varieties to grow

The fiber hemp grown in the United States by the early colonists was of European origin; but our present hemp, commonly known as Kentucky or domestic hemp, is of Chinese origin. Few importations of hempseed have been made in recent years for commercial plantings, as imported seed has not proved as productive under domestic conditions as Kentucky hemp.

7

Enemies

In the United States there are no hemp diseases of economic importance, and hemp has not been seriously attacked by insects. The European corn borer and similar stem-boring insects occasionally kill a hemp stem. However, they have not proved important, perhaps because hemp has not been grown to any extent in the sections of the United States where the European corn borer is a serious pest. Seedling plants are frequently attacked by cutworms and white grubs after spring plowing of sod land.

Broom rape is a small weed 6 to 15 inches high that is parasitic on the roots of hemp, tobacco, and tomatoes. It usually grows in clumps and has purple flowers, which produce many very small seeds. These adhere to the waxy flower parts surrounding the hempseed and are distributed in this manner. Broom rape can be very serious on hemp if proper control measures are not followed. Only well-cleaned hempseed and seed from fields containing no broom rape should be sown.

Hemp has been recommended as a weed-control crop. Its dense, tall growth helps to kill out many common weeds. The noxious bindweed, a member of the morning-glory family, is checked to some extent by hemp. Unfortunately, bindweed and several other species of morning-glory have seeds so near the same size and weight of hemp seed that mixtures obtained in producing hempseed are carried to the field planted for fiber production. In growing hemp for seed all vine weeds of this type found on the hemp stalks should be removed before the hemp plants begin to produce seed.

Harvesting

Time to Harvest

Hemp is harvested for seed production when the plant on being shaken sheds most of its seed. This occurs when the seeds are fully mature on the middle branches. The seeds will mature on the lower branches first and on the top of the plant last. The common method

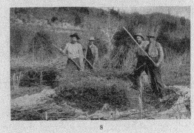

8

of harvesting hemp for seed production is to cut it by hand and shock it to permit more seed to mature and cure before threshing. The harvesting should be in the early morning or on damp days when the seeds do not shatter so much as they do in the warmer and drier part of the day. Threshing of the seed hemp should be done on dry afternoons. In threshing, the seed shocks should be placed on large canvas cloths 24 by 24 feet and then be beaten with long sticks to remove the seed.

Hemp is harvested for fiber production when the male plants are in full flower and are shedding pollen. By harvesting before the male plants die, the retting of both male and female plants is more uniform, as both types of plants are still green and growing. The harvesting period may extend for 2 weeks or longer. Very early harvested hemp may produce a finer and softer fiber than that harvested later, but it is usually weaker. The fiber from hemp that has been harvested so late that many seeds have matured does not possess so good cordage and textile characteristics as fiber from hemp harvested earlier. Hemp stalks should be relatively free of leaves except a few at the very top before harvesting. This is important when hemp is shocked after harvest, as it makes the top of the shock smaller so that less rain can enter the shock.

Machinery

Harvesting methods vary with locality and climate. In Kentucky, hemp may grow to a height of 15 feet or more. These long stalks are difficult to handle with machinery. Self-rake reapers (see below) have been used in harvesting hemp for many years, and they probably do better work with very tall hemp than any other machine now available. A modified rice binder, which cuts and

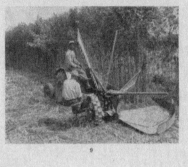

9

binds the hemp into bundles, is also available, although difficulty in handling the very tall hemp may be experienced. This latter type of machine can be used for short hemp in areas, such as Kentucky, where hemp must be shocked within a few days after harvest to avoid sunburn.

In the northern part of the Corn Belt the hemp usually does not grow so tall and therefore can be handled more easily with machines. During the first World War hemp-harvesting machinery was developed. These harvesters (see above) in one operation cut an 8- or 9-foot swath and elevate the stalks to a quarter-circle platform where they are turned automatically and dropped or spread on the ground for retting. The butts of the stems all lie in the same direction and are relatively even. The thickness of the layer of stalks in the swath influences the speed and uniformity of the dew retting. Machines of this type, because of their labor economy, are recommended for use in the Northern States, where hemp can be safely spread for retting when harvested.

Hemp harvesters are usually owned by the hemp mills. They are rented to the individual farmers, who usually furnish the motive power and the labor to run the harvesters.

Retting

Retting is the partial rotting of the hemp stalk. It permits the fiber in the stalk to separate easily in long strands from the woody core. The fiber strands break if unretted stems are bent or broken.

In this country the usual practice is to ret hemp by allowing it to lie on the ground, where it is exposed to rain and dew. This method is called dew retting.

Dew retting is dependent upon dews and rains to furnish the moist conditions necessary for the growth of the molds that cause the retting. In warm, moist weather the retting may require 1 to 2 weeks, but usually 4 to 5 weeks is required for retting in Kentucky and Wisconsin. Hemp has remained spread under snow in Wisconsin until spring without serious injury, but more often hemp left under snow all winter is overretted and ruined.

10

Underretting and Overretting

If hemp stalks are lifted from the ground before they are sufficiently retted, the fiber will not separate easily from the woody hurds (small pieces of the woody core of the plant) in milling. However, if the retting is permitted to go too far, the fiber separates very readily from the core, but the adhesive substance between the individual fiber cells in the long strand breaks down and the fiber is weak. Hemp further overretted produces mostly short broken strands of fiber called tow fiber, which is less valuable than the long parallel strands of fiber called line fiber.

Nowhere in the growing or processing of hemp is good judgment more needed than in determining the time to end the ret. Experience and good judgment are necessary to determine just when the hemp stalks should be lifted from the field and bundled. The lifting and shocking stops the retting action. The value of the fiber can be cut in half or entirely lost by several days' overretting in warm weather.

Sunburning

In Kentucky, hemp spread immediately to ret after harvest is apt to sunburn, or sunscald. It is common belief that the hot, bright days in August and September in some way cause deterioration of the fiber if spread for retting. Sunburned fiber is uneven in color, usually has less strength, and possibly is drier and more harsh than fiber not sunburned. In order to avoid sunscalding, the hemp is shocked after being harvested and not spread for retting until the cooler days of November. In locations having climatic conditions similar to those prevailing in Wisconsin, sunscald of hemp is rare.

Turning Stalks

In dew retting the spread stalks should be turned once or more during the retting period. This aids in bleaching the stalks and results in fiber of more uniform color and quality. The turning is

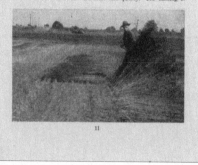

11

done by workmen using bent poles approximately 8 to 10 feet in length. The poles are pushed under the head ends of stalks in the swath, and the stalks are turned over without moving the butt ends.

In turning the straw the workmen start in the middle of the field, turning the first swath into vacant center space. The second swath will be turned to lie where the first swath had been, and so on.

Care should be exercised in turning to prevent the stalks from tangling. The more hemp is handled, the more tangled the stalks may become. Tangled hemp is more difficult to process and produces a high proportion of tangled, short, tow fiber.

Testing the End Point of the Ret

A few days too long in the field may make the difference between retting and rotting. Therefore, it is most important that inexperienced farmers obtain the assistance of the hemp-mill superintendent or an experienced grower in determining when to stop the retting.

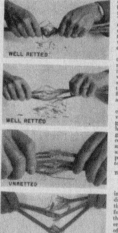

WELL RETTED

WELL RETTED

UNRETTED

UNRETTED

Dry hemp stalks should be tested when possible to determine the degree of retting. Three to six stalks are taken in both hands and bent back and forth to perform the break test. If properly retted, the fiber should not break when the woody core breaks. The hurds should fall free of the fiber in the breaking and shaking between one's hands. If the hemp is only partly retted, some hurds will adhere to the loosened fiber. Unretted hemp fiber is usually green or light yellow. Dew-retted hemp is usually slate gray or black.

After the fiber is broken free, its strength should be tested by break-

12

ing a small strand between the fingers. A small strand of fiber not twisted and about $\frac{1}{32}$ inch wide should break with great difficulty and with a decided snap. If it is very weak and breaks with little or no snap the hemp is probably badly overretted or may have been grown under unfavorable cultural conditions. (See p. 3.)

An indication that the retting end point is near is that the hemp makes "bowstrings." In a small percentage of the stems, less than 1 to 5 percent under certain conditions, the middle of the stalks appears to ret first. The fiber comes free from the middle and forms a string fastened at the top and bottom of the stem, not unlike a bowstring. If bowstring occurs as fixed, a sample of the hemp should be taken to the hemp-mill superintendent as soon as possible for verification of the retting end point. The bowstring condition is only a supplementary aid in determining when to stop the retting, and it may or may not occur in properly dew-retted hemp.

Some experienced hemp producers use the peeling test for determining the degree of retting. This is accomplished by peeling the fiber away from the butt ends of the stems. If properly retted, the fiber should peel freely from the woody core of the stem. If the hemp is not sufficiently retted, the fiber will break after a few inches have been peeled. This free-peeling stage is desirable for breaking hemp on hand breaks. Where hemp is to be processed by machinery the retting need not progress quite so far as is necessary for hand breaking.

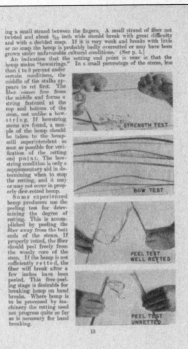

STRENGTH TEST

BOW TEST

PEEL TEST
WELL RETTED

PEEL TEST
UNRETTED

13

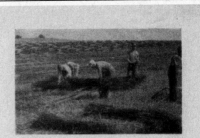

Picking Up the Retted Stalks

Hemp stalks may be picked up by hand. This method has been used from early times and is satisfactory where labor is plentiful. However, in this country it is being replaced by machine pick-up binders.

In picking up the straw by hand, small sticks about 5 feet long with a single steel or wooden hook on the end are used. The hemp is raked into bunches with these implements, and usually tied. Hemp-fiber bands are used in tying the bundles. An inexpensive "buck" (see above) may be used to bunch the hemp, or it may be bunched with a pitchfork.

The most efficient method is to use the pick-up binder. These machines, drawn by tractors, cover about an acre an hour. They

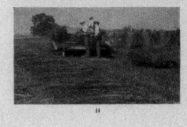

14

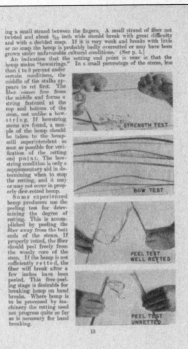

pick up the retted hemp stalks and tie them into bundles in one operation. The machines are part of the modern hemp-mill equipment and are rented to farmers.

Dew-retted hemp is usually shocked after being picked up. The hemp remains in the shock until it is transported to the mill.

Extra Care Insures Extra Profits

The farmer's job is done when he delivers the hemp to the mill. All further processing to prepare the fiber is part of the milling operation. However, it is of interest to both farmers and mill operators to attempt to keep the hemp stalks and fiber well butted. This means keeping the butt ends of the stalks or fiber in a bundle all even. Every time the hemp stalks are handled, care should be taken to see that this is done. If the hemp stalks are well butted in the bundle when processed, the milling operations can be carried out more economically. Tangled, uneven bundles are more difficult and require more time to handle. The yield of high-value long-life fiber is much greater if the stalks are well butted.

Hemp stalks are considered most desirable if they are less than half an inch in diameter. The thickness of a pencil is frequently used to illustrate the size of desirable stalks. The larger diameter stalks have a lower percentage of fiber than finer stems, are harder to break, and produce more tow fiber.

Hemp stalks grown on unproductive soil usually contain a lower percentage of fiber, and this fiber may be coarse, harsh, and of low strength, so that it breaks into tow in milling.

Stalks underretted frequently must be run through the mill breaker a second or third time to remove the remaining hurds. This increases the milling labor costs, and the resultant fiber may be reduced to a low grade. On the other hand, overretted hemp must be milled as little as possible, with less pressure exerted on the rollers and a slower speed of the scutcher wheel to keep from making an excess amount of tow fiber.

15

Yields

Hemp yields have been extremely variable when this crop has been planted in new areas by inexperienced farmers. In Wisconsin and Kentucky, where only experienced farmers have grown the crop in recent years, the yields have not varied a great deal. The crop has been reasonably dependable and has not often been injured by storms or droughts.

The average yields per acre for experienced farmers are approximately $2\frac{1}{4}$ to $2\frac{1}{2}$ tons of air-dry retted hemp stalks; 850 pounds total fiber. Under the Wisconsin machine-milling system the yields may average 450 pounds line fiber and 400 pounds tow fiber; under the Kentucky hand-breaking system they may average 775 pounds Kentucky rough and 75 pounds tow.

If hemp is planted for seed production, the average yield per acre are approximately 15 bushels or 660 pounds, on bottom land, and 12 bushels on uplands.

16

U. S. GOVERNMENT PRINTING OFFICE: 1952

For sale by the Superintendent of Documents, U. S. Government Printing Office
Washington 25, D. C. - Price 15 cents

19

Hemp for Nutrition!

Okay, so we've established that if we're serious about restoring the environment and if we're serious about rebuilding our economy, we should be growing hemp. We should also be growing hemp for its nutritional value. In the USDA's 1964 Yearbook of Agriculture, our government refers to hemp as a vegetable:

> HEMP (Cannabis sativa) is nearly as old as flax and is nearer like flax than any of the other vegetable fibers.[1]

So I will continue to state that hemp is a vegetable. Before I get into the nutritional facts, I want to revisit a few issues from chapter 18, namely the DEA and Hemp for Victory.

Get this: the USDA denied making *Hemp for Victory!* until two VHS copies were donated to the Library of Congress in 1989 by Jack Herer, the author of *The Emperor Wears No Clothes,* which is the encyclopedia of all things cannabis. The Zapruder film opened many people's eyes to the conspiracy behind JFK's assassination, and *Hemp for Victory!* opened a lot of people's eyes to the government's convenient double standard on a plant.

The unofficial story goes like this: Jack Herer was given an original copy of *Hemp for Victory!* by William Conde (a marijuana activist), and Conde received it from a reporter at the Miami Herald.[2] Conde met Jack Herer during the 1984

Oregon Marijuana Initiative. Yes, Oregon has been trying since the '80s to legalize marijuana! (In case you didn't know, the state legalized limited medical marijuana in 1998,[3] industrial hemp in 2009,[4] and recreational weed on July 1, 2015[5]). Thanks to William Conde and Jack Herer, you can now watch *Hemp for Victory!* all over the Internet, much to the federal government's embarrassment. However, if you try to search for *Hemp for Victory!* in the national archives (www.archives. gov), you'll come up empty handed, even though the national archives contain video footage and still photos from WWII.

If you know your history, then you know why the government didn't want *Hemp for Victory!* to become common knowledge. Did you notice the "Caution" section in the USDA's how-to-grow-hemp instructional manual? The farmer must register with the government to grow hemp and send the IRS a payment fee of $1 in order to be in compliance with the law. Every year, the registration must be renewed if the farmer wants to continue to grow the crop. Well, once the war was over, that application to grow hemp suddenly wasn't issued. The government stopped the farmers from growing hemp by not allowing them to register or re-register to grow it.

A United States Special Tax Stamp issued for a Producer of Marihuana in July 1945. This document is related to the US Hemp for Victory campaign, which allowed production of hemp for the US WWII effort. The government stopped issuing the stamp to farmers at the conclusion of WWII, which also allowed the government to end hemp production seamlessly.

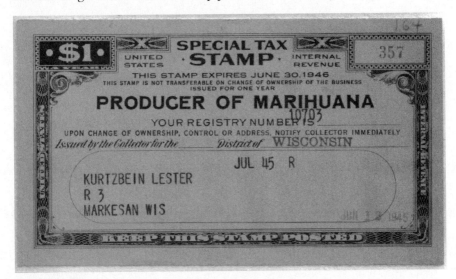

credit: Public domain

Today, that basic principle still applies. Anyone who wants to grow the crop is supposed to contact the DEA and ask for a license to grow it. Yet, nine times out of ten, the DEA refuses to issue licenses for research purposes. And why would they when another research facility would compete with the DEA's own research facility in Ole Miss? Even on its website, the DEA admits it has never once issued a commercial permit for hemp production: "DEA has not in the past granted any registrations for the cultivation of marijuana for industrial purposes."[6] Why is that? Because "the cultivation of the marijuana plant exclusively for commercial/industrial purposes has many associated risks relating to diversion into the illicit drug traffic."[7] Excuse me? Name me one farmer from the Hemp for Victory era who risked his license to grow hemp in order to become a drug trafficker. And while you're at it, quit referring to hemp as marijuana. They are two different plants!

In 1999, the state of North Dakota passed a state law to authorize industrial hemp production, and lawmakers asked the DEA repeatedly for the license to grow it for research purposes, but as of 2016, the state has yet to receive one.[8] Since states know the DEA will not issue the permits, they are going around the agency through the 2014 Farm Bill. Take Oregon, for instance. The state legalized industrial hemp in 2009, but wasn't able to get permits from the DEA, so the state legislatures pretty much said screw it and issued their own licenses in 2015. Currently thirteen farms in Oregon have a license to grow hemp. The licenses are valid for three years, and they were sold for $1,500 apiece.[9]

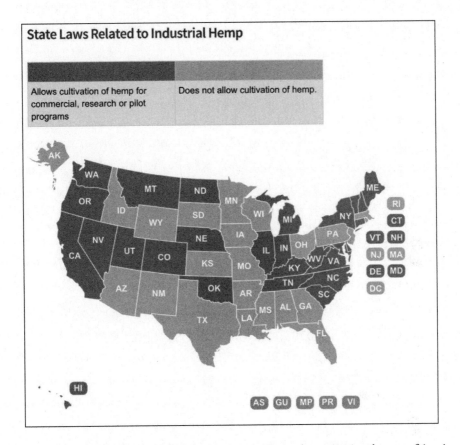

State Laws Related to Industrial Hemp

Allows cultivation of hemp for commercial, research or pilot programs

Does not allow cultivation of hemp.

According to the DEA, the agency is the only entity in charge of issuing licenses under the Controlled Substances Act and the act requires the DEA to make a "determination" if "any such production" of industrial hemp "would be in the public interest."[10] Did you catch that? President Nixon's Controlled Substance Act states that the only agency to determine if industrial hemp is in the public's best interest is the same agency in charge of confiscating it. How the hell is that not a conflict of interest?

This is what the average person has to go through to try to obtain an industrial hemp license from the DEA:[11]

- The DEA application includes a nonrefundable fee, the cost is based on several factors.
- All people employed to grow hemp must go through FBI background checks. No one can have a criminal record relating to marijuana.

- The farmer must set up a "security protocol" at the production site, such as "security fencing around the planting area, a twenty-four-hour monitoring system, controlled access, and possibly armed guard(s) to prevent public access."[12]
- Then that security protocol must be inspected by the DEA and proven effective.
- Other unnamed "factors" are also considered to determine if the operation is for "public health and safety."[13]

This is why the DEA seized imported hemp seeds from Kentucky and Colorado. Congress found a way around the DEA to benefit the economy and the DEA is pissed! You better hope and pray that the 2014 Farm Bill isn't altered in any way moving forward.

According to a Congressional Research Report from February 2015, here are the states on the DEA's most wanted list:[14]

- Eighteen states have laws to provide for industrial hemp production and research, as described by the 2014 Farm Bill: California, Colorado, Hawaii, Indiana, Kentucky, Maine, Minnesota, Montana, Nebraska, New York, North Dakota, Oregon, South Carolina, Tennessee, Utah, Vermont, Washington, and West Virginia.
- Twenty-eight states and Puerto Rico have introduced or carried over industrial hemp legislation: Alabama, Arizona, California, Colorado, Connecticut, Delaware, Hawaii, Illinois, Indiana, Kentucky, Maryland, Massachusetts, Michigan, Minnesota, Mississippi, Missouri, Nebraska, New Hampshire, New Jersey, New York, Oklahoma, South Carolina, South Dakota, Tennessee, Utah, Washington, West Virginia, and Wisconsin.
- Several states have passed hemp resolutions, such as listing hemp as an agricultural crop, including California, Colorado, Illinois, Maine, Montana, New Hampshire, New Mexico, North Dakota, Oregon, Vermont, and Virginia.
- Several states have passed bills to create commissions and authorize research studies, including Hawaii, Kentucky, Maryland, Arkansas, Illinois, Maine, Minnesota, New Mexico, North Carolina, North Dakota, and Vermont. Other states have done studies without a legislative directive.

As of 2016, industrial hemp has been growing "legally" in states like Colorado, Kentucky, Oregon, and Vermont.[15]

Just like medical and recreational marijuana has its own groups of activists and lobbyists, there are national organizations standing up for hemp. These organizations have written to the president, to the attorney general, even to the DEA and Congress in the hopes that this crop will become legal:[16]

- The National Farmers Union (NFU) updated its 2013 farm policy to urge the president, attorney general, and Congress to "direct the US Drug Enforcement Administration (DEA) to reclassify industrial hemp as a noncontrolled substance and adopt policy to allow American farmers to grow industrial hemp under state law without affecting eligibility for USDA benefits." Previously NFU's policy advocated that the DEA "differentiate between industrial hemp and marijuana and adopt policy to allow American farmers to grow industrial hemp under state law without requiring DEA licenses."

- The National Association of State Departments of Agriculture (NASDA) "supports revisions to the federal rules and regulations authorizing commercial production of industrial hemp," and has urged USDA, DEA, and the Office of National Drug Control Policy to "collaboratively develop and adopt an official definition of industrial hemp that comports with definitions currently used by countries producing hemp." NASDA also "urges Congress to statutorily distinguish between industrial hemp and marijuana and to direct the DEA to revise its policies to allow USDA to establish a regulatory program that allows the development of domestic industrial hemp production by American farmers and manufacturers."

- In 2014, the American Farm Bureau Federation, from efforts led by the Indiana Farm Bureau, endorsed a policy to support the "production, processing, commercialization, and utilization of industrial hemp," and reportedly also passed a policy resolution to oppose the "classification of industrial hemp as a controlled substance." Previously, in 1995, the Farm Bureau had passed a resolution supporting "research into the viability and economic potential of industrial hemp production in the United

States . . . [and] further recommend that such research includes planting test plots in the United States using modern agricultural techniques."

- Regional farmers' organizations also have policies regarding hemp. For example, the North Dakota Farmers Union (NDFU), as part of its federal agricultural policy recommendations, has urged "Congress to legalize the production of industrial hemp." The Rocky Mountain Farmers Union (RMFU) has urged "Congress and the USDA to re-commit and fully fund research into alternative crops and uses for crops" including industrial hemp; also, they "support the decoupling of industrial hemp from the definition of marijuana" under the CSA and "demand the president and the attorney general direct the US Drug Enforcement Agency (DEA) to differentiate between industrial hemp and marijuana and adopt a policy to allow American farmers to grow industrial hemp under state law without requiring DEA licenses," to "legalize the production of industrial hemp as an alternative crop for agricultural producers."

- In California, ongoing efforts to revise the definition of marijuana to exclude "industrial hemp" are supported by the State's Sheriffs' Association. Previous efforts in 2011 to establish a pilot program to grow industrial hemp were supported by the county farm bureau and two sheriff's offices, but Governor Brown vetoed them. (Remember, Brown is bought by the private prison industry, among other special interest groups opposed to hemp.)

I'm sure you're not surprised that the majority of law enforcement groups are not advocating for industrial hemp. For example, the California Narcotic Officer's Association claims "allowing for industrial hemp production would undermine state and federal enforcement efforts to regulate marijuana production," because hemp and marijuana "are not distinguishable through ground or aerial surveillance," so local law enforcement agencies "would require costly and time-consuming lab work to be conducted" on hemp farms to ensure no marijuana plants were being grown.[17]

Really? That's what we've come to? When it's legal in California to grow medical marijuana in your house, this is the answer law enforcement is giving us in regards to hemp? Look, I could be farming corn in Nebraska and I could be growing pot plants in the center of my cornfield. I'm sure there's a farmer somewhere in America doing that right now. If someone wants to risk their hemp license to grow marijuana on the side, then that person is going to break the law and grow marijuana. That person is probably growing marijuana right now anyway, so what's the difference?

Look, farmers in Kentucky are growing hemp right now. Kentucky has extremely strict marijuana laws—just ask Navy veteran Raymond Schwab from chapter 12. Do you really think a law-abiding person is going to risk his entire livelihood—his entire farm—to break the law and grow pot? If you're growing hemp, you already have a target on your back. Why the hell would you want to cause anyone to pull the trigger? Yet this is the justification we hear from law enforcement time and time again.

Law enforcement isn't interested in the fact that hemp is a superfood. They're not interested in the fact that the USDA refers to hemp as a vegetable. Meanwhile, studies have proven that hemp has significant health benefits. Hemp has an excellent content of omega-3 and omega-6 fatty acids, which are crucial for cardiovascular health, brain development, and memory retention.

A 2010 study by the University of Manitoba and Institute of Cardiovascular Sciences in Canada and the Cardiovascular Research Division of the V. I. Lenin Universitary Hospital in Cuba observed the following:[18]

- The omega-6 concentration in hempseed can prevent strokes due to the way it inhibits clot formation in blood platelets. In other words, it reduces inflammation, which may decrease the risk of strokes and heart disease.
- When rabbits that were fed a high-cholesterol diet were given a 10 percent hempseed supplement to their high-cholesterol diet, blood platelets responsible for heart attacks and clogged arteries "normalized." In other words, the rabbits were at a high risk of developing a clogged artery or a heart attack due to the high concentration of cholesterol in their diet. With a small amount of hempseed, that risk greatly diminished.
- Higher dosages of hempseed can actually lower a person's cholesterol levels naturally. Hempseed contains linoleic acid, which has been known to lower both LDL-C and HDL-C levels of cholesterol.
- Hempseed can also prevent and control high blood pressure.
- The study concluded that "hempseed has the potential to beneficially influence heart disease."[19]

Hemp seeds are also high in fiber, iron, phosphorus, potassium, calcium, zinc, vitamin E, and magnesium—"a mineral that helps with relaxation, blood sugar control, blood pressure, and potentially osteoporosis."[20] It contains all twenty amino acids, including the nine of the essential amino acids our bodies cannot produce.[21] The nutritional benefits of hemp seeds are similar to chia seeds, quinoa, and flaxseeds. However, hemp provides 50 to 75 percent more protein than flax or chai.[22] Hemp seeds taste similar to pine nuts, and most people sprinkle them on salads or in yogurt.

Three tablespoons of hulled hemp seeds contain 10 g of protein, 14 g of healthy fat (from omega-3 and omega-6 fats), and 2 g of fiber.[23] This is why hemp protein is often found in powdered protein supplements or protein shakes. If you want to compare hemp seeds to animal protein, about seven tablespoons of hemp seeds can provide the same amounts of protein as what's found in a 3 oz., single-serving size of beef or lamb.

1 Tablespoon	Flax	Chia	Hemp
Total Fat	4.5	4g	4.6
Omega-3s	2300 mg	2340 mg	1000 mg
Omega-6	600 mg	800 mg	2500 mg
Protein	2 g	25 g	35
Fiber	3g	5g	0.3g
Calories	55	60	57

Hemp seeds are also easier to digest than grains, nuts, and legumes like peanuts. If you want to get the most nutritional value out of hemp, then go with whole hemp seeds over hulled hemp seeds. Whole hemp seeds are a good source of both soluble (20 percent) and insoluble (80 percent) fiber.[24] Soluble fiber helps with digestion, and it is also linked to reducing blood sugar and regulating cholesterol levels. Insoluble fiber helps our digestive system and our gut expel more waste.[25] It is also linked to reducing the risk of diabetes, particularly type 2 diabetes.[26]

Overall, hemp seeds are incredibly good for you and they have also been known to:

- Benefit skin disorders, such as eczema due to the three-to-one ratio of omega-6 and omega-3. A 2005 study in Finland compared dietary hempseed oil and olive oil in a twenty-week randomized, single-blind crossover study. The study proved that hempseed oil improved skin dryness and itchiness. The patients also decreased their usual dosage of dermal medication because the oil "caused significant changes" in their dermatitis.[27]

- Relieve PMS symptoms. Gamma-linolenic acid (GLA) is found in hemp seeds and it produces prostaglandin E1, which reduces the effects of prolactin. (Prolactin is what causes PMS.) A 2011 study in Brazil found that women who received a dose of 210 mg of GLA per day plus 1 g of fatty acid saw significant decreases in PMS symptoms.[28] Irritability, depression, and other mood-related symptoms were also alleviated.[29] What's hemp seed made out of? GLA and fatty acid (omega-3 and omega-6).

- Reduce menopause symptoms. In a 2010 veterinary study in Iran, hempseed was given to twenty female rats in different dosages. In each case, the hempseed regulated hormone imbalances and inflammation associated with menopause, and even elevated calcium levels.[30]

- Enhance calcium absorption and increase calcium deposition in bone. A 1998 study in South Africa administered GLA for eighteen months to women with the mean age of 79.5. These women had a low calcium diet and markers of bone degradation. Patients saw lumbar spine density increase in a rage of 3.1 to 4.7 percent. The study proved that GLA has "beneficial effects on bone" for "elderly patients" and it is "safe to administer for prolonged periods of time."[31]

- Improvements in skin quality, stronger fingernails, and thicker hair due to "modest daily usage" of hemp oil. According to doctors, "such improvements are considered as good indications of general health."[32] By simply removing oil and butter from your diet and supplementing hemp oil, you'll see improvements in skin quality within two and four weeks; fingernails within two and four months; and thicker hair within six and eight months.

- Rapid healing properties. A recent clinical study took patients recovering from eye, nose, and throat surgery and topically applied hempseed oil to demonstrate a faster rate of healing and recovery.

Hempseed oil is better than Neosporin to help heal simple cuts and burns. It also elevates allergic reactions.[33]

- Strengthen the immune system. Hempseed "has been used to treat nutritional deficiencies brought on by tuberculosis, a severe nutrition blocking disease that causes the body to waste away."[34]

How can one little seed do so much? Well, hemp seeds contain essential fatty acids (EFAs), such as polyunsaturated fatty acids (PUFAs), that the human body is not able to produce on its own, but relies on for proper health and development. These fatty acids are fundamental for strengthening our immune system and our overall health.

A 2004 study from the University of Kuopio, in Finland, explains why Americans are at a huge disadvantage for not utilizing hemp:

Hempseed is an excellent source of nutrition. Indications from traditional Chinese medicine, recent anecdotal reports and modern human clinical trials agree that hempseed has health promoting properties that are supported by results from nutritional analyses of the seed, oil and seed meal. In particular, the healing properties of hempseed can be attributed to high levels of EFAs and other PUFAs in the oil, in addition to a rich source of important amino acids in an easily digested protein. Recent feeding trials with fish, hens and ruminants, in addition to empirical observations over thousands of years, have effectively demonstrated that hempseed and its derivatives are useful in animal feed as well. Subjective concerns over THC in hemp foods are not supported by scientific evidence.[35]

Did you get that last part? There isn't any THC in hemp foods. Not even 0.3 percent THC—which is what is produced in most industrial hemp plants—is transferred to the seed. In China, roasted hempseed is sold as snacks by street venders. In Russia, hempseed oil is used as a substitute for butter and margarine (both are more expensive and less healthy than hempseed oil).[36] Yet, don't our politicians constantly bash on Russia and China for taking away their people's freedoms and rights through communism? Seems to me that the people of Russia and China are at a significant health advantage. Meanwhile, our leaders are obstructing our freedom by continuing to classify a superfood containing vegetable protein as a Schedule I narcotic.

And just so you know, there is a way to remove that 0.3 percent THC from hemp plants. The makers of Charlotte's Web have already created a strain with less than 0.3 percent THC. Due to request from its government, the Ukrainian Institute of Bast Crops has also reduced THC to 0.1 percent or less in the hemp grown in Ukraine.[37] They started doing this in 1988, so that tells you the hemp used at Chernobyl had 0.1 percent THC or less. Folks, you cannot get high off of 0.3 percent THC and you certainly cannot get high off of 0.1 percent THC. But, in either case, THC isn't transferred to hemp seeds or any of the goods manufactured from industrial hemp, so there's no need to panic if you ingest hemp foods, wear hemp products, or apply lotion containing hemp oil.

Since hempseed is such a commodity, most American health food stores now sell imported hemp seeds from Canada. You might have to order hemp oil online, as that's not commonly found in stores, but if you're really interested in doing so, you can also purchase hemp milk and hempseed butter (otherwise known as hempspread), which is similar to peanut butter. The best part about these products is that if you have severe food allergies—from peanuts to lactose intolerance to soy—hemp can be a natural alternative that provides you with a similar source of protein.[38] All that and more is sold on sites like Amazon, and if you do a simple Google search, you'll notice that for the very first time since the Marijuana Tax Act and *Hemp for Victory!* you can find small businesses and family farms that are making these products right here in the USA and shipping them across the country—thanks to the 2014 Farm Bill.

20

Cooking with Cannabis—Hemp and Marijuana

People have been cooking and baking with hemp and marijuana for centuries. Ever since states have legalized marijuana in some form, marijuana dispensaries have been selling food with CBD, THC, and hemp. Food containing CBD and/or THC is referred to as edibles—and you can get just about anything with CBD and/or THC in it. There are even restaurants that cook with cannabis and cater to medical marijuana patients. What many people might find surprising is that different strains of marijuana have different effects. For instance, if you have chronic pain, there are certain strains that target that pain better than others.

So why would you eat your medicine instead of smoke it? Some people just don't like smoking, but whatever the personal preference, the effects from smoking and eating marijuana are different. When a person eats marijuana, the effects are typically stronger and felt for a longer period of time. This is because of the process of digestion. Our livers metabolize cannabis by turning delta-9 THC into 11-hydroxy-THC.[1] When this happens, 11-hydroxy-THC passes the blood-brain barrier more rapidly and there's a stronger effect than what is felt when a person smokes or vaporizes cannabis. Essentially, because the liver doesn't get involved when marijuana is smoked or vaped, the effects are not the same.

When someone smokes marijuana, the effects kick in much faster, and a person can feel the sensation in a matter of minutes, if not seconds. With each puff, the body receives more THC at a faster and higher concentration. The "peak" concentration from THC can happen in five to ten minutes. However, as I mentioned earlier, when a person eats marijuana, it takes longer for the medication to kick in but the effects last much longer. Ingested THC can kick in at thirty minutes or it can hit you two hours later, and it can last for six to ten hours.[2] Meanwhile, a person would have to smoke much more throughout the day to sustain the edible effects of THC. [3]

When it comes to figuring out a recommended dosage, smoking marijuana is much easier to measure. The effects are almost instant, and even a person smokes a little too much, the effects wear off more quickly than if a person ingests marijuana, so it's easier to compensate. Most dispensaries state the ratio of THC and CBD in the strains of marijuana they sell, so the customer has a general sense of how much or how little to smoke at one time, and how to gradually increase the dosage if necessary, depending on how much THC is in a particular bud of weed.

The problem with edibles is that the concentration isn't always standardized. Most edibles are made from leftover scraps, so there can be several different types of strains in one edible. Since each strain of marijuana has different levels of THC, it's difficult to judge the exact dosage in each edible—especially since the effects don't kick in for quite some time. Most people tend to overestimate the dose because of this reason. However, if you come across an edible made with cannabis oil from the buds of the marijuana plant, that edible is much more potent than one made from scraps.

Marijuana dispensaries are now trying to standardize edibles as much as they can by listing serving suggestions. For example, 10 mg of THC or CBD is considered a standard dose that delivers mild effects.[4] A cookie typically has much more THC than 10 mg, so a serving suggestion could be to eat a quarter of the cookie at a time and monitor the results. Even so, each batch of cookies—and each cookie—could be a slightly different dosage depending on what weed is being used. Remember, each strain has a general percentage of THC, but depending on where the plant was grown and what kind of nutrients the plant received, each plant can contain a slightly different amount of THC. It's very difficult (and expensive) to test each batch of cookies to find out exactly how many milligrams of THC is in each one.

Plus, THC affects everyone differently in general. One person might not feel much of an effect from 10 mg of THC and another person might feel a psychedelic buzz. The same goes for CBD. That's why some people take 2 drops of CBD per day to manage seizures and some people have to take more. Not to go too much off topic, but it always amazes me that pharmaceutical drugs and over the counter drugs have the same dosage for everyone. If you're an adult and you have a headache, you take two pills. It doesn't matter your age, your weight, if you're a woman or a man. Meanwhile, we know that everyone's body is different—some people have more body fat percentage than others—and these pills do affect everyone differently. It's no secret that men and women have different metabolisms. For example, the FDA has done many studies that prove women respond differently than men to aspirin, sleeping pills, and anesthesia.[5] What researchers have discovered is that women are usually given too strong of a dose and therefore have more severe side effects than men do—often, these side effects aren't caught right away because they are affecting internal organs. Case in point: in 2013, the FDA recommended that women taking sleeping pills with zolpidem in them, like Ambien and Intermezzo, take half of whatever dosage a doctor would prescribe because women "eliminate zolpidem from their bodies more slowly than men."[6] Intermezzo actually has two pills—a recommended dosage for men and one for women.[7] So when people say we need more research on THC and CBD because they affect everyone differently, I have to laugh. The FDA is approving drugs all the time that affect people differently due to many factors, yet we very rarely see anything but universal dosages for everyone.

So when it comes to picking the right dosage and the right strain of marijuana to cook with, the options can seem overwhelming at first. There's *Cannabis indica* and *Cannabis sativa*. There are strains that supposedly taste sweet and those that supposedly taste tart. Then there are indica and sativa hybrids with all sorts of creative names, like Girl Scout Cookies, Purple Diesel, Pineapple Express, and OG Kush. Some hybrids can be indica dominant, some can be sativa dominant. Plus, even when people prefer to use a specific strain to cook with, they are often at the mercy of what's available and what's in season.

Leafly.com is a great place to turn as a new medical marijuana patient. The website lists every strain available, and it's easy to find what's available nearby. Patients can even search by medical necessity. So if a patient has symptoms of arthritis, migraines, depression, eye pressure, seizures, or what have you, it's easy to find what strains work best for those conditions. Plus, marijuana patients often rate their experiences with the strains, like a Yelp review, so a new patient gets reliable feedback from actual users.

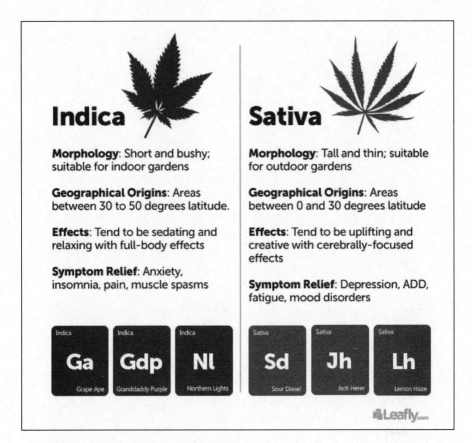

When it comes to cooking with cannabis, I would recommend finding out exactly how much THC is in the strain you're planning on cooking with because that will dictate how much weed to use:

- Most strains have about 10 percent THC
- Strains with 15–20 percent of THC are above average
- Strains with 21 percent THC or higher are exceptionally strong
- When cooking with marijuana, always double check with your local dispensary to find out the THC percentage in a certain strain if you aren't sure.

Once you know that, you can figure out how much marijuana to include in your meal by doing some math:

- Every 1 g of cannabis bud has 1,000 mg of dry weight.

- If a strain has about 10 percent THC, ten percent of 1,000 mg would be 100 mg. So for cooking or baking at home, it is safe to assume that a gram of cannabis contains at least 100 mg THC.

- Take the weighed amount of ground marijuana, convert it to milligrams and divide it by the recipe yield to determine a per-serving dose of THC.

- For example, 3 g of ground marijuana equals 300 mg THC (3 g x 100 mg = 300 mg THC). Then divide 300 mg by the recipe yield to find out how much mg will be in each serving. For example, if a recipe makes 60 cookies, then 300 mg ÷ 60 cookies = 5 mg. That means you'll have 5 mg THC per cookie. If you want less THC, then simply use less ground marijuana in the recipe and you'll decrease the amount.

- Keep in mind that a starting dosage for beginners is 5 mg per serving (the Colorado-mandated serving size for marijuana-infused edibles is 10 mg THC).[8]

- To avoid getting overly intoxicated when eating the finished product, make sure you already have some food in your stomach. Eating cannabis on an empty stomach exacerbates the effects.

- If you find that you've consumed too much, don't eat more food (particularly fats and proteins) because this can actually increase the amount of THC in your bloodstream.

- Instead, do your best to breathe slowly and relax. You can drink fruit juice (which raises your blood sugar naturally and might make you feel more stable) or eat an orange or other citrus fruit, which can also lower the effects of THC. If you have CBD oil handy, a few drops of that can balance out the THC. Remember, CBD naturally counteracts THC. The best solution to overdoing the dosage is within the plant itself!

When figuring out the dosage, it's also important to consider what you're cooking. If you're putting cannabis into a fatty, protein-rich food—such as a marinade on a steak, then the effects will last longer. If you're putting cannabis into candy, then the effects won't last quite as long.[9] Today, there are many websites and cookbooks that offer all kinds of meals—from smoothies to breakfast to lunch to dinner to dessert. It seems every marijuana website out there—from *High Times* to Herb.co—on cooking with cannabis and offers unique recipe ideas.

Since cannabis has a distinct taste, most recipes focus on how to mask it so each meal doesn't taste the same. Most of the bad taste in edibles is likely due to phytol, chlorophyll, and oxidized plant fats. The trick to decrease the potency of that taste is to cook the weed at just the right temperature before adding it to the rest of the food—some people do this through a process called decarboxylation. Most recipes also mask the taste with ingredients like cinnamon, cardamom, black pepper, nutmeg, and citrus zest.

Decarboxylation is a simple process:

1. Preheat the oven to 240° F. / 115° C.

2. Break up cannabis flowers and buds into smaller pieces with your hands. We use one ounce, but you can elect to do more or less.

3. Put the pieces in one layer on a rimmed baking sheet. Make sure the pan is the correct size so there is not empty space on the pan.

4. Bake the cannabis for 30 to 40 minutes, stirring every 10 minutes so that it toasts evenly.

5. When the cannabis is darker in color, a light to medium brown, and has dried out, remove the baking sheet and allow the cannabis to cool. It should be quite crumbly when handled.

6. In a food processor, pulse the cannabis until it is coarsely ground (you don't want a superfine powder). Store it in an airtight container and use as needed to make extractions

Now, you don't have to decarboxylate your weed beforehand, but here's why some chefs prefer to do so: in the 1970s, US government researchers discovered that heating cannabis to about 200 degrees Fahrenheit actually increases THC and CBD percentages.[10] Think of how hot the temperature of weed is when you smoke it. The cannabis actually heats up to a certain temperature to lose a CO_2 molecule, thereby heightening the THC content. Decarboxylating weed prior to cooking achieves the same goal—it makes the cannabis far more potent. People decant red wine for a similar reason: they want the wine to "open up" and be as favorable as possible. You can obviously drink red wine without decanting it, but it's preferred to do so. With decarboxylation, you get the strongest levels of THC in your cooking weed, and therefore the most for your money. Here's how to do it, from Herb.co, formerly known as TheStonersCookBook.com[11]:

Cooking with Marijuana

I must admit that I'm not an expert when it comes to edibles or cooking them. But the basic principle is this: marijuana isn't water soluble, so to cook with it, it must be added in fat-soluble ingredient such as butter or oil. When a recipe requires butter or oil, simply add butter or oil-infused with marijuana. You can find several butter and oil recipes online—the process is simple, but typically time consuming.

That being said, you're going to thank me for this one: here's a great oil recipe for a beginner—or anyone who can't commit to a full day of cooking or baking—a twenty-minute cannabis-infused olive oil by Chris Kilham. Chris Kilham is on the Medical Advisory Board for *The Dr. Oz Show* and writes about cannabis frequently in his weekly *Fox News* column. He is the author of fourteen books on holistic health and botanical medicines. He has been referred to as the "Indiana Jones of natural medicine."

To make his oil, Chris stirs together a quarter ounce of ground, cured cannabis flowers, and a quarter cup of extra-virgin olive oil for about twenty minutes and strains it. That's it. This easy, versatile staple can be stirred into pasta sauce, brushed on bruschetta, and used in many recipes that call for extra-virgin olive oil.

TWENTY-MINUTE CANNABIS OLIVE OIL

Ingredients: Makes about ¼ cup of oil (THC per cup: 283.5 mg)

¼ oz. cured cannabis flowers, finely ground (can be decarboxylated)
¼ cup organic extra-virgin olive oil
coffee grinder/food processor
fine mesh strainer
cheesecloth
saucepan

Directions

1. Place cannabis into a coffee grinder or food processor and grind until powdered. The cannabis will stick to the insides of the grinder, so scrape it out thoroughly.
2. Place oil into a 6" diameter shallow frying pan or saucepan. Using a wooden spoon, continuously stir cannabis into oil over very low simmer for 10 to 20 minutes.
3. Remove from heat and let cool.

4. Line a fine mesh strainer with cheesecloth and place over a bowl, wide-mouth jar, or measuring cup. Twist cannabis with cheesecloth, squeezing out every last drop of oil. Discard cannabis solids.
5. Use oil immediately or transfer oil to a clean clear or dark bottle or jar with a lid or cork. Label with the type of oil and date. Store in a cool, dry place for up to a year.

Wasn't that easy? Ready to try a cannabis butter recipe?

Herb Seidel (otherwise known as Mota, a Spanish term for marijuana) was one of the first chefs to step up and publically teach people how to make great-tasting cannabis foods in the early 2000s. Mota's recipes have been featured in marijuana magazines and cook books. He's perfected a gourmet butter recipe for beginners that has less green flavor than the typical recipes available online. Here's his butter recipe that can be incorporated into literally anything—but to do it right, it takes two days to complete the process. Why two days? Most butter recipes either overcook the butter or break down the structure of the butter, but this technique allows the cannabis butter to mimic traditional butter as closely as possible.

BEGINNER'S BUTTER

Ingredients: Makes about 2 cups (THC per cup: 70.9 mg)

2 cups water
½ oz. cannabis, finely ground (can be decarboxylated)
½ lb. butter
fine mesh strainer
cheesecloth
airtight containers

Directions

1. Combine cannabis and water in a saucepan and bring to a boil. Simmer for 1 hour. If moisture reduces, add up to 2 cups of water.
2. Remove from heat, cover, and let cool to room temperature (about 2 hours). Return to stove and simmer for about 1 hour. Cover and refrigerate overnight. The next morning, return to saucepan and bring to simmer. Stir. Remove from flame, cover, and let cool to room temperature.

3. Line a fine mesh strainer with cheesecloth and place over a bowl, wide-mouth jar, or measuring cup. Pour butter through strainer to strain out cannabis. Twist cannabis with cheesecloth, squeezing out every last drop of oil. Discard cannabis solids.

4. Transfer butter into airtight container. Refrigerate overnight. Butter will separate from water. The next morning, run a knife around edges of container to loosen butter. Use knife to remove butter that has separated from water in bottom of container.

5. Line a fine mesh strainer with cheesecloth and strain remaining butter.

6. Place butter in airtight containers, label, and store in the refrigerator for up to two months or the freezer for up to six months.

Cooking with Hash

You can also use hash or hash oil to create edibles. Hash tastes less like pot because the green plant material has been removed. Be prepared though: this process includes a slow-simmer in a slow cooker and takes several hours. Hash is also much stronger than decarboxylated weed, so you might get more for your money as well.

Here's a recipe to make hash coconut oil by Matt Davenport, a sustainable cannabis grower and the founder of Permalos Consulting. Matt Davenport makes it possible to grow commercial cannabis without fertilizers, synthetic pesticides, GMOs, insecticides, hormones, herbicides, fungicides, and commercial bagged potting soil.[12]

SOLVENTLESS HASH AND COCONUT OIL

Ingredients: Makes 1 cup of oil (200 mg of THC per cup)

10–14 g of bubble hash and/or dry sift, finely ground
1 pt. organic, unrefined coconut oil, melted
2–3 pt. purified water
slow cooker or double boiler
candy thermometer
fine mesh strainer
cheesecloth
deep pan, such as a cake or brownie pan, to place the mixture in until fully cooled
mason or Ball jar for storing final product

Directions

1. Crumble dry hash with your hands until finely ground.
2. If you choose to decarboxylate hash, heat hash in oven at 200°F to 220°F for about 30 to 40 minutes. The material will turn a bit darker and release a slight aroma, much milder than the aroma of roasting flowers.
3. Melt coconut oil in slow cooker or double boiler.
4. Stir in bubble hash and/or dry sift. Continue stirring as hash melts into oil.
5. Add 3 to 4 cups of water. You can add more water as it evaporates during heating.
6. Set temperature on slow cooker or double boiler. Use a candy thermometer to ensure that the temperature remains between 220°F and 240°F and cook for 2 to 3 hours for decarboxylated hash or 6 to 7 hours for hash that wasn't decarboxylated. Stir occasionally.
7. Remove liquid from heat. Wait until liquid cools slightly, then pour into large pan through a fine mesh strainer or cheesecloth to remove any clumps or hash residue. The liquid can then be placed in a jar.
8. Place jar into refrigerator for up to 8 hours (until liquid is fully cooled). When cooled, the oil and water will separate, leaving oil on top.
9. To remove water from bottom, take jar out of the refrigerator and use a knife to poke a hole in the oil layer and pour water out. Dispose of the water, and store the remaining coconut oil in refrigerator for up to six months.

Cooking with Hemp

Cannabis sativa L—otherwise known as hemp—can be used for making everything from bread to pasta to cookies to protein shakes to milk. Remember, there is no THC in hemp, so you can add as much hemp seed as you want to your favorite meals. This is also why hempseed tastes entirely different from the mother cannabis plant.

Here are two simple hemp recipes from my co-author, Jen Hobbs, whose family recently started a medical marijuana farm in California called Hobbs Greenery. Both recipes are non-dairy, vegan, and gluten free.

HEMP MILK

Ingredients

1 cup shelled hemp seeds
3 to 4 cups filtered or spring water (3 cups for thicker milk, and up to 4 cups for thinner)

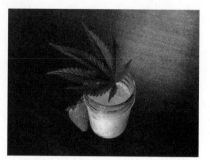

2 tbsp. of coconut oil
2 tbsp. of honey or agave or maple syrup
½ tbsp. of organic vanilla powder OR 1½ tbsp. of vanilla bean paste
A pinch of Himalayan pink salt (or other unprocessed sea salt)
½ tsp nutmeg
A few drops of hazelnut extract (optional)

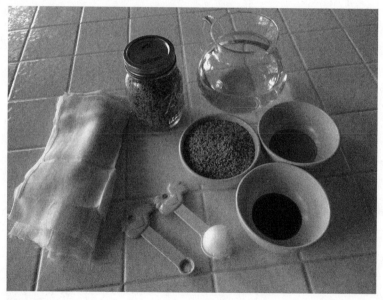

Directions

1. In a high-speed blender, add hemp and water. (A lot of people prefer Vitamix blenders, but any high-speed blender will do.)
2. Blend on high for about two minutes, until fully liquefied.
3. Optional: Strain the liquid into a bowl through a milk bag, nut bag, cheese bag, or fine strainer by squeezing the milk through the bag or by pushing it out of the strainer with a spoon.

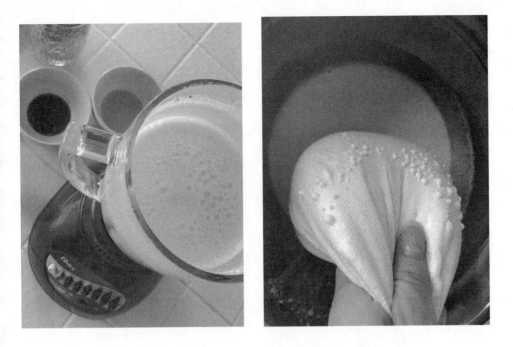

4. Discard the hemp fibers from the bag/strainer. Rinse the blender and pour the milk back into the blender from the bowl.
5. Add coconut oil, honey (or agave or maple syrup), vanilla, nutmeg, and salt. Blend briefly. Add hazelnut to taste.

Hemp milk will keep in the refrigerator for 3 to 4 days. It can also be frozen.

TO STRAIN OR NOT TO STRAIN HEMP MILK

This is really up to personal preference. Some people prefer to strain hemp milk because it tastes less earthy and it isn't as grainy, which means the consistency of the end result is much closer to actual milk. The straining process will give you a sweeter flavor with less texture because the pulp of the hempseed is strained out.

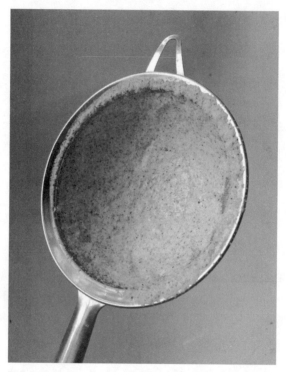

Photo credit for all hemp milk/hemp sorbet images © 2016 by Jen Hobbs.

Personally, I prefer not to strain because then I'm getting all the nutrition from the hempseed. But if you find the nutty flavor is too much, you can strain the milk after you've added all the ingredients. And if you want an even smoother consistency after straining, you can put the strained milk back into the blender, add a tablespoon of soy or sunflower seed lecithin (lecithin is incredibly nutritious), and blend briefly.

Whether you strain your hemp milk or don't, it is a great base for smoothies and shakes. I find that the nutmeg and hazelnut help detract from the hempseed taste, but you might want to consider forgoing both ingredients if you're adding this to a smoothie with fruits and vegetables. But if you wanted to make chocolate milk or hot chocolate with the hemp milk, I'd leave the nutmeg and hazelnut in.

STRAWBERRY HEMP SEED SORBET

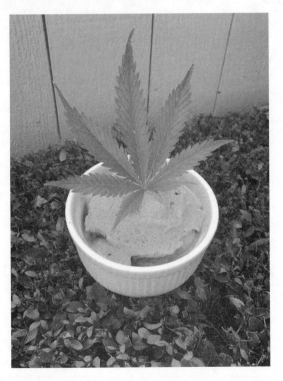

Ingredients

9 leveled tbsp. of hulled hemp seeds

2 pt. (2 lbs.) of strawberries
1¼ cup of water
½ tsp. ground raw vanilla bean OR vanilla bean paste
6 pitted dates
1 tbsp. of lecithin powder (as a natural emulsifier)

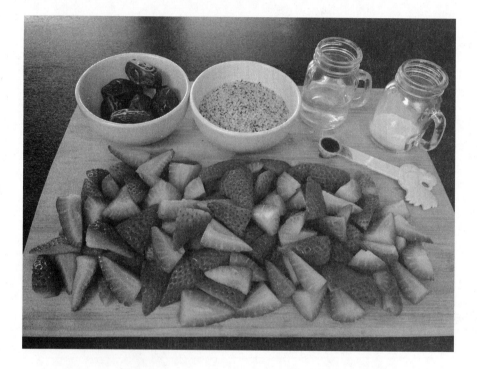

Directions

1.   In a high-speed blender, add all ingredients, blend for about 2 minutes.
2.   Pour into ice cream machine. Makes approximately 1½ quarts of sorbet.
     If you don't have an ice cream machine, you can also use this recipe as a

strawberry smoothie. The strawberries completely mask the flavor of the hemp seeds, so it tastes exactly like a strawberry smoothie.

Cannabis Cookbooks

If you've perfected your cannabis butter and oil, there are many cookbooks out there to choose from that offer cannabis recipes for breakfast, lunch, dinner, dessert, snacks, and even alcoholic beverages. Cannabis cuisine from Matt Davenport, Herb Seidel, Chris Kilham, and other gourmet chefs is available in *The Cannabis Kitchen Cookbook: Feel-Good Food for Home Cooks*, by Robyn Griggs Lawrence.

Afterword
It's High Time to End Prohibition

Our country's dry crusade came to an end on December 5, 1933. That was eighty-three years ago. I don't consider that day as the end of Prohibition because we never really ended Prohibition in this country. We just replaced alcohol with marijuana. Case in point: the same president who repealed alcohol prohibition was the same president who signed the Marijuana Tax Act.

Alcohol prohibition failed because there was no possible way to fully enforce sobriety. The program actually wound up costing billions.[1] According to the May 1930 issue of *Popular Science Monthly*, the Prohibition Commissioner estimated that in 1919 (the year before the Volstead Act became law) the average drinking American spent $17 per year on alcoholic beverages. By 1930—because law enforcement diminished the supply and because the risk involved in obtaining alcohol increased the price—the average drinking American spent $35 per year. It's interesting to note that there was no inflation in America during this period, so the price literally went up $18 due to Prohibition.

As a result of Prohibition, the illegal alcohol beverage industry made an average of $3 billion per year in untaxed income.[2] That was $3 billion that did not go to the US government. Franklin D. Roosevelt ran for president and won because he vowed to overturn the Volstead Act and repeal the Eighteenth Amendment. And he had three major reasons for doing so.

Reason number one was the Great Depression. Americans needed jobs, and by legalizing the alcohol industry, there would be a whole new job market immediately available. The second reason was tax dollars. During the Great Depression, Americans were willing to spend money to acquire alcohol, and since alcohol was illegal, they were buying it tax-free. That meant the government was losing money at a time it could not afford to. The third reason was common sense. FDR didn't think it was the government's job to control the people's temperance. That was up to a person's personal beliefs and convictions.

FDR addressed this third reason in a campaign speech on August 27, 1932:

> We all agree that temperance is one of the cardinal virtues. . . . But the methods adopted since the World War with the purpose of achieving a greater temperance by the forcing of Prohibition have been accompanied in most parts of the country by complete and tragic failure. I need not point out to you that general encouragement of lawlessness has resulted; that corruption, hypocrisy, crime and disorder have emerged, and that instead of restricting, we have extended the spread of intemperance. This failure has come for this very good reason: we have depended too largely upon the power of governmental action instead of recognizing that the authority of the home and that of the churches in these matters is the fundamental force on which we must build.[3]

Roosevelt admitted that the government meant well by outlawing alcohol, but it was never the government's job to do so. The government actually increased all the negative aspects of alcohol by outlawing it, and spent massive amounts of money in the process. Roosevelt realized that if a person is going to drink, that person will find a way to do so—even if that means breaking the law—and he knew this because he was one of those people who drank during Prohibition. Well, the same logic easily applies to marijuana and the War on Drugs!

The Netherlands and Portugal have decriminalized drugs. When you read world news, tell me, are the Netherlands and Portugal endangering any other country? Do they have a massive heroin epidemic, like we do in the United States? Are they exporting drugs all over the world? Or have their policies actually helped drug addicts by taking criminality out of the act? In the Netherlands and in Portugal, if a citizen has a drug problem, that citizen goes to rehab, not jail. Drug use is a medical issue, not a criminal issue, and these aren't the only two countries that view it that way.

In 2013, Uruguay completely legalized marijuana to end the criminal black market. This meant that cannabis users could grow weed at home or join a cannabis club to obtain weed.[4] Uruguay's Minister of Defense Eleuterio Fernandez said this of the country's new marijuana laws: "We think the prohibition of some drugs is creating more problems to society than the drug itself."[5] Finally! Common sense prevails!

The new marijuana law was ratified under President José Mujica, who donates 90 percent of his presidential salary to charity.[6] Could you imagine if any of our politicians actually did that? This is what President Mujica had to say about the end of Uruguay's marijuana prohibition:

> We had eighty deaths from drug-related violence last year [in 2012], and only three or four deaths from drug overdoses. So what is worse: drug trafficking, or drug consumption? Isn't it too much to allow each Uruguayan to buy 30 [grams of] marijuana cigarettes each month? And the advantage [of Uruguay's legalization policy] is that we can identify who is consuming. If we identify consumers, we can help them. If we criminalize them and keep them underground, we steer them towards drug dealers and wash our hands of responsibility.[7]

This is coming from a man who never tried pot. President Mujica sees marijuana prohibition the way President Roosevelt saw alcohol prohibition, and it makes sense to see it that way. The only difference between them is that President Roosevelt understood those who were breaking the law to consume alcohol because he was guilty of the same crime. President Mujica has never done any drugs, but he can still understand how best to help a citizen in his country who uses them.

Think about all of the police measures we've undertaken in the last forty-five years in the War on Drugs. If you've read this book, then you already know all we've got to show for our "tough on drugs" policies is the overwhelming number of Americans in jail. The United States hasn't stopped drugs from spreading and if anything, we've created more violence through the War on Drugs.

Case in point: Mexico made marijuana illegal in 1920, which is seventeen years before the Marijuana Tax Act of 1937.[8] Mexico began "bootlegging" marijuana seventeen years before it became illegal in the United States. Then when we needed a source of weed, we looked to our southern neighbors, just like we did during alcohol prohibition. The only difference is that we never ended the war on marijuana, and so we've been funding the Mexican criminals for approximately ninety-six years!

President Nixon started the War on Drugs in 1971, and six years later, President Jimmy Carter wanted to see some serious changes. President Carter addressed Congress on August 2, 1977, and had this to say about drug abuse:

> Penalties against possession of a drug should not be more damaging to an individual than the use of the drug itself; and where they are, they should be changed. . . . Therefore, I support legislation amending federal law to eliminate all federal criminal penalties for the possession of up to 1 oz. of marihuana. . . . No government can completely protect its citizens from all harm not by legislation, or by regulation, or by medicine, or by advice. Drugs cannot be forced out of existence; they will be with us for as long as people find in them the relief or satisfaction they desire. But the harm caused by drug abuse can be reduced. We cannot talk in absolutes—that drug abuse will cease, that no more illegal drugs will cross our borders—because if we are honest with ourselves we know that is beyond our power. But we can bring together the resources of the federal government intelligently to protect our society and help those who suffer. . . . Drug addiction can be cured; but we must not only treat the immediate effects of the drugs, we must also provide adequate rehabilitation, including job training, to help the addict regain a productive role in society.[9]

It seems other countries have gone this route, but ours has yet to follow. Even our neighbor to the north has legalized industrial hemp and medical marijuana. Remember, since 1998, Canada has been developing its hemp industry. In the first four months of 2015, Canada exported $34 million worth of hemp seeds and oil.[10] People, the United States has all that to gain and more if our damn representatives stop bending to the will of the DEA! Canada is currently considering legalizing recreational marijuana, as the majority of citizens want it to be legal. Cannabis as a whole is a new industry that our country could be profiting off of! Do we really need to see another Great Depression or another World War to get our acts together?

All I know is that our current laws—both for and against marijuana legalization—need to be amended nationwide. If I live in California and fly to Florida, my medical conditions come with me. If my doctor prescribed me a pharmaceutical pill for chronic back pain, I take that medication in the same dosage, whether I'm in my home state or in Florida. It makes no sense that I can be a law-abiding citizen for utilizing medical marijuana in California and I then become a criminal for doing the same exact thing in Florida. If my doctor prescribed marijuana for chronic back pain, what right does a Florida lawmaker have to get into my medical history and make an assessment? And recreational marijuana is the same principle. Why are people getting fired for doing something completely legal? All these idiotic laws do is make the United States look foolish to our allies.

As Thomas Jefferson once said, "Hemp is of first necessity to the wealth and protection of the country." That fact hasn't changed. If anything, the case is stronger now than ever before to end the prohibition on cannabis. We have the ability leave our children a better world than what we inherited. Cannabis built this great nation, and it can save this nation now in its time of need. As my personal hero Muhammad Ali once said: "He who is not courageous enough to take risks will accomplish nothing in life." I truly believe this applies to what we need to do as a nation to legalize cannabis. A man by the name of Steve Kubby had the courage to stand up against the government and pass California's Prop 215, the first and most inclusive medical marijuana measure to-date in the US. We the People are powerful enough to stand against the DEA, against the special interest groups, against our elected officials and demand that the day has come to end prohibition. The question is, will we be vigilant enough to do so?

Endnotes

A NOTE TO THE READER FROM JESSE VENTURA

1 Jennifer De Pinto, Fred Backus, Kabir Khanna, and Anthony Salvanto, "Marijuana Legalization Support at All-Time High," *CBS News*, April 20, 2017, http://www.cbsnews.com/news/support-for-marijuana-legalization-at-all-time-high/.

CHAPTER 1: MEXICO SAYS *SÍ* TO RECREATIONAL WEED

1 http://www.chicagotribune.com/lifestyles/health/ct-americans-alcohol-deaths-20151222-story.html

2 Rafa Fernandez De Castro, "Will Mexico Say Sí to Weed Legalization by the End of October?" *Fusion*, October 23, 2015, http://fusion.net/story/220008/will-mexico-say-si-to-weed-legalization-by-the-end-of-october/.

3 Arturo Zaldívar Lelo de Larrea, "Mexico's Supreme Court Ruling on Cannabis—English Translation," Scribd, November 4, 2015, https://www.scribd.com/doc/289159427/Mexico-s-Supreme-Court-Ruling-on-Cannabis-English-Translation.

4 Associted Press, "Mexico's Supreme Court Opens Door to Recreational Pot Use," *CBS News*, November 4, 2015, http://www.cbsnews.com/news/mexico-supreme-court-opens-door-to-recreational-pot-use/.

5 Agence France-Presse, "Mexico Issues First Permit to Grow and Use Marijuana," *Raw Story*, December 11, 2015, http://www.rawstory.com/2015/12/mexico-issues-first-permit-to-grow-and-use-marijuana/.

6 Associated Press, "Mexico Issues First Permit for Growing and Possessing Marijuana," *CBS News*, December 11, 2015, http://www.cbsnews.com/news/mexico-issues-first-permits-for-growing-and-possessing-marijuana/.

7 Edward Delman, "Is Smoking Weed a Human Right?" *The Atlantic*, November 9, 2015, http://www.theatlantic.com/international/archive/2015/11/mexico-marijuana-legal-human-right/415017/.

8 Ibid.

9 Associated Press, "Mexico Issues First Permit for Growing and Possessing Marijuana," *CBS News*, December 11, 2015, http://www.cbsnews.com/news/mexico-issues-first-permits-for-growing-and-possessing-marijuana/.

10 Associated Press, "Mexican President Opposes Marijuana Legalization," *CBS News*, November 9, 2015, http://www.cbsnews.com/news/mexican-president-opposes-marijuana-legalization/.

11 Sofia Miselem, "Mexico Senator Proposes Legalizing Medical Marijuana," *Yahoo! News*, November 10, 2015, http://news.yahoo.com/two-thirds-mexicans-oppose-pot-legalization-poll-232519556.html.

12 Seth Motel, "6 Facts about Marijuana," *Pew Research Center*, April 14, 2015, http://www.pewresearch.org/fact-tank/2015/04/14/6-facts-about-marijuana/.

13 "Retail Marijuana Use within the City of Denver," *Colorado Official State Web Portal*, accessed May 12, 2016, https://www.colorado.gov/pacific/marijuanainfodenver/residents-visitors.

14 Delfin Rodriguez-Layva and Grant N. Pierce, "The Cardiac and Haemostatic Effects of Dietary Hempseed," *Nutr Metlab* 7, no. 32 (2010): 1–9, http://www.ncbi.nlm.nih.gov/pmc/articles/PMC2868018/.

CHAPTER 2: How to Win the War on Drugs

1 Ioan Grillo, "Mexico's New Drug Law May Set and Example," *TIME*, August 26, 2009, http://content.time.com/time/world/article/0,8599,1918725,00.html.

2 Florence Keen, "Report Hightlights Mexico's Failed Drug Decriminalization Law," July 31, 2014, http://www.talkingdrugs.org/mexico-failed-drug-decriminalization-law.

3 Centro de Investigación y Docencia Económicas, "Resultados de la Primera Encuesta Realizada a Población Interna en Centros Federales de Readaptación Social," *Public Economics*, 2012, https://publiceconomics.files.wordpress.com/2013/01/encuesta_internos_cefereso_2012.pdf.

4 Florence Keen, "Report Hightlights Mexico's Failed Drug Decriminalization Law," July 31, 2014, http://www.talkingdrugs.org/mexico-failed-drug-decriminalization-law.

5 Jason M. Breslow, "The Staggering Death Toll of Mexico's Drug War," *Frontline*, July 27, 2015, http://www.pbs.org/wgbh/frontline/article/the-staggering-death-toll-of-mexicos-drug-war/.

6 "Mexico Drug War Fast Facts," *CNN*, May 9, 2016, http://www.cnn.com/2013/09/02/world/americas/mexico-drug-war-fast-facts/.

7 Jason M. Breslow, "The Staggering Death Toll of Mexico's Drug War," *Frontline*, July 27, 2015, http://www.pbs.org/wgbh/frontline/article/the-staggering-death-toll-of-mexicos-drug-war/.

8 "Operation Iraqi Freedom" and "Operation Enduring Freedom/Afghanistan," iCasualties. org, accessed May 12, 2016, http://icasualties.org/.

9 Catherine E. Shoichet, "Mexico Reports More than 26,000 Missing," *CNN*, February 27, 2013, http://www.cnn.com/2013/02/26/world/americas/mexico-disappeared/.

10 US Department of Homeland Security, "United States of America–Mexico: Bi-national Criminal Proceeds Study," ICE.gov, https://www.ice.gov/doclib/cornerstone/pdf/cps-study.pdf.

11 Deborah Bonello, "Mexican Marijuana Farmers See Profits Tumble as US Loosens Laws," *Los Angeles Times*, December 30, 2015, http://www.latimes.com/world/mexico-americas/la-fg-mexico-marijuana-20151230-story.html.

12 Ibid.

13 Ibid.

14 Ibid.

15 Ibid.

16 Ricardo Baca, "Check Your Stash: Are You Consuming Pesticide-Peppered Pot? Full Recall List," *The Cannabist*, December 4, 2015, http://www.thecannabist.co/2015/12/04/pesticide-pot-recall-list-marijuana/44711/.

17 Patrick Radden Keefe, "Cocaine Incorporated," *New York Times*, June 15, 2012, http://www.nytimes.com/2012/06/17/magazine/how-a-mexican-drug-cartel-makes-its-billions.html?_r=0.

18 Deborah Bonello, "Mexican Marijuana Farmers See Profits Tumble as US Loosens Laws," *Los Angeles Times*, December 30, 2015, http://www.latimes.com/world/mexico-americas/la-fg-mexico-marijuana-20151230-story.html.

19 Patrick Radden Keefe, "Cocaine Incorporated," *New York Times* magazine, June 15, 2012, http://www.nytimes.com/2012/06/17/magazine/how-a-mexican-drug-cartel-makes-its-billions.html?_r=1.

20 Ibid.

21 Stuart Ramsay, "Inside Mexico's Infamous Meth 'Super Labs,'" *Sky News*, July 9, 2015, http://news.sky.com/story/1515628/inside-mexicos-infamous-meth-super-labs.

22 PBS, "Frequently Asked Questions," *Frontline*, accessed May 12, 2016, http://www.pbs.org/wgbh/pages/frontline/meth/faqs/.

23 Ibid.

24 Ibid.

25 US Department of Justice Drug Enforcement Administration, "2015 National Drug Threat Assessment Summary," Scribd, accessed May 12, 2016, http://www.scribd.com/doc/288524161/DEA-Report.

26 PBS, "Frequently Asked Questions," *Frontline*, accessed May 12, 2016, http://www.pbs.org/wgbh/pages/frontline/meth/faqs/.

27 Ibid.

28 Patrick Radden Keefe, "Cocaine Incorporated," *New York Times* magazine, June 15, 2012,

http://www.nytimes.com/2012/06/17/magazine/how-a-mexican-drug-cartel-makes-its-billions.html?_r=1.

29 Ibid.

30 Ibid.

31 Ibid.

32 Associated Press, "AP Impact: After 40 Years, $1 Trillion, US War on Drugs has Failed to Meet Any of Its Goals," *Fox News*, May 13, 2010, http://www.foxnews.com/world/2010/05/13/ap-impact-years-trillion-war-drugs-failed-meet-goals.html.

33 Sofia Miselem, "Mexico Senator Proposes Legalizing Medical Marijuana," *Yahoo! News*, November 10, 2015, http://news.yahoo.com/two-thirds-mexicans-oppose-pot-legalization-poll-232519556.html.

CHAPTER 3: Ross Ulbricht and the Silk Road Conspiracy

1 Madison Pauly, "A DEA Agent Who Helped Take Down Silk Road Is Going to Prison for Unbelievable Corruption," *Mother Jones*, October 19, 2015, http://www.motherjones.com/mixed-media/2015/10/silk-road-investigator-sentencing-corruption-force.

2 https://freeross.org/wp-content/uploads/AppealBriefFinal-1.pdf?v=f96d936325f0

3 Ibid.

4 Ibid.

5 https://freeross.org/wp-content/uploads/EFF-Letter-Amicus.pdf?v=f96d936325f0

6 "Snowden: NSA Was Involved in Silk Road Investigation," YouTube video, 2:14, posted by Free Ross, March 17, 2016, https://www.youtube.com/watch?time_continue=134&v=yKu3KHkqf5w.

7 Madison Pauly, "A DEA Agent Who Helped Take Down Silk Road Is Going to Prison for Unbelievable Corruption," *Mother Jones*, October 19, 2015, http://www.motherjones.com/mixed-media/2015/10/silk-road-investigator-sentencing-corruption-force.

8 Nicky Woolf, "Ex-secret Service Agent Who Stole $800,000 in Bitcoin Newly Arrested," *The Guardian*, February 1, 2016, http://www.theguardian.com/us-news/2016/feb/01/ex-secret-service-agent-shaun-bridges-bitcoin-arrest.

9 Madison Pauly, "A DEA Agent Who Helped Take Down Silk Road Is Going to Prison for Unbelievable Corruption," *Mother Jones*, October 19, 2015, http://www.motherjones.com/mixed-media/2015/10/silk-road-investigator-sentencing-corruption-force.

10 Alistair Charlton, "Silk Road Cop Shaun Bridges Gets 71 Months in Jail for Stealing Bitcoins from Dark Web Drug Site," *International Business Times*, December 8, 2015, http://www.ibtimes.co.uk/silk-road-cop-shaun-bridges-gets-71-months-jail-stealing-bitcoins-dark-web-drug-site-1532336.

11 Ibid.

12 ibid.

13 Nicky Woolf, "Ex-secret Service Agent Who Stole $800,000 in Bitcoin Newly Arrested," *The Guardian*, February 1, 2016, http://www.theguardian.com/us-news/2016/feb/01/ex-secret-service-agent-shaun-bridges-bitcoin-arrest.

14 http://freeross.org/the-case-the-goal-and-why-this-matters-2/

15 Kate Vinton, "Corrupt DEA Agent Pleads Guilty to Extorting Bitcoin from Silk Road Creator Ross Ulbricht," *Forbes*, July 1, 2015, http://www.forbes.com/sites/katevinton/2015/07/01/corrupt-dea-agent-pleads-guilty-to-extorting-bitcoin-from-silk-road-creator-ross-ulbricht/2/.

16 Fran Berkman, "Feds Say Ross Ulbricht Ordered Six Murders, Kept a Silk Road Journal," Mashable, November 21, 2013, http://mashable.com/2013/11/21/ross-ulbricht-silk-road-murder-journal/#YrfsEoasjPq6.

17 Mike Masnick, "Second Silk Road Indictment Details Ulbright's Attempt to Have Former Silk Road Employee Killed," *TechDirt*, October 2, 2013, https://www.techdirt.com/articles/20131002/17220924733/second-silk-road-indictment-details-ulbrights-attempt-to-have-former-silk-road-employee-killed.shtml.

18 Fran Berkman, "Feds Say Ross Ulbricht Ordered Six Murders, Kept a Silk Road Journal," Mashable, November 21, 2013, http://mashable.com/2013/11/21/ross-ulbricht-silk-road-murder-journal/#YrfsEoasjPq6.

19 "Former DEA Agent Sentenced to 6.5 Years in Prison for Corruption in Silk Road Probe," CBS SFBayArea, October 20, 2015, http://sanfrancisco.cbslocal.com/2015/10/20/former-dea-agent-sentenced-to-6-5-years-in-prison-for-corruption-in-silk-road-probe/.

20 http://freeross.org/the-case-the-goal-and-why-this-matters-2/

21 "Lord Acton Quote Archive," Acton Institute for the Study of Religion and Liberty, accessed May 12, 2016, http://www.acton.org/research/lord-acton-quote-archive.

22 https://freeross.org/wp-content/uploads/AppealBriefFinal-1.pdf?v=f96d936325f0

23 https://freeross.org/wp-content/uploads/AppealBriefFinal-1.pdf?v=f96d936325f0

24 https://freeross.org/wp-content/uploads/AppealBriefFinal-1.pdf?v=f96d936325f0

25 https://freeross.org/wp-content/uploads/AppealBriefFinal-1.pdf?v=f96d936325f0

26 http://freeross.org/who-is-ross-2/who-is-ross-really/

27 Kevin Johnson, "Review: Cartel Funded Sex Parties of DEA Agents," *USA Today*, March 26, 2015, http://www.usatoday.com/story/news/nation/2015/03/26/dea-brothel-prostitutes/70482964/.

CHAPTER FOUR: Why and How the DEA is Rigging the Drug War4

1 "DEA History," United States Drug Enforcement Administration, accessed May 12, 2016, http://www.dea.gov/about/history.shtml.

2 "DEA Staffing and Budget," United States Drug Enforcement Administration, accessed May 12, 2016, http://www.dea.gov/about/history/staffing.shtml.

3 "DEA Fact Sheet," Drug Enforcement Administration, accessed May 12, 2016, http://www.dea.gov/docs/factsheet.pdf.

4 Kevin Johnson, "Review: Cartel Funded Sex Parties of DEA Agents," *USA Today*, March 26, 2015, http://www.usatoday.com/story/news/nation/2015/03/26/dea-brothel-prostitutes/70482964/.

5 Ibid.

6 Ibid.

7 Ibid.

8 Ibid.

9 Maggie Ybarra, "No DEA Agents Fired for Colombia Prostitute Parties, Internal Report Reveals," *Washington Times*, April 14, 2015, http://www.washingtontimes.com/news/2015/apr/14/none-dea-agents-who-partied-prostitutes-were-fired/?page=all.

10 Ibid.

11 Ibid.

12 Ibid.

13 Ibid.

14 "2010 PR Cases," PDF on DocumentCloud.org, posted by Brad Heath, accessed on May 12, 2016, https://www.documentcloud.org/documents/2434230-150824164300-0001.html.

15 Brad Heath and Meghan Hoyer, "DEA Agents Kept Jobs Despite Serious Misconduct," *USA Today*, September 27, 2015, http://www.usatoday.com/story/news/2015/09/27/few-dea-agents-fired-misconduct/72805622/.

16 Ibid.

17 Ibid.

18 "2010 PR Cases," PDF on DocumentCloud.org, posted by Brad Heath, accessed on May 12, 2016, https://www.documentcloud.org/documents/2434230-150824164300-0001.html.

19 Brad Heath and Meghan Hoyer, "DEA Agents Kept Jobs Despite Serious Misconduct," *USA Today*, September 27, 2015, http://www.usatoday.com/story/news/2015/09/27/few-dea-agents-fired-misconduct/72805622/.

20 Ibid.

21 Ibid.

22 Ibid.

23 Ibid.

24 Nick Wing, "DEA Steals $16,000 In Cash from Young Black Man, Because He Must Be a Drug Dealer," Huffpost Politics, *Huffington Post*, May 8, 2015, http://www.huffingtonpost.com/2015/05/07/dea-asset-forfeiture-joseph-rivers_n_7231744.html?utm_hp_ref=tw.

25 Ibid.

26 Scott Shane and Colin Moynihan, "Drug Agents Use Vast Phone Trove, Eclipsing NSA's," *New York Times*, September 1, 2013, http://www.nytimes.com/2013/09/02/us/drug-agents-use-vast-phone-trove-eclipsing-nsas.html?pagewanted=all&_r=1.

27 James Ball, "US Drug Agency Partners with AT&T for Access to 'Vast Database' of Call Records," *The Guardian*, September 2, 2013, http://www.theguardian.com/world/2013/sep/02/nsa-dea-at-t-call-records-access.

28 John Shiffman and Kristina Cooke, "Exclusive : US Directs Agents to Cover Up Program Used to Investigate Americans," *Reuters*, August 5, 2013, http://www.reuters.com/article/us-dea-sod-idUSBRE97409R20130805.

29 Brad Heath and Kevin Johnson, "Crimes by ATF and DEA Informants Not Tracked by Feds," *USA Today*, October 7, 2012, http://www.usatoday.com/story/news/2012/10/07/informants-justice-crime/1600323/.

30 Rich Lord, "Court Files Reveal Million-Dollar Informants," Telling for Dollar$, *Pittsburgh Post-Gazette*, April 26, 2014, http://www.post-gazette.com/news/nation/2014/04/27/Telling-for-Dollars-Court-files-reveal-DEA-million-dollar-informants/stories/201404270144.

31 Nick Wing, "The DEA Once Turned a 14-Year-Old into a Drug Kingpin. Welcome to the War on Drugs," Huffpost Politics, *Huffington Post*, October 24, 2014, http://www.huffingtonpost.com/2014/10/24/dea-war-on-drugs_n_6030920.html.

32 Rich Lord, "Court Files Reveal Million-Dollar Informants," Telling for Dollar$, *Pittsburgh Post-Gazette*, April 26, 2014, http://www.post-gazette.com/news/nation/2014/04/27/Telling-for-Dollars-Court-files-reveal-DEA-million-dollar-informants/stories/201404270144.

33 David Rosenzweig, "Judge Frees 3 Men in Drug Case," *Los Angeles Times*, May 10, 2004, http://articles.latimes.com/2004/may/10/local/me-informant10.

34 Ibid.

35 Joseph Kolb, "New Mexico Man Says Federal Agents Gave Him Crack Cocaine," *Reuters*, July 16, 2014, http://www.reuters.com/article/us-usa-newmexico-lawsuit-idUSKBN0FL2RI20140716.

36 Ibid.

37 Yolanda Gonzalez Gomez, trans. Elena Shore and Yoland Gonzalez Gomez, "Double Crossed by the DEA: The Story of an Undocumented Informant," Immigration, *New American Media*, March 03, 2014, http://newamericamedia.org/2014/03/from-the-frying-to-the-fire-the-story-of-an-undocumented-dea-informant.php.

38 Department of Justice Office of Public Affairs, "David Coleman Headley Sentenced to 35 Years in Prison for Role in India and Denmark Terror Plots," news release, January 24, 2013, http://www.justice.gov/opa/pr/david-coleman-headley-sentenced-35-years-prison-role-india-and-denmark-terror-plots.

39 Sebastian Rotella, "The American Behind India's 9/11—And How US Botched Chances to Stop Him," Pakistan's Terror Connections, *ProPublica*, January 24, 2013, http://www.propublica.org/article/david-headley-homegrown-terrorist.

40 Seth Ferranti, "Why Is This Man Still in Jail," *The Fix*, January 20, 2013, https://www.thefix.com/content/story-white-boy-rick-richard-wershe-detroit-corruption70041.

41 C. J. Ciaramella, "Why Is White Boy Rick Still Serving Life in Prison?" *Vice*, July 31, 2014, http://www.vice.com/read/why-is-white-boy-rick-still-serving-life-in-prison.

42 Laura Sager, "Michigan Enacts Reform of '650-Lifer' Law," News Briefs, *National Drug Strategy Network*, February 1998, http://www.ndsn.org/julaug98/sent.html.

43 Pete Brady, "The Murder of Ashley," *Cannabis Culture*, October 8, 2003, http://www.cannabisculture.com/content/2003/10/8/2998.

44 Thomas Avina; Rosalie Avina; B.F. A., a minor; B.S.A., a minor v. United States of America, (9th Cir. 2012), http://cdn.ca9.uscourts.gov/datastore/opinions/2012/06/12/11-55004.pdf.

45 Ibid.

46 Tim Brown, "Obama Admin Defended Agents Putting Gun to Little Girl's Head," *Reclaim Our Republic*, January 12, 2013, https://reclaimourrepublic.wordpress.com/2013/01/12/obama-admin-defended-agents-putting-gun-to-little-girls-head/.

47 Christopher Ingraham, "Federal Court Tells the DEA to Stop Harassing Medical Marijuana Providers," Wonkblog, *The Washington Post*, October 15, 2015, https://www.washingtonpost.com/news/wonk/wp/2015/10/20/federal-court-tells-the-dea-to-stop-harassing-medical-marijuana-providers/.

48 Consolidated and Further Continuing Appropriations Act of 2015, H.R. 83, 113th Cong. (2015), https://www.congress.gov/bill/113th-congress/house-bill/83/text.

49 Ibid.

50 Patty Merkamp Stemler to All Federal Prosecutors, memorandum, 27 February 2015, on Scribd, posted by tomangell, accessed May 12, 2016, http://www.scribd.com/doc/273620932/Depart-of-Justice-Says-Medical-Marijuana-Law-Doesn-t-Impact-Prosecutions.

51 United States of America v. Marin Alliance for Medical Marijuana, and Lynette Shaw.

52 Office of the Inspector General, "A Review of ATF's Operation Fast and Furious and Related Matters," United States Department of Justice, September 2012, https://oig.justice.gov/reports/2012/s1209.htm.

53 Brad Heath and Kevin Johnson, "Crimes by ATF and DEA Informants Not Tracked by Feds," *USA Today*, October 7, 2012, http://www.usatoday.com/story/news/2012/10/07/informants-justice-crime/1600323/.

54 Mark J. Perry, "Milton Friedman Interview from 1991 on America's War on Drugs," AEIdeas, *American Enterprise Institute*, accessed on May 12, 2016, https://www.aei.org/publication/milton-friedman-interview-from-1991-on-americas-war-on-drugs/.

CHAPTER FIVE: The American Historical Significance of Cannabis

1 "Drug War Today," The House I Live *In*, accessed on May 12, 2016, http://www.thehouseilivein.org/get-involved/drug-war-today/.

2 https://www.gpo.gov/fdsys/pkg/STATUTE-84/pdf/STATUTE-84-Pg1236.pdf

3 Dan Eggen, "Marijuana Becomes Focus of Drug War," *Washington Post*, May 4, 2005, http://www.washingtonpost.com/wp-dyn/content/article/2005/05/03/AR2005050301638.html.

4 "History of Marijuana," Narconon, accessed on May 12, 2016, http://www.narconon.org/drug-information/marijuana-history.html.

5 PBS, "Marijuana Timeline," *Frontline*, accessed May 12, 2016, http://www.pbs.org/wgbh/pages/frontline/shows/dope/etc/cron.html.

6 Brent Moore, *The Hemp Industry in Kentucky* (Lexington, KY: James E. Hughes, 1905), 12.

7 G. M. Herndon, "Hemp in Colonial Virginia," *Agricultural History* 37 (1963): 93.

8 Jack Herer, *The Emperor Wears No Clothes: Hemp and the Marijuana Conspiracy* (Austin, TX: Ah Ha Publishing, 2007), 1.

9 Larry Sloman, *Reefer Madness: A History of Marijuana* (Indianapolis, IN: Bobbs-Merrill, 1979), 21.

10 "Industrianl Hemp in Virginia," ReeferMadnessMuseum.org, accessed May 12, 2016, http://reefermadnessmuseum.org/chap04/Virginia/VA_IndHempP3.htm.

11 Victor Selden Clark, *History of Manufactures in the United States* (New York: McGraw-Hill, 1929), 34.

12 Brent Moore, *The Hemp Industry in Kentucky* (Lexington, KY: James E. Hughes, 1905), 17.

13 Jack Herer, *The Emperor Wears No Clothes: Hemp and the Marijuana Conspiracy* (Austin, TX: Ah Ha Publishing, 2007), 79.

14 Clement Eaton, *A History of the Old South* (New York: Macmillan, 1966), 229.

15 Larry Sloman, *Reefer Madness: A History of Marijuana* (Indianapolis, IN: Bobbs-Merrill, 1979), 22.

16 Ibid., 26.

17 Ibid.

18 Ibid., 30.

19 "Schlihchten Papers," *InnVista*, accessed on May 12, 2016, http://www.innvista.com/health/foods/hemp/schlichten-papers/.

20 Jack Herer, *The Emperor Wears No Clothes: Hemp and the Marijuana Conspiracy* (Austin, TX: Ah Ha Publishing, 2007), 17.

21 Louis Fisher, "Destruction of the Maine (1898)," The Law Library of Congress, accessed on May 12, 2016, https://www.loc.gov/law/help/usconlaw/pdf/Maine.1898.pdf.

22 Ibid.

23 Jack Herer, *The Emperor Wears No Clothes: Hemp and the Marijuana Conspiracy* (Austin, TX: Ah Ha Publishing, 2007), 31.

24 Ibid.

25 Ibid.

26 Ibid., 31.

27 Ibid., 33.

28 Ibid., 32.

29 Ryan Grim, *This is Your Country on Drugs: The Secret History of Getting High in America* (New Jersey: John Wily & Sons Inc., 2009), 47.

30 Ibid.

31 Ibid.

32 Alicia Williamson, *The Everything Marijuana Book* (Blue Ash, OH: F+W Media, 2010), 18.

33 Ibid., 19.

34 "#14 Du Pont family," America's Richest Families, Forbes, accessed on May 12, 2016, http://www.forbes.com/profile/du-pont/.

35 *Wikipedia*, s.v. "DuPont," last modified May 8, 2016, https://en.wikipedia.org/wiki/DuPont.

36 "Investor Relations," DuPont website, accessed on May 12, 2016, http://investors.dupont.com/investor-relations/overview/default.aspx.

37 Megha Bahree, "The World's Richest 1% Just Got a Lot Richer, While Everyone Else Didn't," Forbes Asia, Forbes, January 19, 2016, http://www.forbes.com/sites/meghabahree/2016/01/19/the-worlds-richest-1-just-got-a-lot-richer-while-everyone-else-didnt/#2715e4857a0b1f25ed424586.

38 Ibid.

39 Larry Elliott and Ed Pilkington, "New Oxfam Report Says half of Global Wealth Held by the 1%," *The Guardian*, January 19, 2015, http://www.theguardian.com/business/2015/jan/19/global-wealth-oxfam-inequality-davos-economic-summit-switzerland.

CHAPTER SIX: America's Marijuana Hypocrisy

1 Fiorello LaGuardia, "Foreword," *The LaGuardia Report*, accessed May 12, 2016, http://www.druglibrary.org/schaffer/library/studies/lag/foreword.htm.

2 Alicia Williamson, *The Everything Marijuana Book* (Blue Ash, OH: F+W Media, 2010), 20.

3 Rebekah Metzler, "On Marijuana: What Hillary Clinton and Bernie Sanders Would Do," *CNN*, October 14, 2015, http://www.cnn.com/2015/10/13/politics/pot-hillary-clinton-bernie-sanders/.

4 Jack Herer, *The Emperor Wears No Clothes: Hemp and the Marijuana Conspiracy* (Austin, TX: Ah Ha Publishing, 2007), 35.

5 Jack Herer, *The Emperor Wears No Clothes: Hemp and the Marijuana Conspiracy* (Austin, TX: Ah Ha Publishing, 2007), 35.

6 PBS, "Marijuana Timeline," *Frontline*, accessed May 12, 2016, http://www.pbs.org/wgbh/pages/frontline/shows/dope/etc/cron.html.

7 A. L. Ash, *"Hemp—Production and Utilization,"* (1948), *Economic Botany* 2 (1948): 158–169.

8 John Roulac, *Industrial Hemp Practical Products: Paper to Fabric to Cosmetics* (St. Petersburg, FL: Hemptech, 1996), 13.

9 Ibid., 11.

10 "BMW i3 Saves Weight Using Hemp Fibers," *EV World*, August 5, 2013, http://evworld.com/news.cfm?newsid=30943.

11 Jack Herer, *The Emperor Wears No Clothes: Hemp and the Marijuana Conspiracy* (Austin, TX: Ah Ha Publishing, 2007), 97.

12 Arturo Garcia, "'This Is Hypocrisy': Sanjay Gupta Tells Anderson Cooper about the Federal Medical Marijuana Patent," *Raw Story*, August 14, 2013, http://www.rawstory.com/2013/08/this-is-hypocrisy-sanjay-gupta-tells-anderson-cooper-about-the-federal-medical-marijuana-patent/.

13 "Cannabinoids as Antioxidants and Neuroprotectants," *Internet Archive Wayback Machine*, accessed on May 12, 2016, http://web.archive.org/web/20120317122506/http://www.patentstorm.us/patents/6630507.html.

14 "US Government's Medical Marijuana Patent," *Patents for Medical Cannabis*, accessed on May 12, 2016, https://patients4medicalmarijuana.wordpress.com/medical-use-of-cannabis-video/the-government-holds-a-patent-for-medical-marijuana/.

15 "Drug Scheduling," *United States Drug Enforcement Administration*, accessed on May 12, 2016, http://www.dea.gov/druginfo/ds.shtml.

16 Larry Sloman, *Reefer Madness: A History of Marijuana* (Indianapolis, IN: Bobbs-Merrill, 1979), 21.

17 *The Criminal Law Reporter*, (Arlington, VA: Bureau of National Affairs, 1976), 2300.

18 Mohamed Ben Amar, "Cannabinoids in Medicine: A Review of Their Therapeutic Potential," *Journal of Ethnopharmacology* 105 (2006): 1–25, accessed May 12, 2016, http://www.doctordeluca.com/Library/WOD/WPS3-MedMj/CannabinoidsMedMetaAnalysis06.pdf.

19 "Free Pot? Federal Program Ships Marijuana to Four," CBS News, accessed May 12, 2016, http://www.cbsnews.com/pictures/free-pot-federal-program-ships-marijuana-to-four/.

20 *Wikipedia*, s.v. "Compassionate Investigational New Drug Program," last modified March 29, 2016, https://en.wikipedia.org/wiki/Compassionate_Investigational_New_Drug_program#cite_note-BenAmar2006-2.

21 "Drug War Statistics," DrugPolicy.org, accessed May 12, 2016, http://www.drugpolicy.org/drug-war-statistics.

22 "Quick Facts: Federal Offenders in Prison, January 2015," *United States Sentencing Commission*, accessed May 12, 2016, http://www.ussc.gov/sites/default/files/pdf/research-and-publications/quick-facts/Quick-Facts_BOP.pdf.

23 "Drug War Statistics," DrugPolicy.org, accessed May 12, 2016, http://www.drugpolicy.org/drug-war-statistics.

24 Steve Nelson, "Police Made One Marijuana Arrest Every 42 Seconds in 2012," *US News and World Report*, September 16, 2013, http://www.usnews.com/news/articles/2013/09/16/police-made-one-marijuana-arrest-every-42-seconds-in-2012.

25 Fareed Zakaria, "Incarceration Nation," *TIME*, April 2, 2012, http://content.time.com/time/magazine/article/0,9171,2109777,00.html.

26 "Drug War Statistics," DrugPolicy.org, accessed May 12, 2016, http://www.drugpolicy.org/drug-war-statistics.

27 "The Cost of a Nation of Incarcertaion," CBS News, April 23, 2012, http://www.cbsnews.com/news/the-cost-of-a-nation-of-incarceration/.

28 "Fate by Weight: Examining Marijuana Felonies across the United States," DrugTreatment. com, accessed May 12, 2016, http://www.drugtreatment.com/expose/marijuana-felony-amounts-by-state/.

29 Matt Ferner, "No, Colorado Isn't Releasing People Imprisoned for Pot Crimes. But Why the Hell Not?" Huffpost Politics, *Huffington Post*, February 25, 2014, http://www.huffingtonpost. com/2014/02/25/colorado-releasing-marijuana-prisoners_n_4854244.html.

30 "210,000 Marijuana Possession Arrests in Colorado," Marijuana-Arrests.com, accessed May 12, 2016, http://marijuana-arrests.com/docs/210,000-Marijuana-Arrests-In-Colorado.pdf.

31 "Drug War Statistics," DrugPolicy.org, accessed May 12, 2016, http://www.drugpolicy.org/ drug-war-statistics.

32 Travis Waldron, "California Spends Six Times More on Prison Inmates Than on College Students," Justice, *ThinkProgress*, April 5, 2012, http://thinkprogress.org/ justice/2012/04/05/458148/california-spends-six-times-more-on-prison-inmates-than-on-college-students/.

33 "Drug War Statistics," DrugPolicy.org, accessed May 12, 2016, http://www.drugpolicy.org/ drug-war-statistics.

CHAPTER SEVEN: Marijuana Is NOT a Schedule I Narcotic

1 "Drug Scheduling," *United States Drug Enforcement Administration*, accessed May 12, 2016, http://www.dea.gov/druginfo/ds.shtml.

2 Kimberly Leonard, "Heroin Use Skyrockerts in U.S.," *US News and World Report*, July 7, 2015, http://www.usnews.com/news/blogs/data-mine/2015/07/07/heroin-use-skyrockets-in-us-cdc-says.

3 "Opioid Addiction: 2016 Facts and Figures," *American Society of Addiction Medicine*, accessed May 12, 2016, http://www.asam.org/docs/default-source/advocacy/opioid-addiction-disease-facts-figures.pdf.

4 Benedict Carey, "Prescription Painkillers Seen as a Gateway to Heroin," *New York Times*, February 10, 2014, http://www.nytimes.com/2014/02/11/health/prescription-painkillers-seen-as-a-gateway-to-heroin.html.

5 "Today's Heroin Epidemic," Centers for Disease Control and Prevention, accessed May 12, 2016, http://www.cdc.gov/vitalsigns/heroin/.

6 "Opioid Addiction: 2016 Facts and Figures," *American Society of Addiction Medicine*, accessed May 12, 2016, http://www.asam.org/docs/default-source/advocacy/opioid-addiction-disease-facts-figures.pdf.

7 Kimberly Leonard, "Heroin Use Skyrockerts in U.S.," *US News and World Report*, July 7, 2015, http://www.usnews.com/news/blogs/data-mine/2015/07/07/heroin-use-skyrockets-in-us-cdc-says.

8 Barnini Chakraborty, "'Heroin in a Capsule'? Lawmakers Step Up Fight against FDA-Approved Painkiller Zohydro," Politics, *Fox News*, May 3, 2014, http://www.foxnews.com/ politics/2014/05/03/heroin-in-capsule-lawmakers-step-up-fight-against-fda-approved-painkiller.html.

9 Mike Adams, "Controversial 'HeroinPill' Hits the Market This Month," *High Times*, May 7, 2014, http://www.hightimes.com/read/controversial-heroin-pill-hits-market-month.

10 Tod H. Mikuriya, "Marijuana in Medicine: Past, Present, and Future," *California Medicine* 110, no. 1 (1969): 34–40, http://www.ncbi.nlm.nih.gov/pmc/articles/PMC1503422/pdf/califmed 00019-0036.pdf.

11 Mary E. Lynch and Alexander J. Clark, "Cannabis Reduces Opioid Dose in the Treatment of Chronic Non-cancer Pain," *Journal of Pain and Symptom Management* 25, no. 6 (2003): 496–498, http://www.jpsmjournal.com/article/S0885-3924(03)00142-8/fulltext.

12 Thomas J. O'Connell and Ché B. Bou-Matar, "Long Term Marijuana Users Seeking Medical Cannabis in California (2001–2007): Demographics, Social Characteristics, Patterns of

Cannabis and Other Drug Use of 4,117 Applicants," *Harm Reduction Journal* 4, no. 16 (2007), doi: 10.1186/1477-7517-4-16.

13 "Active Ingredient in Cannabis Eliminates Morphine Dependence in Rats," Scien*ce Daily*, accessed May 12, 2016, http://www.sciencedaily.com/releases/2009/07/090706090440.htm.

14 Amanda Reiman, "Cannabis as a Substitute for Alcohol and Other Drugs," Harm *Reduction Journal* 6, no. 35 (2009), doi: 10.1186/1477-7517-6-35.

15 S. Oilère, A. Joliette-Riopel, S. Potvin, and D. Jutras-Aswad, "Modulation of the Endocannabinoid System: Vulnerability Factor and New Treatment Target for Stimulant Addiction," *Front Psychiatry* 23, no. 4 (2013): 109, doi: 10.3389/fpsyt.00109.

16 Daniel J. Liput, Dana C. Hammell, Audra L. Stinchcomb, and Kimberly Nixon, "Transdermal Delivery of Cannabidiol Attenuates Binge Alcohol-Induced Neurodegeneration in a Rodent Model of an Alcohol Use Disorder," *Pharmacology Biochemistry and Behavior* 111 (2013): 120–127, http://www.sciencedirect.com/science/article/pii/S0091305713002104.

17 http://archinte.jamanetwork.com/article.aspx?articleid=1898878

18 Tod H. Mikuriya, "Marijuana in Medicine: Past, Present, and Future," *California Medicine* 110, no. 1 (1969): 34–40, http://www.ncbi.nlm.nih.gov/pmc/articles/PMC1503422/pdf/califmed00019-0036.pdf.

19 R. Benyamin, A. M. Trescot, S. Datta, R. Buenaventura, R. Adlaka, N. Sehgal, S. E. Glaser, and R. Vallejo, "Opiod Complications and Side Effects," *Pain Physician* 11, no. 2 (2008): 105–120, http://www.ncbi.nlm.nih.gov/pubmed/18443635.

20 Tod H. Mikuriya, "Marijuana in Medicine: Past, Present, and Future," *California Medicine* 110, no. 1 (1969): 34–40, http://www.ncbi.nlm.nih.gov/pmc/articles/PMC1503422/pdf/califmed00019-0036.pdf.

21 PBS, "Marijuana Timeline," *Frontline*, accessed May 12, 2016, http://www.pbs.org/wgbh/pages/frontline/shows/dope/etc/cron.html.

22 Sunil Aggarwal, "Cannabis: A Commonwealth Medicinal Plant, Long Suppressed, Now at Risk of Monopolozation," *Denver University Law Review* 88 (2010): 1–12, http://www.cannabinologist.org/Documents/Aggarwal-Macroed1.pdf.

23 PBS, "Marijuana Timeline," *Frontline*, accessed May 12, 2016, http://www.pbs.org/wgbh/pages/frontline/shows/dope/etc/cron.html.

24 Ibid.

25 Lisa Leff, "Pot-Based Mouth Spray Medicine Looks for U.S. Approval," USA Today, January 27, 2012, http://usatoday30.usatoday.com/money/industries/health/story/2012-01-29/pot-based-prescription-drug/52826376/1.

26 http://www.druglibrary.org/olsen/MEDICAL/YOUNG/young1.html

27 "A Brief History of the Drug War," DrugPolicy.org, accessed May 12, 2016, http://www.drugpolicy.org/new-solutions-drug-policy/brief-history-drug-war.

28 PBS, "Marijuana Timeline," *Frontline*, accessed May 12, 2016, http://www.pbs.org/wgbh/pages/frontline/shows/dope/etc/cron.html.

29 Ibid.

30 Rick Doblin, "The Medicinal Use of Marijuana," Newsletter of the Multidisciplinary Association *for Psychedelic Studies (MAPS)* 5, no. 1 (1994), http://www.maps.org/news-letters/v05n1/05111mmj.html.

31 "Medicinal Marijuana: The Struggle for Legalization," *CNN Interactive*, accessed May 12, 2016, https://web.archive.org/web/20070608185133/http://www.cnn.com:80/HEALTH/9702/weed.wars/issues/background/.

32 Jeff Stein, "The Clinton Dynasty's Horrific Legacy: More Drug War, More Prisons," Drugs, *Alternet*, April 13, 2015, http://www.alternet.org/drugs/clinton-dynasty-horrific-legacy-more-drug-war-more-prisons.

33 "Medicinal Marijuana: The Struggle for Legalization," *CNN Interactive*, accessed May 12, 2016, https://web.archive.org/web/20070608185133/http://www.cnn.com:80/HEALTH/9702/weed.wars/issues/background/.

34 http://www.fda.gov/ohrms/dockets/dockets/05n0479/05N-0479-emc0004-04.pdf

35 "Drug Scheduling," United States Drug Enforcement Administration, accessed May 12, 2016, http://www.dea.gov/druginfo/ds.shtml.

36 Ibid.

37 http://www.fda.gov/ohrms/dockets/dockets/05n0479/05N-0479-emc0004-04.pdf

38 Anna Edney, "Marijuana Considered for Looser Restrictions by U.S. FDA," *Bloomberg*, June 20, 2014, http://www.bloomberg.com/news/articles/2014-06-20/drug-regulators-study-easing-u-s-marijuana-restrictions.

39 Ibid.

40 "Number of legal Medical Marijuana Patients," ProCon.org, last updated March 3, 2016, http://medicalmarijuana.procon.org/view.resource.php?resourceID=005889.

41 "U.S. and World Population Clock," United States Census Bureau, accessed May 12, 2016, http://www.census.gov/popclock/.

CHAPTER EIGHT: Marijuana Is a Medication

1 "Where Is Marijuana Legal?" *New Health Guide*, accessed May 12, 2016, http://www.newhealthguide.org/Where-Is-Marijuana-Legal.html.

2 Christopher Ingraham, "Why Hardly Anyone Dies from a Drug Overdose in Portugal," *Washington Post*, June 5, 2015, https://www.washingtonpost.com/news/wonk/wp/2015/06/05/why-hardly-anyone-dies-from-a-drug-overdose-in-portugal/.

3 Hampton Sides, "Science Seeks to Unlock Marijuana's Secrets," *National Geographic*, June 2015, http://ngm.nationalgeographic.com/2015/06/marijuana/sides-text.

4 *WebMD*, s.v. "marijuana," accessed May 12, 2016, http://www.webmd.com/vitamins-supplements/ingredientmono-947-marijuana.aspx?activeingredientid=947&activeingredientname=marijuana.

5 Hampton Sides, "Science Seeks to Unlock Marijuana's Secrets," *National Geographic*, June 2015, http://ngm.nationalgeographic.com/2015/06/marijuana/sides-text.

6 Di Marzo, Vincenzo; Sepe, Nunzio; De Petrocellis, Luciano; Berger, Alvin; Crozier, Gayle; Fride, Ester; Mechoulam, Raphael,"*Trick or treat from food endocannabinoids?* (1998), *Nature* 396 (6712): 636–7.

7 Jonathan Benson, "Cannabinoids, Like Those Found in Marijuana, Occur Naturally in Human Breast Milk," *Natural News*, July 20, 2012, http://www.naturalnews.com/036526_cannabinoids_breast_milk_THC.html.

8 Kevin Bonsor and Nicholas Gerbis, "How Marijuana Works," *HowStuffWorks*, accessed May 12, 2016, http://science.howstuffworks.com/marijuana4.htm.

9 Igor Grant and B. Rael Cahn, "Cannabis and Endocannabinoid Modulators: Therapeutic Promises and Challenges," *Clinical Neuroscience Research* 5, no. 2–4 (2005): 185–199, http://www.ncbi.nlm.nih.gov/pmc/articles/PMC2544377/.

10 Angelique Chrisafis, "French Drug Trial Leaves One Brain Dead and Five Critically Ill," *The Guardian*, January 15, 2016, http://www.theguardian.com/world/2016/jan/15/french-drug-trial-one-person-in-coma-and-five-critically-ill?CMP=fb_gu.

11 Sewell Chan, "6 Hospitalized, One of Them Brain-Dead, After Drug Trial in France," *New York Times*, January 15, 2016, http://www.nytimes.com/2016/01/16/world/europe/french-drug-trial-hospitalization.html?_r=0.

12 Robert C. Randall and Alice M. O'Leary, *Marijuana RX: The Patients' Fight for Medicinal Pot* (New York: Thunder's Mouth Press, 1998), ix–x.

13 Jordan Bechtold et al., "Chronic Adolescent Marijuana Use as a Risk Factor for Physical and Mental Health Problems in Young Adult Men," *Psychology of Addictive Behaviors* 29, no. 3 (2015): 552–563, http://www.apa.org/pubs/journals/releases/adb-adb0000103.pdf.

14 Igor Grant and B. Rael Cahn, "Cannabis and Endocannabinoid Modulators: Therapeutic Promises and Challenges," *Clinical Neuroscience Research* 5, no. 2–4 (2005): 185–199, http://www.ncbi.nlm.nih.gov/pmc/articles/PMC2544377/.

15 "Drug Facts: Marijuana," *National Institute on Drug Abuse*, last updated March 2016, http://www.drugabuse.gov/publications/drugfacts/marijuana.

16 Paul Armentano, "Breathe, Push, Puff? Pot Use and Pregnancy: A Review of the Literature," *Norml*, accessed May 12, 2016, http://norml.org/about/item/breathe-push-puff-pot-use-and-pregnancy-a-review-of-the-literature.

17 "Brain Maturity Extends Well Beyond Teen Years," *Tell Me More*, podcast audio, October 10, 2011, http://www.npr.org/templates/story/story.php?storyId=141164708.

18 Alina Bradford, "What Is THC?" Live Science, April 7, 2015, http://www.livescience.com/24553-what-is-thc.html.

19 Jordan Bechtold et al., "Chronic Adolescent Marijuana Use as a Risk Factor for Physical and Mental Health Problems in Young Adult Men," *Psychology of Addictive Behaviors* 29, no. 3 (2015): 552–563, http://www.apa.org/pubs/journals/releases/adb-adb0000103.pdf.

20 Prakash Nagarkatti et al., "Cannabinoids as Novel Anti-inflammatory Drugs," *Future Medicinal Chemistry* 1, no. 7 (2009): 1333–1349, http://www.ncbi.nlm.nih.gov/pmc/articles/PMC2828614/.

21 "Are There Any Negative Side Effects to CBD Rich Strains of Cannabis/Marijuana?" *Quora*, accessed May 12, 2016, https://www.quora.com/Are-there-any-negative-side-effects-to-CBD-rich-strains-of-cannabis-marijuana.

22 Mateus Machado Bergamaschi et al., "Safety and Side Effects of Cannabidiol, a *Cannabis sativa* Constituent," *Current Drug Safety* 6, no. 4 (2011): 1–13, http://www.medicinalgenomics.com/wp-content/uploads/2013/01/Bergamaschi_2011.pdf.

23 Ibid.

24 Ibid.

25 Ibid.

26 Joshua Gowin, "Long Term Effects of Marijuana on the Brain," *Psychology Today*, September 18, 2014, https://www.psychologytoday.com/blog/you-illuminated/201409/long-term-effects-marijuana-the-brain.

27 "Drug Facts: Marijuana," *National Institute on Drug Abuse*, last updated March 2016, http://www.drugabuse.gov/publications/drugfacts/marijuana.

28 Ibid.

29 "Caffeine Withdrawal Symptoms: Top Fifteen," Caffeine Informer, accessed May 12, 2016, http://www.caffeineinformer.com/caffeine-withdrawal-symptoms-top-ten.

30 Ibid.

31 Johns Hopkins University, "Caffeine Dependence," *Behavioral Pharmacology Research Unit (BPRU) Fact Sheet*, accessed May 12, 2016, http://www.hopkinsmedicine.org/psychiatry/research/BPRU/docs/Caffeine_Dependence_Fact_Sheet.pdf.

32 Patrick Hruby, "American Caffeine Addiction Races Full Speed Ahead," *Washington Times*, January 17, 2012, http://www.washingtontimes.com/news/2012/jan/17/amp-up-america/?page=all.

33 *Medline*Plus, s.v. "opiate and opioid withdrawal," accessed May 12, 2016, https://www.nlm.nih.gov/medlineplus/ency/article/000949.htm.

34 "Methamphetamine: What Are the Long-Term Effects of Methamphetamine Abuse?" *National Institute on Drug Abuse*, accessed May 12, 2016, http://www.drugabuse.gov/publications/research-reports/methamphetamine/what-are-long-term-effects-methamphetamine-abuse.

35 Ibid.

36 "Setting the Record Straight on the Phrase 'Gateway Drug,'" All Things Considered, April 18, 2015, podcast audio, http://www.npr.org/2015/04/18/400658693/setting-the-record-straight-on-the-phrase-gateway-drug.

37 Jayne O'Donnell and Laura Ungar, "CVS Stops Selling Tobacco, Offers Quit-Smoking Programs," *USA Today*, September 3, 2014, http://www.usatoday.com/story/news/nation/2014/09/03/cvs-steps-selling-tobacco-changes-name/14967821/.

38 Chris D'Angelo, "Hawaii Becomes First State to Raise Smoking Age to 21," Huffpost Politics, *Huffington Post*, December 31, 2015, http://www.huffingtonpost.com/entry/hawaii-becomes-first-state-raise-smoking-age-to-21_us_568577d5e4b0b958f65ba00b.

39 Marvin Fong, "More Than 100 U.S. Cities Raise Smoking Age to 21," Cleveland.com, accessed May 12, 2016, http://tobacco21.org/wp-content/uploads/2015/12/cleveland.com-More-than-100-US-cities-raise-smoking-age-to-21.pdf.

40 "Health Effects of Cigarette Smoking," *Centers for Disease Control and Prevention*, last modified October 1, 2015, http://www.cdc.gov/tobacco/data_statistics/fact_sheets/health_effects/effects_cig_smoking/.

41 Donald P. Tashkin, "Effects of Marijuana Smoking on the Lung," *Annals of American Thoracic Society* 10, no. 3 (2013): 239–247, http://www.atsjournals.org/doi/abs/10.1513/AnnalsATS.201212-127FR#.VqQDOJMrJE5.

42 Stephen C. Webster, "Yale Study: Alcohol's Gateway Effect Much Larger Than Marijuana," *Raw Story*, August 22, 2012, http://www.rawstory.com/2012/08/yale-study-alcohols-gateway-effect-much-larger-than-marijuanas/.

43 "Drug harms in the UK: A Multicriteria Decision Analysis," *The Lancet* 376, no. 9752 (2010): 1558–1565, http://www.thelancet.com/journals/lancet/article/PIIS0140-6736(10)61462-6/fulltext.

44 Tristan Kirby and Adam E. Barry, "Alcohol as a Gateway Drug: A Study of US 12th Graders," *Journal of School Health* 82, no. 8 (2012): 371–379, http://onlinelibrary.wiley.com/doi/10.1111/j.1746-1561.2012.00712.x/abstract.

45 "Medical Marijuana as Treatment for Alcoholism and Addiction," *United Patients Group*, July 26, 2012, http://www.unitedpatientsgroup.com/blog/2012/07/26/medical-marijuana-as-treatment-for-alcoholism-addiction/.

46 *MedilinePlus*, s.v. "alcohol withdrawal," last modified February 8, 2015, https://www.nlm.nih.gov/medlineplus/ency/article/000764.htm.

47 "Nicotine Withdrawal Symptoms and Recovery," QuitSmokingSupport.com, accessed May 12, 2016, http://www.quitsmokingsupport.com/withdrawal1.htm.

48 Thomas J. O'Connell and Ché B. Bou-Matar, "Long Term Marijuana Users Seeking Medical Cannabis in California (2001–2007): Demographics, Social Characteristics, Patterns of Cannabis and Other Drug Use of 4,117 Applicants," *Harm Reduction Journal* 4, no. 16 (2007), doi: 10.1186/1477-7517-4-16.

49 Sabrina Tavernise, "FDA Commissioner Leaving after Six Years of Breakneck Changes," *New York Times*, February 5, 2015, http://www.nytimes.com/2015/02/06/health/margaret-hamburg-fda-commissioner-stepping-down.html.

50 Sabrina Tavernise, "Robert Califf, FDA Nominee, Queried on Industry Ties," *New York Times*, November 17, 2015, http://www.nytimes.com/2015/11/18/health/robert-califf-fda-nomination.html?_r=0.

51 "FDA Commissioner's Page," *United States Food and Drug Administration*, accessed May 12, 2016, http://www.fda.gov/AboutFDA/CommissionersPage/.

52 "Candidate to Lead FDA Has Close Ties to Big Pharma," *Fortune*, February 19, 2015, http://fortune.com/2015/02/19/candidate-to-lead-fda-has-close-ties-to-big-pharma/.

53 Kelly Riddell, "Marijuana Addiction Drug Research Gets $3 Million Grant as Obama Encourages Legalization," *Washington Times*, June 25, 2015, http://www.washingtontimes.com/news/2015/jun/25/marijuana-addiction-drug-research-gets-3-million-g/?page=1.

54 "Marijuana: Is Marijuana Addictive?" *National Institute on Drug Abuse*, accessed May 12, 2016, http://www.drugabuse.gov/publications/research-reports/marijuana/marijuana-addictive.

55 Ibid.

56 "Popping Pills: Prescription Drug Abuse in America," National Institute on *Drug Abuse*, accessed May 12, 2016, http://www.drugabuse.gov/related-topics/trends-statistics/infographics/popping-pills-prescription-drug-abuse-in-america.

57 Daniel Perdomo, "100,000 Americans Die Each Year from Prescription Drugs, While Pharma Companies Get Rich," Personal Health, *AlterNet*, June 24, 2010, http://www.alternet.org/story/147318/100,000_americans_die_each_year_from_prescription_drugs,_while_pharma_companies_get_rich.

58 Donald W. Light, "New Prescription Drugs: A Major Health Risk with Few Offsetting Advantages," *Edmond J. Safra Center for Ethics* (blog), June 27, 2014, http://ethics.harvard.edu/blog/new-prescription-drugs-major-health-risk-few-offsetting-advantages.

59 Ibid.

CHAPTER NINE: The Truth about Marijuana and Big Pharma

1 Patrick Stack and Claire Suddath, "A Brief History of Medical Marijuana," *TIME*, October 21, 2009, http://content.time.com/time/health/article/0,8599,1931247,00.html.

2 PBS, "Marijuana Timeline," Frontline, accessed May 12, 2016, http://www.pbs.org/wgbh/pages/frontline/shows/dope/etc/cron.html.

3 Jacob Sullum, "Bill Bennett's Marijuana Gateway Theory (and Harry Anslinger's)," *Forbes*, February 10, 2015, http://www.forbes.com/sites/jacobsullum/2015/02/10/bill-bennetts-marijuana-gateway-theory-and-harry-anslingers/#48b84239215c.

4 Center on Addiction and Substance Abuse, "CASA Releases Report: Non-medical Marijuana—Rite of Passage or Russian Roulette?" news release, July 13,1999.

5 Jacob Sullum, *Saying Yes: In Defense of Drug Use,* (New York: Penguin, 2004), 54–55.

6 "Drunk Driving Statistics," *MADD*, accessed May 12, 2016, http://www.madd.org/drunk-driving/about/drunk-driving-statistics.html?referrer=https://www.google.com/.

7 "2013 Tables: Ilicit Drug Use," *Substance Abuse and Mental Health Service Administration (SAMHSA)*, accessed May 12, 2016, http://www.samhsa.gov/data/sites/default/files/NSDUH-DetTabsPDFWHTML2013/Web/HTML/NSDUH-DetTabsSect1peTabs1to46-2013.htm.

8 Jacob Sullum, "Bill Bennett's Marijuana Gateway Theory (and Harry Anslinger's)," *Forbes*, February 10, 2015, http://www.forbes.com/sites/jacobsullum/2015/02/10/bill-bennetts-marijuana-gateway-theory-and-harry-anslingers/#48b84239215c.

9 "Marijuana Arrests by the Numbers," *American Civil Liberties Union (ACLU)*, accessed May 12, 2016, https://www.aclu.org/gallery/marijuana-arrests-numbers.

10 David Turbert and Dayle Kern, "Does Marijuana Help Treat Glaucoma?" *American Academy of Ophthalmology*, June 27, 2014, http://www.aao.org/eye-health/tips-prevention/medical-marijuana-glaucoma-treament.

11 "Glaucoma Medications and Their Side Effects," Glaucoma Research Foundation, accessed May 12, 2016, http://www.glaucoma.org/treatment/glaucoma-medications-and-their-side-effects.php.

12 Henry Jampel, "Position Statement on Marijuana and the Treatment of Glaucoma," *American Glaucoma Society*, August 10, 2009, http://www.americanglaucomasociety.net/patients/position_statements/marijuana_glaucoma.

13 "Opioid Painkiller Prescribing," Centers for Disease *Control and Prevention*, accessed May 12, 2016, http://www.cdc.gov/vitalsigns/opioid-prescribing/.

14 Darren McCollester, "Study Shows 70 Percent of Americans Take Prescription Drugs," *CBS News*, June 20, 2013, http://www.cbsnews.com/news/study-shows-70-percent-of-americans-take-prescription-drugs/.

15 Saundra Young, "Marijuana Stops Child's Severe Seizures," *CNN*, August 7, 2013, http://www.cnn.com/2013/08/07/health/charlotte-child-medical-marijuana.

16 "Charlotte Figi's Ongoing Story with Medical Marijuana," *Healthy Hemp Oil*, accessed May 12, 2016, https://healthyhempoil.com/charlotte-figi-2/#.Vq6l35MrJE4.

17 Saundra Young, "Marijuana Stops Child's Severe Seizures," *CNN*, August 7, 2013, http://www.cnn.com/2013/08/07/health/charlotte-child-medical-marijuana.

18 Ibid.

19 Ibid.

20 Ibid.

21 Anne-Marie O'Connor, "Israeli Medical Marijuana Creates Buzz but No High—Will It Go Global?" *Washington Post*, February 1, 2015, https://www.washingtonpost.com/world/middle_east/israeli-medical-marijuana-creates-buzz-but-no-high-will-it-go-global/2015/01/31/558fe072-a19a-11e4-9f89-561284a573f8_story.html.

22 Natalya M. Kogan et al., "Cannabidiol, a Major Non-psychotropic Cannabis Constituent Enhances Fracture Healing and Stimulates Lysyl Hydroxylase Activity in Osteoblasts," *Journal of Bone and Mineral Research* 30, no. 10 (2015): 1905–1913, http://onlinelibrary.wiley.com/doi/10.1002/jbmr.2513/abstract;jsessionid=DBEF56DB42BCE5AEDD3BB6A9D3D0B03B.f03t02.

23 Wilborn P. Nobles III, "Another Medical Use for Pot: Healing Broken Bones," *Washington Post*, July 20, 2015, https://www.washingtonpost.com/news/morning-mix/wp/2015/07/20/can-pot-heal-broken-bones-the-answer-is-yes-study-finds/.

24 http://nof.org/articles/22

25 Kate Pickert, "Finally, Some Hard Science on Medical Marijuana for Epilepsy Patients," *TIME*, September 3, 2014, http://time.com/3264691/medical-marijauna-epilepsy-research-charlottes-web-study/.

26 Ibid.

27 Fred Vogelstein, "One Man's Desperate Quest to Cure His Son's Epilepsy—With Weed," *Wired*, July 2015, http://www.wired.com/2015/07/medical-marijuana-epilepsy/.

28 Amy Nordrum, "Medical Marijuana: Early Test Results of Epidiolex Show Promise for Epilepsy Patients," *International Business Times*, April 13, 2015, http://www.ibtimes.com/medical-marijuana-early-test-results-epidiolex-show-promise-epilepsy-patients-1879515.

29 Carly Schwartz, "Groundbreaking Research Suggests Medical Marijuana Could Reduce Seizures in Children," Huffpost Healthy Living, *Huffington Post*, April 14, 2015, http://www.huffingtonpost.com/2015/04/13/epidiolex_n_7055784.html.

30 Amy Nordrum, "Medical Marijuana: Early Test Results of Epidiolex Show Promise for Epilepsy Patients," *International Business Times*, April 13, 2015, http://www.ibtimes.com/medical-marijuana-early-test-results-epidiolex-show-promise-epilepsy-patients-1879515.

31 Ibid.

32 Ibid.

33 Ibid.

34 Trevor Hughes, "Study Gives Hope Marijuana Extract Can Treat Seizures," *USA Today*, April 13, 2015, http://www.usatoday.com/story/news/nation/2015/04/13/marijuana-extract-seizure-study/25725381/.

35 Carly Schwartz, "Groundbreaking Research Suggests Medical Marijuana Could Reduce Seizures in Children," Huffpost Healthy Living, *Huffington Post*, April 14, 2015, http://www.huffingtonpost.com/2015/04/13/epidiolex_n_7055784.html.

36 "Charlotte's Web," *Leafly*, accessed May 12, 2016, https://www.leafly.com/sativa/charlottes-web.

37 Hampton Sides, "Science Seeks to Unlock Marijuana's Secrets," *National Geographic*, June 2015, http://ngm.nationalgeographic.com/2015/06/marijuana/sides-text.

38 *eMC*, s.v. "Sativex Oromucosal Spray," last updated May 20, 2015, http://www.medicines.org.uk/emc/medicine/23262.

39 Ibid.

40 Ibid.

41 Rick Simpson, "Home Page," *Phoenix Tears*, accessed May 12, 2016, http://phoenixtears.ca/.

42 Rick Simpson, "Nature's Answer for Cancer," *Phoenix Tears*, accessed May 12, 2016, http://phoenixtears.ca/natures-answer-for-cancer/.

CHAPTER TEN: The US Government's Marijuana Patent Conspiracy

1 Lisa Leff, "Pot-Based Mouth Spray Medicine Looks for US Approval," *USA Today*, January 27, 2012, http://usatoday30.usatoday.com/money/industries/health/story/2012-01-29/pot-based-prescription-drug/52826376/1.

2 Aidan J. Hampson, Julius Axelrod, and Maurizio Grimaldi, "Cannabinoids as Antioxidants and Neuroprotectants," US Patent 6,630,507 B1, filed April 21, 1999, and issued October 7, 2003, http://www.google.ca/patents/US6630507.

3 *Patent Genius*, s.v. "Mechoulam, Raphael," accessed May 12, 2016, http://www.patentgenius.com/inventor/MechoulamRaphael.html.

4 "Food and Drug Administration," US Department of Health and Human Services, last modified March 18, 2016, http://www.hhs.gov/ohrp/humansubjects/fda/.

5 Matthew Herper, "Solving the Drug Patent Problem," *Forbes*, May 2, 2002, http://www.forbes.com/2002/05/02/0502patents.html.

6 Yardena Schwartz, "The Outsourcing of American Marijuana Research," Tech and Science, News*week*, December 17, 2015, http://www.newsweek.com/2015/12/25/outsourcing-american-marijuana-research-406184.html?rx=us.

7 Anne-Marie O'Connor, "Israeli Medical Marijuana Creates Buzz but No High—Will It Go Global?" *Washington Post*, February 1, 2015, https://www.washingtonpost.com/world/middle_east/israeli-medical-marijuana-creates-buzz-but-no-high-will-it-go-global/2015/01/31/558fe072-a19a-11e4-9f89-561284a573f8_story.html.

8 Ibid.

9 Anthony Wile, "Dr. Raphael Mechoulam: The Promise of Cannabis," *The Daily Bell*, October 19, 2014, http://www.thedailybell.com/exclusive-interviews/35732/Anthony-Wile-Dr-Raphael-Mechoulam-The-Promise-of-Cannabis/.

10 Ido Efrati, "Preliminary Results from Israeli Study: Cannabis Delays Cancer Development," *HAARETZ*, April 11, 2015, http://www.haaretz.com/israel-news/culture/health/.premium-1.651249.

11 www.cannabics.com

12 M. M. Caffarel et al., "JunD Is Involved in the Antiproliferative Effect of Delta9-tetrahydrocannabinol on Human Breast Cancer Cells," *Oncogene* 27, no. 37 (2008): 5033-5044, http://www.ncbi.nlm.nih.gov/pubmed/18454173.

13 Pál Pacher and George Kunos, "Modulating the Endocannabinoid System in Human Health and Disease: Successes and Failures," *FEBS Journal* 280, no. 9 (2013): 1918–1943, http://www.ncbi.nlm.nih.gov/pmc/articles/PMC3684164/pdf/nihms460242.pdf.

14 Yardena Schwartz, "The Outsourcing of American Marijuana Research," Tech and Science, *Newsweek*, December 17, 2015, http://www.newsweek.com/2015/12/25/outsourcing-american-marijuana-research-406184.html?rx=us.

15 *Newsweek Special Issue: Weed 2.0* (New York: Media Lab Publishing, 2016).

16 Lizzie Parry, "How Cannabis Can Help Cancer Patients: Drug Kills Cancer and Shrinks Brain Tumours, Report Reveals," *Daily Mail*, April 13, 2015, http://www.dailymail.co.uk/health/article-3036667/How-cannabis-help-cancer-patients-Drug-kills-cancer-cells-shrinks-brain-tumours-report-reveals.html.

17 Alex Rogers, "Uncle Sam Will Buy $69 Million Worth of Pot from Ole Miss," *TIME*, March 23, 2015, http://time.com/3755253/university-mississippi-marijuana/.

18 Steven Nelson, "The End of Ole Miss' Pot Monopoly?" *US News and World Report*, August 28, 2014, http://www.usnews.com/news/articles/2014/08/28/the-end-of-ole-miss-pot-monopoly.

19 Evan Halper, "Mississippi, Home to Federal Government's Official Stash of Marijuana," *Los Angeles Times*, May 28, 2014, http://www.latimes.com/nation/la-na-pot-monopoly-20140529-story.html#page=1.

20 Ibid.

21 GW Pharmaceuticals, "GW Pharmaceuticals Receives Orphan Drug Designation by FDA for Epidiolex in the Treatment of Lennox-Gastaut Syndrome," news release, February 28, 2014, http://www.gwpharm.com/LGS%20Orphan%20Designation.aspx.

22 "Dravet Syndrome," *Epilepsy Foundation*, accessed May 12, 2016, http://www.epilepsy.com/learn/types-epilepsy-syndromes/dravet-syndrome.

23 GW Pharmaceuticals, "GW Pharmaceuticals Receives Orphan Drug Designation by FDA for Epidiolex in the Treatment of Lennox-Gastaut Syndrome," news release, February 28, 2014, http://www.gwpharm.com/LGS%20Orphan%20Designation.aspx.

24 Ibid.

25 Mike Adams, "Federal Lawmakers Concerned the FDA Is Sustaining a Painkiller Epidemic, Pot Prohibition," *High Times*, January 14, 2016, http://www.hightimes.com/read/federal-lawmakers-concerned-fda-sustaining-painkiller-epidemic-pot-prohibition.

26 http://www.gwpharm.com/GW%20Pharmaceuticals%20plc%20Announces%20US

27 Debra Borchardt, "How the US Government Makes Money on Cannabis," *The Street*, June 13, 2014, http://www.thestreet.com/story/12743192/1/how-the-us-government-makes-money-on-cannabis.html.

28 http://www.keystoneedge.com/innovationnews/kannalife0711.aspx

29 Paul J. Lim, "7 Marijuana Stocks for a Buzzworthy (But Risky) Pot-folio," *Money*, July 8, 2014, http://time.com/money/2965556/7-marijuana-stocks-for-a-buzzworthy-but-risky-pot-folio/.

30 Debra Borchardt, "How the US Government Makes Money on Cannabis," *The Street*, June 13, 2014, http://www.thestreet.com/story/12743192/1/how-the-us-government-makes-money-on-cannabis.html.

31 "Could Marijuana Treat Concussions for Professional Athletes?" *Marijuana Stocks*, October 5, 2015, http://marijuanastocks.com/tag/cannatol/.

32 http://www.keystoneedge.com/innovationnews/kannalife0711.aspx

33 www.cannatol.com

34 http://www.keystoneedge.com/innovationnews/kannalife0711.aspx

35 https://www.kannalife.com/cnbc-small-business-cannabis-concussions/

36 Eddie Pells, "'Concussion' Doctor Aiding Marijuana-Based Research Company," *The Big Story*, November 3, 2015, http://bigstory.ap.org/article/f10a8575925e4bb8b64f6e7877175fac/concussion-doctor-aiding-marijuana-based-research-company.

37 https://www.kannalife.com/cnbc-small-business-cannabis-concussions/

38 MedlinePlus, s.v. "loss of brain function—liver disease," last modified August 14, 2015, https://www.nlm.nih.gov/medlineplus/ency/article/000302.htm.

39 Jim Doyle, "KV Boosts Pernatal Drug Price 100-Fold," Business, *St. Louis Post-Dispatch*, March 10, 2011, http://www.stltoday.com/business/local/article_55dbaf88-4ab0-11e0-ad73-0017a4a78c22.html.

40 Michael Hiltzik, "Congress Made Martin Shkreli Look Like a Jerk, but It Bears Responsibility for High Drug Prices," *Los Angeles Times*, February 4, 2016, http://www.latimes.com/business/hiltzik/la-fi-mh-shkreli-looked-like-a-jerk-20160204-column.html.

CHAPTER ELEVEN: Marijuana Invades Americana with Contradictions All Around

1 Trevor Hughes, "Feds Ask Supreme Court to Stay Out of Lawsuit Over Colorado Marijuana," *USA Today*, December 17, 2015, http://www.usatoday.com/story/news/2015/12/16/feds-ask-supreme-court-stay-out-lawsuit-over-colorado-marijuana/77457652/.

2 Ricardo Baca, "Professor: Why Nebraska, Oklahoma Have a Right to Kill Colorado's Legal Pot," *The Cannabist*, June 26, 2015, http://www.thecannabist.co/2015/06/26/nebraska-oklahoma-colorado-marijuana-pot/36873/.

3 Christ Casteel, "Colorado Not Hurting Oklahoma and Nebraska with Pot Laws, Administration Says," *NewsOK*, December 17, 2015, http://newsok.com/article/5467342.

4 https://assets.documentcloud.org/documents/2648064/U-S-Solicitor-General-response-to-Colorado.pdf

5 Jesse Ventura's Off the Grid, "Supreme Court Denies Case Against Colorado's Marijuana Legalization," *Ora*, March 24, 2016, http://www.ora.tv/offthegrid/article/2016/3/24/supreme-court-denies-case-against-colorados-marijuana-legalization.

6 "Just Plain False," *Monsanto*, accessed May 12, 2016, http://www.monsanto.com/newsviews/pages/myths-about-monsanto.aspx.

7 Kit O'Connell, "Did Monsanto Really Just Get a Patent for GMO Marijuana?" *MintPress News*, April 17, 2015, http://www.mintpressnews.com/did-monsanto-really-just-get-a-patent-for-gmo-marijuana/204480/.

8 Dana Mattioli, "High Hopes at Miracle-Gro in Medical Marijuana Field," *Wall Street Journal*, June 14, 2011, http://www.wsj.com/articles/SB10001424052702304665904576383832249741032.

9 Jack Kaskey, "Lawn-Care Giant Targets a New Weed as Pot Industry Grows," *Bloomberg*, April 16, 2015, http://www.bloomberg.com/news/articles/2015-04-16/lawn-care-giant-looks-to-another-kind-of-weed.

10 Kit O'Connell, "Did Monsanto Really Just Get a Patent for GMO Marijuana?" *MintPress News*, April 17, 2015, http://www.mintpressnews.com/did-monsanto-really-just-get-a-patent-for-gmo-marijuana/204480/.

11 Fezisa Mdibi, "War on Dagga Puts Rural People at Toxic Risk, Specialists Warn," *Mail and Guardian*, March 19, 2015, Kit O'Connell, "Did Monsanto Really Just Get a Patent for GMO Marijuana?" *MintPress News*, April 17, 2015, http://www.mintpressnews.com/did-monsanto-really-just-get-a-patent-for-gmo-marijuana/204480/.

12 Derrick Broze, "World Health Organization Won't Back Down from Study Linking Monsanto to Cancer," *The Anti-Media*, March 30, 2015, http://theantimedia.org/world-health-organization-wont-back-down-from-study-linking-monsanto-to-cancer/.

13 Cannabis Sativa Inc., "Cannabis Sativa Inc. Signs Purchase Agreement for Patent Pending Hybrid, Marijuana Strain CTA and Option to Acquire KUSH for $1 Million," news release, January 2, 2014, https://globenewswire.com/news-release/2014/01/02/599901/10062731/en/Cannabis-Sativa-Inc-Signs-Purchase-Agreement-for-Patent-Pending-Hybrid-Marijuana-Strain-CTA-and-Option-to-Acquire-KUSH-for-1-Million.html?parent=647863.

14 Paul J. Lim, "7 Marijuana Stocks for a Buzzworthy (But Risky) Pot-Folio," *Money*, July 8, 2014, http://time.com/money/2965556/7-marijuana-stocks-for-a-buzzworthy-but-risky-pot-folio/.

15 Sam Kamin and Joel Warner, "Your Money Stinks," *Slate*, January 31, 2014, http://www.slate.com/articles/news_and_politics/altered_state/2014/01/colorado_marijuana_businesses_have_a_big_problem_banks_won_t_take_their.html.

16 Ibid.

17 Alan Pyke, "Big Banks Balk, So Colorado Has Created a Credit Union for the Marijuana Industry," ThinkProgress, December 9, 2014, http://thinkprogress.org/economy/2014/12/09/3601055/colorado-marijuana-credit-union/.

18 "Editorial: Congress Must Act on Marijuana Banking, Allow Access to System," BizWest, January 22, 2016, http://bizwest.com/congress-must-act-on-marijuana-banking-allow-access-to-system/.

19 "Why the Fourth Corner CU Is Suing NCUA, Fed," *CUToday*, October 24, 2015, http://www.cutoday.info/THE-feature/Why-The-Fourth-Corner-CU-Is-Suing-NCUA-Fed.

20 "Editorial: Congress Must Act on Marijuana Banking, Allow Access to System," *BizWest*, January 22, 2016, http://bizwest.com/congress-must-act-on-marijuana-banking-allow-access-to-system/.

21 Marijuana Businesses Access to Banking Act of 2015, H.R. 2076, 114th Cong. (2015).

22 "Subcommittee on Crime, Terrorism, Homeland Security, and Investigations," *House of Representatives Judiciary Committee*, accessed May 12, 2016, http://judiciary.house.gov/index.cfm/subcommittee-on-crime-terrorism-homeland-security-and-investigations.

23 *OnTheIssues*, s.v. "James Sensenbrenner on Drugs," accessed May 12, 2016, http://www.ontheissues.org/House/James_Sensenbrenner_Drugs.htm.

24 Jennifer Kaplan, "Where to Stash Cannabis Cash? Tribal Nations Make Bid to Bank It," Technology, *Bloomberg*, October 11, 2015, http://www.bloomberg.com/news/articles/2015-10-11/where-to-stash-cannabis-cash-tribal-nations-make-bid-to-bank-it.

25 Ibid.

26 www.cannanative.com

27 Tom Huddleston Jr., "The Marijuana Industry's Battle against the IRS," *Fortune*, April 15, 2015, http://fortune.com/2015/04/15/marijuana-industry-tax-problem/.

28 Robert W. Wood, "Big Court Defeat for Marijuana Despite Record Tax Harvests," Taxes, *Forbes*, July 13, 2015, http://www.forbes.com/sites/robertwood/2015/07/13/big-court-defeat-for-marijuana-despite-record-tax-harvests/#4f1ac4d27c7e.

29 Terrence McCoy, "How the IRS and Congress Cripple the Marijuana Industry with an Obscure, Decades-Old Law," Morning Mix, *Washington Post*, November 5, 2014, https://www.washingtonpost.com/news/morning-mix/wp/2014/11/05/how-the-irs-and-congress-cripple-the-marijuana-industry-with-an-obscure-decades-old-law/.

30 Tom Huddleston Jr., "The Marijuana Industry's Battle against the IRS," *Fortune*, April 15, 2015, http://fortune.com/2015/04/15/marijuana-industry-tax-problem/.

31 Matthew Villmer, "Tax Creativity Keeps Pot Industry Out of IRS Hot Water," Law360.*com*, March 4, 2014, http://www.law360.com/articles/513633/tax-creativity-keeps-pot-industry-out-of-irs-hot-water.

32 John Hudak, "Who's Right on Marijuana? Justice or the IRS?" Opinion, *Newsweek*, July 19, 2015, http://www.newsweek.com/whos-right-marijuana-justice-or-irs-354975.

33 Tanya Basu, "Colorado Raised More Tax Revenue from Marijuana Than from Alcohol," *TIME*, September 16, 2015, http://time.com/4037604/colorado-marijuana-tax-revenue/.

34 John Frank, "Colorado to Offer One-Day Tax Holiday on Marijuana," *Denver Post*, June 4, 2015, http://www.denverpost.com/news/ci_28252221/colorado-offer-one-day-tax-holiday-marijuana.

35 Kit O'Connell, "New Schools, Less Crime: Colorado Sees Benefits of Marijuana Legalization," *MintPress News*, August 19, 2015, http://www.mintpressnews.com/new-schools-less-crime-colorado-sees-benefits-of-marijuana-legalization/208751/.

36 Trevor Hughes, "Colo. Pot Users Helping Build Schools with Tax Dollars," *USA Today*, February 17, 2015, http://www.usatoday.com/story/news/nation/2015/02/17/colorado-marijuana-revenues/23565543/.

37 Masuma Ahuja, "College Paid for by Marijuana," *CNN*, November 6, 2015, http://www.cnn.com/2015/11/06/us/colorado-marijuana-college-scholarship/.

38 "Status Report: Marijuana Legalization in Colorado after One Year of Retail Sales and Two Years of Decriminalization," *Drug Policy Alliance*, accessed May 12, 2016, https://www.drugpolicy.org/sites/default/files/Colorado_Marijuana_Legalization_One_Year_Status_Report.pdf.

39 Ibid.

40 Substance Abuse and Mental Health Services, "State Estimates of Nonmedical Use of Prescription Pain Relievers," *The NSDUH Report*, January 8, 2013, http://www.samhsa.gov/data/sites/default/files/NSDUH115/NSDUH115/sr115-nonmedical-use-pain-relievers.htm.

41 Will Yakowicz, "Why Legal Marijuana Could Be a $6 Billion Industry in 2016," *MoneyBox*, February 5, 2016, http://www.slate.com/blogs/moneybox/2016/02/05/sales_of_legalized_cannabis_projected_to_hit_6_7_billion_in_2016.html.

42 "How Long Does THC Stay in Your System?" *Leaf Science*, April 22, 2014, http://www.leafscience.com/2014/04/22/how-long-thc-stay-system/.

43 psmith, "South Dakota Law Can Get You Busted for Using Marijuana in Another State," StopTheDrugWar.org, November 11, 2015, http://stopthedrugwar.org/chronicle/2015/nov/11/south_dakota_law_can_get_you_bus.

44 http://legis.sd.gov/Statutes/Codified_Laws/DisplayStatute.aspx?Type=Statute&Statute=22-42-15

45 "South Dakota 'Internal Possession' Drug Law Upheld," StopTheDrugWar.org, February 27, 2004, http://stopthedrugwar.org/chronicle-old/326/southdakota.shtml.

46 "South Dakota: Home of the Most Draconian Weed Laws in the US," *PanAm Post*, November 18, 2015, http://blog.panampost.com/guillermo-jimenez/2015/11/18/south-dakota-home-of-the-most-draconian-weed-laws-in-the-us/.

47 Neal Augenstein, "Weed in DC—What's Legal, What's Not," *WTOP*, February 26, 2015, http://wtop.com/dc/2015/02/weed-in-d-c-whats-legal-whats-not/.

48 Will Yakowicz, "Why Legal Marijuana Could Be a $6 Billion Industry in 2016," *MoneyBox* (blog), February 5, 2016, http://www.slate.com/blogs/moneybox/2016/02/05/sales_of_legalized_cannabis_projected_to_hit_6_7_billion_in_2016.html.

49 Jen Rini, "How to Get on Delaware's Medical Marijuana List," *Delaware Online*, November 1, 2015, http://www.delawareonline.com/story/news/health/2015/11/01/how-get-dels-marijuana-list/74812436/.

50 *Centers for Disease Control and Prevention*, s.v. "autism spectrum disorder (ASD)," accessed May 12, 2016, http://www.cdc.gov/ncbddd/autism/treatment.html.

51 Joe Stone, "Part Three: Practical Approach to Cannabis Based ASD Therapies," *Medical Jane*, June 17, 2015, http://www.medicaljane.com/2015/06/17/part-three-practical-approach-to-cannabis-based-asd-therapies/.

52 Joe Stone, "Part One: the Endocannabinoid System and Autism Spectrum Disorder (ASD)," *Medical Jane*, June 17, 2015, http://www.medicaljane.com/2015/06/17/is-the-endocannabinoid-system-involved-in-the-progression-of-asd/.

53 Ibid.

CHAPTER TWELVE: Marijuana and Post-Traumatic Stress Disorder

1 David Olinger, "Kansas Holds Children of Colorado Veteran Who Uses Medical Marijuana," *Brush News-Tribune*, January 13, 2016, http://www.brushnewstribune.com/ci_29387805/kansas-holds-children-colorado-veteran-who-uses-medical.

2 Ibid.

3 Josiah Hesse, "US Veteran's Children Taken Away over His Use of Medical Marijuana," *The Guardian*, February 1, 2016, http://www.theguardian.com/society/2016/feb/01/medical-marijuana-use-colorado-kansas-veteran-custody-battle.

4 David Olinger, "Kansas Holds Children of Colorado Veteran Who Uses Medical Marijuana," *Brush News-Tribune*, January 13, 2016, http://www.brushnewstribune.com/ci_29387805/kansas-holds-children-colorado-veteran-who-uses-medical.

5 Josiah Hesse, "US Veteran's Children Taken Away over His Use of Medical Marijuana," *The Guardian*, February 1, 2016, http://www.theguardian.com/society/2016/feb/01/medical-marijuana-use-colorado-kansas-veteran-custody-battle.

6   Bob Knudsen, "Kansas Declares War on Veterans and Families in the Name of Prohibition, *Examiner*, January 14, 2016, http://www.examiner.com/article/kansas-declares-war-on-veterans-and-families-the-name-of-prohibition.

7   "PTSD-Afflicted Veteran Deprived of His 5 Children over Medical Marijuana Use," *RT*, January 15, 2016, https://www.rt.com/usa/329060-ptsd-veteran-marijuana-children/.

8   Josiah Hesse, "US Veteran's Children Taken Away over His Use of Medical Marijuana," *The Guardian*, February 1, 2016, http://www.theguardian.com/society/2016/feb/01/medical-marijuana-use-colorado-kansas-veteran-custody-battle.

9   "Parental Drug Use as Child Abuse: State Statutes Current through April 2015," *Child Welfare Information Gateway*, accessed May 12, 2016, https://www.childwelfare.gov/pubPDFs/drugexposed.pdf.

10   "18 Most Famous Lenny Bruce Quotes," NLCATP.org, December 1, 2014, http://nlcatp.org/18-most-famous-lenny-bruce-quotes/.

11   Julia Wright, "How Anti-cannabis Laws Victimize Vets and Their Families," *Civilized*, February 8, 2016, https://www.civilized.life/veterans-families-ptsd-cannabis-laws-1591565152.html.

12   "Post-traumatic Stress Syndrome (PTSD)," *Veterans for Compassionate Care*, accessed May 12, 2016, http://veteransforcompassionatecare.org/ptsd.asp.

13   T. Kid, "Why Aren't American Veterans Allowed to Treat Their PTSD with Medical Marijuana," *Vice*, January 26, 2015, http://www.vice.com/read/when-will-americas-war-veterans-with-ptsd-get-weed-126.

14   "Report on VA Facility Specific Operation Enduring Freedom (OEF), Operation Iraqi Freedom (OIF), and Operation New Dawn (OND) Veterans Coded with Potential PTSD—Revised," *Department of Veteran Affairs*, accessed May 12, 2016, http://www.publichealth.va.gov/docs/epidemiology/ptsd-report-fy2012-qtr3.pdf.

15   "US Military Veteran Suicides Rise, One Dies Every 65 Minutes," *Reuters*, February 1, 2013, http://www.reuters.com/article/us-usa-veterans-suicide-idUSBRE9101E320130202.

16   Leo Sher, María Dolores Braquehais, and Miquel Casas, "Posttraumatic Stress Disorder, Depression, and Suicide in Veterans," *Cleveland Clinic Journal of Medicine* 79, no. 2 (2012): 92–97, http://www.ccjm.org/cme/cme/article/posttraumatic-stress-disorder-depression-and-suicide-in-veterans/9599364d492ae6090d035c25ff18e884.html.

17   "Treatments for PTSD," TraumaCenter.org, accessed May 12, 2016, http://www.traumacenter.org/resources/pdf_files/PTSD_Treatments.pdf.

18   "24 Legal Medical Marijuana States and DC," ProCon.org, last modified March 14, 2016, http://medicalmarijuana.procon.org/view.resource.php?resourceID=000881.

19   Bailey Rahn, "Qualifying Conditions for Medical Marijuana by State," *Leafly*, January 31, 2014, https://www.leafly.com/news/health/qualifying-conditions-for-medical-marijuana-by-state.

20   "24 Legal Medical Marijuana States and DC," ProCon.org, last modified March 14, 2016, http://medicalmarijuana.procon.org/view.resource.php?resourceID=000881.

21   Bailey Rahn, "Qualifying Conditions for Medical Marijuana by State," *Leafly*, January 31, 2014, https://www.leafly.com/news/health/qualifying-conditions-for-medical-marijuana-by-state.

22   Emily Lane, "Medical Marijuana in Louisiana: Who Will Get Access?" *NOLA*, June 30, 2015, http://www.nola.com/politics/index.ssf/2015/06/medical_marijuana_louisiana_wh.html.

23   April M. Short, "Medical Marijuana Industry Sprouts Up in Israel," *AlterNet*, September 12, 2013, http://www.alternet.org/drugs/medical-marijuana-industry-sprouts-israel.

24   Ido Efrati, "Medical Marijuana Is Legal for PTSD in Israel, but Good Luck Getting It," *Haaretz*, December 8, 2015, http://www.haaretz.com/israel-news/.premium-1.690611.

25 Shira Rubin, "A Flourishing $40 Million Medical Marijuana Industry Helps Israelis Forget," *Tablet*, July 12, 2013, http://www.tabletmag.com/jewish-news-and-politics/137423/medical-marijuana-kibbutz.

26 April M. Short, "Medical Marijuana Industry Sprouts Up in Israel," *AlterNet*, September 12, 2013, http://www.alternet.org/drugs/medical-marijuana-industry-sprouts-israel.

27 Ido Efrati, "Medical Marijuana Is Legal for PTSD in Israel, but Good Luck Getting It," *Haaretz*, December 8, 2015, http://www.haaretz.com/israel-news/.premium-1.690611.

28 Ibid.

29 Thor Benson, "More and More US Veterans Are Smoking Weed to Treat Their PTSD," *Vice*, November 7, 2013, http://www.vice.com/read/more-and-more-us-veterans-are-smoking-weed-to-treat-their-ptsd.

30 Raphael Mechoulam, "General Use of Cannabis for PTSD Symptoms," *Veterans for Medical Cannabis Access*, accessed May 12, 2016, http://veteransformedicalmarijuana.org/content/general-use-cannabis-ptsd-symptoms.

31 P. Roitman, R. Mechoulam, R. Cooper-Kazaz, and A. Shalev, "Preliminary, Open-Label, Pilot Study of Add-On Oral Delta9-tetrahydrocannabinol in Chronic Post-traumatic Stress Disorder," *Clinical Drug Investigating* 34, no. 8 (2014): 587–591, http://www.ncbi.nlm.nih.gov/pubmed/24935052.

32 George R. Greer, Charles S. Grob, and Adam L. Halberstadt, "PTSD Syptom Reports of Patients Evaluated for the New Mexico Medical Cannabis Program," *Journal of Psychoactive Drugs* 46, no. 1 (2014): 73–77, http://www.tandfonline.com/doi/pdf/10.1080/02791072.2013.873843.

33 http://www.vice.com/read/when-will-americas-war-veterans-with-ptsd-get-weed-126

34 http://www.denverpost.com/2016/04/22/dea-gives-approval-to-colorado-funded-study-on-marijuana-and-ptsd/

35 http://www.militarytimes.com/story/veterans/2016/04/21/dea-approves-ptsd-marijuana-study/83356604/

36 http://www.newsweek.com/pot-and-ptsd-358139

37 http://www.maps.org/news/media/6141-press-release-dea-approves-first-ever-trial-of-medical-marijuana-for-ptsd-in-veterans

38 http://www.newsweek.com/pot-and-ptsd-358139

39 http://www.phoenixnewtimes.com/news/dea-approves-pot-study-in-arizona-and-colorado-aimed-at-helping-veterans-with-ptsd-8238610

40 http://www.maps.org/news/media/4603-ptsd-relief-in-israel-through-mdma-and-cannabis-research

41 http://www.sciencedirect.com/science/article/pii/S0278584615000603

42 http://www.nbcnews.com/health/health-news/pot-researcher-firing-unleashes-rising-veteran-backlash-n167691

43 http://www.nbcnews.com/health/health-news/pot-researcher-firing-unleashes-rising-veteran-backlash-n167691

44 http://www.denverpost.com/2016/04/22/dea-gives-approval-to-colorado-funded-study-on-marijuana-and-ptsd/

45 http://blazenow.com/article/dea-finally-approves-study-on-cannabis-and-ptsd

46 http://www.ptsd.va.gov/professional/co-occurring/marijuana_use_ptsd_veterans.asp

47 Department of Veterans Affairs, "Access to Clinical Programs for Veterans Participating in State-Approved Marijuana Programs," Veterans Health Administration, January 31, 2011, http://veteransforcompassionatecare.org/resources/VA-access-to-marijuana-programs.pdf.

48 Leafly, "Senate Approves Funding Bill Allowing Medical Marijuana for Veterans," *MintPress News*, November 12, 2015, http://www.mintpressnews.com/senate-approves-funding-bill-allowing-medical-marijuana-for-veterans/211222/.

49 Christina Marcos, "House Rejects Proposal to Let VA Doctors Recommend Medical Marijuana," *Floor Action* (blog), April 30, 2015, http://thehill.com/blogs/floor-action/house/240731-house-rejects-allowing-va-doctors-to-recommend-medical-marijuana.

50 Consolidated Appropriations Act of 2016, H. R. 2029, 114th Cong. (2016), https://www.congress.gov/bill/114th-congress/house-bill/2029.

51 Kirsten Gillibrand, "Gillibrand, Daines, Merkley, Blumenauer, Titus, and Rohrabacher Lead Bipartisan Effort Urging the Department of Veterans Affairs to Change Its Current Policy, Allow VA Doctors to Discuss and Recommend Medical Marijuana in States Where It Is Legal," news release, January 27, 2016, https://www.gillibrand.senate.gov/newsroom/press/release/gillibrand-daines-merkley-blumenauer-titus-and-rohrabacher-lead-bipartisan-effort-urging-the-department-of-veterans-affairs-to-change-its-current-policy-allow-va-doctors-to-discuss-and-recommend-medical-marijuana-in-states-where-it-is-legal.

52 http://www.drugpolicy.org/news/2016/04/senate-appropriations-committee-approves-veterans-access-medical-marijuana

53 http://www.drugpolicy.org/news/2016/04/senate-appropriations-committee-approves-veterans-access-medical-marijuana

54 Matthew Daly and Terry Tang, "VA chief: 18 Vets Left oOff Waiting List Have Died," *Associated Press*, June 6, 2014, http://bigstory.ap.org/article/senate-moves-toward-vote-va-health-care.

CHAPTER THIRTEEN: Jury Nullification—How to Fight Back against Marijuana Prohibition

1 Aaron McKnight, "Jury Nullification as a Tool to Balance the Demands of Law and Justice," *BYU Law Review* 4 (2013): 1103–1132, http://digitalcommons.law.byu.edu/cgi/viewcontent.cgi?article=2890&context=lawreview.

2 James Joseph Duane, "Jury Nullification: The Top Secret Constitutional Right," *Litigation* 22, no. 4 (1996): 6–60, http://www.constitution.org/2ll/2ndschol/131jur.pdf.

3 "West Virginia Bill Would Require Courts to Inform Jurors of Their Right to Nullify," *Tenth Amendment Center*, January 22, 2016, http://blog.tenthamendmentcenter.com/2016/01/west-virginia-bill-would-require-courts-to-inform-jurors-of-their-right-to-nullify/.

4 Steven Nelson, "Ex-Pastor Faces Felony for Preaching Jury Nullification," *US News and World Report*, December 2, 2015, http://www.usnews.com/news/articles/2015/12/02/ex-pastor-faces-felony-for-preaching-jury-nullification.

5 Eugene Volokh, "Felony Prosecution for Distributing Pro-jury-nullification Leaflets Outside Courthouse," The Volokh Conspiracy, *Washington Post*, December 2, 2015, https://www.washingtonpost.com/news/volokh-conspiracy/wp/2015/12/02/felony-prosecution-for-distributing-pro-jury-nullification-leaflets-outside-courthouse/.

6 Ibid.

7 JRank.org, s.v. "Jury: Legal Aspects—Jury Nullification," accessed May 12, 2016, http://law.jrank.org/pages/1440/Jury-Legal-Aspects-Jury-nullification.html.

8 West Virginia Legislature, Fair Trial Act of 2016, H. R. 2600, 82nd Legislature (2016), http://www.legis.state.wv.us/Bill_Status/Bills_history.cfm?input=2600&year=2016&sessiontype=RS&btype=bill.

9 Gina Kolata and Sarah Cohen, "Drug Overdoses Propel Rise in Mortality Rates of Young Whites," Health, *New York Times*, January 16, 2016, http://www.nytimes.com/2016/01/17/science/drug-overdoses-propel-rise-in-mortality-rates-of-young-whites.html?smid=re-share&_r=1.

10 "Race in Prison," DrugWarFacts.org, accessed May 12, 2016, http://www.drugwarfacts.org/cms/Race_and_Prison#sthash.0ifaqssT.fYpnybLJ.dpbs.

11 "Marijuana Profiling," *Los Angeles Times*, October 27, 2010, http://articles.latimes.com/2010/oct/27/opinion/la-ed-arrests-20101027.

12 Robby Soave, "Nixon Invented the Drug War to Decimate Hippies and Black People, Former Adviser Confesses," *Hit and Run* (blog), March 22, 2016, http://reason.com/blog/2016/03/22/nixon-invented-the-drug-war-to-decimate.

13 Dan Baum, "Legalize It All: How to Win the War on Drugs," *Harper's Magazine*, April 2016, https://harpers.org/archive/2016/04/legalize-it-all/.

14 Jesse McKinley, "Montana Jurors Raise Hopes of Marijuana Advocates," *New York Times*, December 23, 2010, http://www.nytimes.com/2010/12/23/us/23pot.html.

15 Gwen Florio, "Missoula District Court: Pot Case 'Mutiny' Leaves Ripples for Other Drug Cases," *Missoulian*, January 2, 2011, http://missoulian.com/special-section/news/medical_cannabis/missoula-district-court-pot-case-mutiny-leaves-ripples-for-other/article_d219f9ee-1638-11e0-b017-001cc4c002e0.html.

16 Eric Olson, *Courting Justice: More Montana Courthouse Tales*, (Indianapolis: Dog Ear Publishing, 2015), 348.

17 Ibid., 349.

18 Justin Gardner, "Colorado Juries Keep Letting People Go for Driving on Weed, Prosecutors and Cops Are Furious," *The Free Thought Project*, November 22, 2015, http://thefreethoughtproject.com/colorado-juries-letting-people-driving-weed-prosecutors-furious/.

19 Justin Gardner, "First of Its Kind Study Finds Virtually No Driving Impairment under the Influence of Marijuana," *The Free Thought Project*, September 30, 2015, http://thefreethoughtproject.com/kind-study-finds-virtually-driving-impairment-influence-marijuana/.

20 Sara Diedrich, "UI Studies Impact of Marijuana on Driving," *Iowa Now*, June 23, 2015, http://now.uiowa.edu/2015/06/ui-studies-impact-marijuana-driving.

21 Nigel Duara, "It's Legal to Smoke Pot in Colorado, but You Can Still Get Fired for It," *Los Angeles Times*, June 15, 2015, http://www.latimes.com/nation/la-na-ff-colorado-high-court-employee-marijuana-20150615-story.html.

22 Ibid.

23 Marcus A. Bachhuber, Brendan Saloner, Chinazo O. Cunningham, and Colleen L. Barry, "Medical Cannabis Laws and Opioid Analgesic Overdose Mortality in the United States, 1999–2010," *JAMA Internal Medicine* 174, no. 10 (2014): 1668–1673, http://archinte.jamanetwork.com/article.aspx?articleid=1898878.

24 Nina Lincoff, "States with Legal Marijuana See 25 Percent Fewer Prescription Painkiller Deaths," *Healthline*, August 26, 2014, http://www.healthline.com/health-news/states-with-legal-marijuana-have-fewer-overdose-deaths-082614.

25 "Employment-at-Will," *Colorado Department of Labor and Employment*, accessed May 12, 2016, https://www.colorado.gov/pacific/cdle/employment-at-will.

26 Ibid.

27 Jacob Sullum, *Saying Yes*, (New York: Penguin, 2004), 116.

28 Wayne Washington, "Palm Beach County's New Pot Law: $100 Fine for Holding about 3/4-ounce," *Palm Beach Post*, December 16, 2015, http://www.mypalmbeachpost.com/news/news/local-govt-politics/palm-beach-countys-new-pot-law-100-fine-for-holdin/npkSC/.

29 Marcie Cipriani, "Law to Decriminalize Marijuana, Hash in Pittsburgh Takes Effect," *Pittsburgh Action News 4*, January 4, 2016, http://www.wtae.com/news/pittsburgh-council-to-hold-hearing-to-decriminalize-pot/36971222.

30 "These 14 Cities in Michigan Have Passed Laws Decriminalizing Marijuana Possession and Use," *Michigan Radio*, November 7, 2014, http://michiganradio.org/post/these-14-cities-michigan-have-passed-laws-decriminalizing-marijuana-possession-and-use#stream/0.

31 Adam Lozier, "Texas County Moving Forward with Decriminalization Law," *Ganjapreneur*, December 29, 2015, http://www.ganjapreneur.com/texas-county-moving-forward-decriminalization/.

CHAPTER FOURTEEN: Inside America's Prison Industrial Complex

1 Nathan James, "CRS Report for Congress," *Congressional Research Service*, July 13, 2007, http://www.fas.org/sgp/crs/misc/RL32380.pdf.

2 Sara Flounders, "The Pentagon and Slave Labor in US Prisons," *Global Research*, June 23, 2011, http://www.globalresearch.ca/the-pentagon-and-slave-labor-in-u-s-prisons/25376.

3 Gina M. Florio, "5 Ways the US Prison Industrial Complex Mimics Slavery," *Bustle*, February 17, 2016, http://www.bustle.com/articles/142340-5-ways-the-us-prison-industrial-complex-mimics-slavery.

4 Ian Urbina, "US Flouts Its Own Advice in Procuring Overseas Clothing," *New York Times*, December 22, 2013, http://www.nytimes.com/2013/12/23/world/americas/buying-overseas-clothing-us-flouts-its-own-advice.html?_r=0.

5 Emily Jane Fox, "Factory Owners: Federal Prisoners Stealing Our Business," *CNN Money*, August 14, 2012, http://money.cnn.com/2012/08/14/smallbusiness/federal-prison-business/index.html?iid=HP_River.

6 Ibid.

7 Ibid.

8 Mike Elk and Bob Sloan, "The Hidden History of ALEC and Prison Labor," *The Nation*, August 1, 2011, http://www.thenation.com/article/hidden-history-alec-and-prison-labor/.

9 Joseph Lemieux, "The Modernized Slave Labor System: Also Known as the Prison Industrial Complex," *MintPress News*, November 28, 2014, http://www.mintpressnews.com/modernized-slave-labor-system-also-known-prison-industrial-complex/199374/.

10 http://abcnews.go.com/Business/foods-suppliers-defend-prison-labor/story?id=34258597

11 Colleen Curry, "Whole Foods, Expensive Cheese, and the Dilemma of Cheap Prison Labor," Crime and Punishment, *Vice*, July 21, 2015, https://news.vice.com/article/whole-foods-expensive-cheese-and-the-dilemma-of-cheap-prison-labor.

12 http://www.npr.org/sections/thesalt/2015/09/30/444797169/whole-foods-says-it-will-stop-selling-foods-made-by-prisoners

13 Victoria Law, "Martori Farms: Abusive Conditions at a Key Wal-Mart Supplier," *Truthout*, June 24, 2011, http://www.truth-out.org/index.php?option=com_k2&view=item&id=1808:martori-farms-abusive-conditions-at-a-key-walmart-supplier.

14 Brian Sumner, "These 7 Household Names Make a Killing Off of the Prison-Industrial Complex," CopBlock.org, February 20, 2016, http://www.copblock.org/154587/these-7-household-names-make-a-killing-off-of-the-prison-industrial-complex/.

15 https://www.prisonlegalnews.org/news/1993/apr/15/att-exploits-prison-labor/http://atlantablackstar.com/2014/10/10/12-mainstream-corporations-benefiting-from-the-prison-industrial-complex/
http://www.truthdig.com/report/item/boycott_divest_and_sanction_corporations_that_feed_on_prisons_20150405
http://usnews.nbcnews.com/_news/2012/01/12/10140493-inside-the-secret-industry-of-inmate-staffed-call-centers

16 "AT&T Exploits Prison Labor," *Prison Legal News*, April 15, 1993, https://www.prisonlegalnews.org/news/1993/apr/15/att-exploits-prison-labor/.

17 Rick Riley, "13 Mainstream Corporations Benefiting from the Prison Industrial Complex," *Atlanta Blackstar*, October 10, 2014, http://atlantablackstar.com/2014/10/10/12-mainstream-corporations-benefiting-from-the-prison-industrial-complex/3/.
http://www.truthdig.com/report/item/boycott_divest_and_sanction_corporations_that_feed_on_prisons_20150405

18 Campbell Robertson, John Schwartz, and Richard Pérez-Peña, "BP to Pay $18.7 Billion for Deepwater Horizon Oil Spill," *New York Times*, July 2, 2015, http://www.nytimes.

com/2015/07/03/us/bp-to-pay-gulf-coast-states-18-7-billion-for-deepwater-horizon-oil-spill.
html.

19 Rick Riley, "13 Mainstream Corporations Benefiting from the Prison Industrial Complex,"
Atlanta Blackstar, October 10, 2014, http://atlantablackstar.com/2014/10/10/12-mainstream-
corporations-benefiting-from-the-prison-industrial-complex/3/.

20 Beth Schwartzapfel, "Your Valentine, Made in Prison," *The Nation*, February 12, 2009, http://
www.thenation.com/article/your-valentine-made-prison/.

21 Rick Riley, "13 Mainstream Corporations Benefiting from the Prison Industrial Complex,"
Atlanta Blackstar, October 10, 2014, http://atlantablackstar.com/2014/10/10/12-mainstream-
corporations-benefiting-from-the-prison-industrial-complex/3/.

22 Caroline Winter, "What Do Prisoners Make for Victoria's Secret?" *Mother Jones*, July/August
2008, http://www.motherjones.com/politics/2008/07/what-do-prisoners-make-victorias-secret.

23 Brian Sumner, "These 7 Household Names Make a Killing Off of the Prison-Industrial
Complex," CopBlock.org, February 20, 2016, http://www.copblock.org/154587/these-7-
household-names-make-a-killing-off-of-the-prison-industrial-complex/.

24 Rania Khalek, "21st-Century Slaves: How Corporations Exploit Prison Labor," *AlterNet*, July
21, 2011, http://www.alternet.org/story/151732/21st-century_slaves%3A_how_corporations_
exploit_prison_labor.

25 Caroline Winter, "What Do Prisoners Make for Victoria's Secret?" *Mother Jones*, July/August
2008, http://www.motherjones.com/politics/2008/07/what-do-prisoners-make-victorias-secret.

26 Joe McGauley, "13 Everyday Items You Never Knew Were Made by Prisoners," *Thrillist*,
accessed May 12, 2016, https://www.thrillist.com/gear/products-made-by-prisoners-clothing-
furniture-electronics.

27 Jan Biles, "Inmates Make Dentures for Patients at Safety Net Clinics," *Topeka Capital-
Journal*, February 1, 2014, http://cjonline.com/life/arts-entertainment/2014-02-01/inmates-
make-dentures-patients-safety-net-clinics#.

28 Max Ehrenfreund, "Why Dentists Are So Darn Rich," *Wonkblog*, July 29, 2015, https://www.
washingtonpost.com/news/wonk/wp/2015/07/29/why-dentists-are-so-darn-rich/.

29 Nathan James, "CRS Report for Congress," *Congressional Research Service*, July 13, 2007,
http://www.fas.org/sgp/crs/misc/RL32380.pdf.

30 Tanzina Vega, "Costly Prison Fees Are Putting Inmates ddeep in Debt," *CNN Money*,
September 18, 2015, http://money.cnn.com/2015/09/18/news/economy/prison-fees-inmates-
debt/.

31 M. Scott Carter and Clifton Adcock, "Prisoners of Debt: Justice System Imposes Steep Fines,
Fees," *Oklahoma Watch*, January 31, 2015, http://oklahomawatch.org/2015/01/31/justice-
system-steeps-many-offenders-in-debt/.

32 Ibid.

33 Ibid.

34 Jim Liske, "Yep, Slavery Is Still Legal: Column," *USA Today*, August 14, 2014, http://www.
usatoday.com/story/opinion/2014/08/14/slavery-legal-exception-prisoners-drugs-reform-
column/14086227/.

35 Nathan James, "CRS Report for Congress," *Congressional Research Service*, July 13, 2007,
http://www.fas.org/sgp/crs/misc/RL32380.pdf.

36 Oliver Roeder, "Releasing Drug Offenders Won't End Mass Incarceration," *FiveThirtyEight*
(blog), July 17, 2015, http://fivethirtyeight.com/datalab/releasing-drug-offenders-wont-end-
mass-incarceration/.

37 "Walmart Gives Tennessee Employees Pay Raise," Wate.com, last modified March 9, 2016,
http://wate.com/2016/02/22/walmart-gives-employees-pay-raise/.

38 Drew Harwell and Jena McGregor, "This New Rule Could Reveal the Huge Gap Between
CEO Pay and Worker Pay," *Washington Post*, August 4, 2015, https://www.washingtonpost.

com/news/on-leadership/wp/2015/08/04/this-new-rule-could-reveal-the-huge-gap-between-ceo-pay-and-worker-pay/.

39 Salary.*com*, s.v. "Wal-mart Stores Inc," accessed May 12, 2016, http://www1.salary.com/Wal-Mart-Stores-Inc-Executive-Salaries.html.

40 "How US Taxpayers Subsidize the Nation's Wealthiest Family," *Jobs with Justice*, April 14, 2014, http://www.jwj.org/how-u-s-taxpayers-subsidize-the-nations-wealthiest-family.

41 http://democrats.edworkforce.house.gov/press-release/low-wages-single-wal-mart-store-cost-taxpayers-about-1-million-every-year-says-new

42 Krissy Clark, "Part II: 'Save Money, Live Better,'" *The Secret Life of a Food Stamp* (blog), April 2, 2014, http://www.marketplace.org/2014/04/02/wealth-poverty/secret-life-food-stamp/part-ii-save-money-live-better.

CHAPTER FIFTEEN: Our Politicians Are Backed by For-Profit Prisons

1 Andy Kroll, "This Is How Private Prison Companies Make Millions Even When Crime Rates Fall," *Mother Jones*, September 19, 2013, http://www.motherjones.com/mojo/2013/09/private-prisons-occupancy-quota-cca-crime.

2 "Private Jails in the United States," FindLaw.com, accessed May 12, 2016, http://civilrights.findlaw.com/other-constitutional-rights/private-jails-in-the-united-states.html.

3 Michael Kranish, "Jeb Bush Shaped by Troubled Phillips Academy Years," *Boston Globe*, February 1, 2015, https://www.bostonglobe.com/news/politics/2015/02/01/tumultuous-four-years-phillips-academy-helped-shape-jeb-bush/q6ccyHNOtP1n6kqDokMBfK/story.html.

4 Associated Press, "Bush Admits to Smoking Pot in Taped Discussion," *Taipei Times*, February 21, 2005, http://www.taipeitimes.com/News/world/archives/2005/02/21/2003224003.

5 George H. W. Bush, September 5, 1989, "Address to the Nation on the National Drug Control Strategy," transcript, *The American Presidency Project*, accessed May 12, 2016, http://www.presidency.ucsb.edu/ws/?pid=17472.

6 Lindsay Abrams, "Why America's fired up about hemp," *Salon*, April 19, 2014, http://www.salon.com/2014/04/19/why_americas_fired_up_about_hemp/.

7 Associated Press, "Former President George H. W. Bush Marks 90th bBirthday with Parachute Jump," Politics, *Fox News*, June 12, 2014, http://www.foxnews.com/politics/2014/06/12/0-year-old-ex-president-to-make-parachute-jump.html.

8 "The Cost of a Nation of Incarceration," *CBS News*, April 23, 2012, http://www.cbsnews.com/news/the-cost-of-a-nation-of-incarceration/.

9 Ibid.

10 PBS, "Thirty Years of America's Drug War," *Frontline*, accessed May 12, 2016, http://www.pbs.org/wgbh/pages/frontline/shows/drugs/cron/.

11 Eric Levitz, "Bill Clinton Admits His Crime Law Made mMass Incarceration 'Worse,'" MSNBC, last modified July 15, 2015, http://www.msnbc.com/msnbc/clinton-admits-his-crime-bill-made-mass-incarceration-worse.

12 "Bill Clinton Regrets 'Three Strikes,' Bill," *BBC*, July 16, 2015, http://www.bbc.com/news/world-us-canada-33545971.

13 Will Cabaniss, "Black Lives Matter Activist Says 'the Clintons' Passed Policy that Led to Mass Incarceration," *PunditFact*, August 25, 2015, http://www.politifact.com/punditfact/statements/2015/aug/25/julius-jones/black-lives-matter-activist-says-clintons-passed-p/.

14 Ibid.

15 Eric Levitz, "Bill Clinton Admits His Crime Law Made mMass Incarceration 'Worse,'" *MSNBC*, last modified July 15, 2015, http://www.msnbc.com/msnbc/clinton-admits-his-crime-bill-made-mass-incarceration-worse.

16 Jeff Stein, "The Clinton Dynasty's Horrific Legacy: How "Tough-on-Crime" Politics Built the World's Largest Prison System," *Salon*, April 13, 2015, http://www.salon.com/2015/04/13/

the_clinton_dynastys_horrific_legacy_how_tough_on_crime_politics_built_the_worlds_largest_prison/.

17 Greg Krikorian, "Federal and State Prison Populations Soared under Clinton, Report Finds," *Los Angeles Times*, February 19, 2001, http://articles.latimes.com/2001/feb/19/news/mn-27373.

18 Anti Drug Abuse Act of 1986, S. 2878, 99th Cong. (1986), https://www.congress.gov/bill/99th-congress/senate-bill/2878.

19 Shane Bauer, "Would Joe Biden Put His Son in Prison for Doing Coke?" *Mother Jones*, October 17, 2014, http://www.motherjones.com/mojo/2014/10/joe-biden-hunter-biden-cocaine.

20 Don Fitch, "Joe Biden: Drug War President 2016? Marijuana Reform Could Take a Step Back," *Marijuana Politics*, August 16, 2015, http://marijuanapolitics.com/joe-biden-drug-war-president-2016-marijuana-reform-could-take-a-step-back/.

21 Greta Jochem, "Joe Biden's Stance on Legal Weed Won't Have Smokers Too Thrilled about His Possible Presidential Campaign," *Bustle*, August 25, 2015, http://www.bustle.com/articles/106513-joe-bidens-stance-on-legal-weed-wont-have-smokers-too-thrilled-about-his-possible-presidential-campaign.

22 Colleen McCain Nelson and Julian E. Barnes, "Biden's Son Hunter Discharged from Navy Reserve after Failing Cocaine Test," *Wall Street Journal*, last modified October 16, 2014, http://www.wsj.com/articles/bidens-son-hunter-discharged-from-navy-reserve-after-failing-cocaine-test-1413499657.

23 "NDI Chairman's Council," *National Democratic Institute*, accessed May 12, 2016, https://www.ndi.org/chairmans-council.

24 http://cnponline.org/?team=r-hunter-biden

25 "Leadership," *US Global Leadership Coalition*, accessed May 12, 2016, http://www.usglc.org/about/our-leadership/.

26 "Board," *Truman National Security Project*, accessed May 12, 2016, http://trumanproject.org/home/about/board-leadership/.

27 http://cnponline.org/?team=r-hunter-biden

28 Adam Taylor, "Hunter Biden's New Job at a Ukrainian Gas Company Is a Problem for US Soft Power," WorldViews, *Washington Post*, May 14, 2014, https://www.washingtonpost.com/news/worldviews/wp/2014/05/14/hunter-bidens-new-job-at-a-ukrainian-gas-company-is-a-problem-for-u-s-soft-power/.

29 http://cnponline.org/?team=r-hunter-biden

30 Eric Levitz, "Bill Clinton Admits His Crime Law Made mMass Incarceration 'Worse,'" *MSNBC*, last modified July 15, 2015, http://www.msnbc.com/msnbc/clinton-admits-his-crime-bill-made-mass-incarceration-worse.

31 Richard A. Oppel Jr., "Private Prisons Found to Offer Little in Savings," *New York Times*, May 18, 2011, http://www.nytimes.com/2011/05/19/us/19prisons.html?pagewanted=1&ref=us&_r=2&mtrref=undefined&gwh=D534A935A56B2B7B090459CDABA9D3CC&gwt=pay.

32 Ibid.

33 Gabrielle Canon, "Here's the Latest Evidence of How Private Prisons Are Exploiting Inmates for Profit," *Mother Jones*, June 17, 2015, http://www.motherjones.com/mojo/2015/06/private-prisons-profit.

34 Beau Hodai, "Marco Rubio's Prison Problem," *In These Times*, February 14, 2011, http://inthesetimes.com/article/6940/marco_rubios_prison_problem.

35 Ibid.

36 Mary Ellen Klas, "The 'Cannibalizing' of Florida's Prison System," Miami Herald, February 28, 2015, http://www.miamiherald.com/news/special-reports/florida-prisons/article11533064.html.

http://vltp.net/inspection-of-kasichs-cca-owned-prison-shows-staff-assaults-up-over-300-thanks-alec/
http://www.truth-out.org/news/item/8875-corrections-corporation-of-america-a-study-in-predatory-capitalism-and-cronyism
http://www.drc.ohio.gov/web/director.htm

37 "Private Prison Monitoring," *Florida Department of Management Services*, accessed May 12, 2016, http://www.dms.myflorida.com/business_operations/private_prison_monitoring.

38 Mary Ellen Klas, "The 'Cannibalizing' of Florida's Prison System," *Miami Herald*, February 28, 2015, http://www.miamiherald.com/news/special-reports/florida-prisons/article11533064.html.

39 Beth Buczynski, "Shocking Facts about America's For-Profit Prison Industry," *Truthout*, February 6, 2014, http://www.truth-out.org/news/item/21694-shocking-facts-about-americas-for-profit-prison-industry.

40 Mary Ellen Klas, "The 'Cannibalizing' of Florida's Prison System," State Politics, Bradenton Herald, March 2, 2015, http://www.bradenton.com/news/politics-government/state-politics/article34803480.html.

41 David M. Reutter, "Florida Provides Lesson in How Not to Privatize State Prisons," *Prison Legal News*, February 15, 2012, https://www.prisonlegalnews.org/news/2012/feb/15/florida-provides-lesson-in-how-not-to-privatize-state-prisons/.

42 Mary Ellen Klas, "The 'Cannibalizing' of Florida's Prison System," State Politics, *Bradenton Herald*, March 2, 2015, http://www.bradenton.com/news/politics-government/state-politics/article34803480.html.

43 Stefan Kamph, "Police Officers Still Cold on Republicans, a Year After "Party to Leave the Party," *Broward Palm Beach New Times*, June 12, 2012, http://www.browardpalmbeach.com/news/police-officers-still-cold-on-republicans-a-year-after-party-to-leave-the-party-6442813.

44 David M. Reutter, "Florida Provides Lesson in How Not to Privatize State Prisons," *Prison Legal News*, February 15, 2012, https://www.prisonlegalnews.org/news/2012/feb/15/florida-provides-lesson-in-how-not-to-privatize-state-prisons/.

45 "GEO Group," FollowTheMoney.org, accessed May 12, 2016, http://beta.followthemoney.org/entity-details?eid=1096.

46 Keegan Hamilton, "How Private Prisons Are Profiting from Locking Up US Immigrants," Vice, October 6, 2015, https://news.vice.com/article/how-private-prisons-are-profiting-from-locking-up-us-immigrants.

47 Josh Gerstein, "Clinton Campaign Gives Private Prison Lobbyist Cash to Charity," *Under the Radar* (blog), February 1, 2016, http://www.politico.com/blogs/under-the-radar/2016/02/clinton-campaign-gives-private-prison-lobbyist-cash-to-charity-218524.

48 "Banking on Bondage: Private Prisons and Mass Incarceration," American Civil Liberties Union, accessed May 12, 2016, https://www.aclu.org/banking-bondage-private-prisons-and-mass-incarceration.

49 Stephanie Mencimer, "Florida Gov. Rakes in Campaign Cash from CEO Who Makes Millions Locking Up Immigrants," Mother Jones, July 18, 2014, http://www.motherjones.com/politics/2014/07/fundraiser-rick-scott-florida-geo-group.

50 Ibid.

51 Bob Ortega, "Arizona Prison Oversight Lacking for Private Facilities," AZCentral.com, August 7, 2011, http://www.azcentral.com/news/articles/2011/08/07/20110807arizona-prison-private-oversight.html?nclick_check=1.

52 Laurie Roberts, "Roberts: Private Prison Contract Goes to Ducey Contributor," AZCentral.com, October 28, 2015, http://www.azcentral.com/story/opinion/op-ed/laurieroberts/2015/10/28/roberts-private-prison-contract-goes-ducey-contributor/74750596/.

53 Craig Harris, "Arizona Awards 20-Year Private-Prison Contract to Only Bidder," AZCentral. com, December 17, 2015, http://www.azcentral.com/story/news/arizona/politics/2015/12/17/ lucrative-private-prison-contract-goes-to-cca/77449748/.

54 Matt Roche, "ACLU: Prison Privatization Is a Bad Deal for Ohioans," *Norwalk Reflector*, February 11, 2016, http://www.norwalkreflector.com/Law-Enforcement/2016/02/11/ACLU. http://www.cleveland.com/open/index.ssf/2011/03/private_corrections_company_wi.html

55 http://legacy.wkyc.com/story/news/investigations/2013/11/26/lake-erie-correctional/3761031/

56 Chris Kirkham, "Lake Erie Correctional Institution, Ohio Private Prison, Faces Concerns about 'Unacceptable' Conditions," Huffpost Business, *Huffington Post*, February 2, 2013, http:// www.huffingtonpost.com/2013/02/02/lake-erie-correctional-institution_n_2599428.html.

57 Ibid.

58 "Banking on Bondage: Private Prisons and Mass Incarceration," *American Civil Liberties Union*, accessed May 12, 2016, https://www.aclu.org/banking-bondage-private-prisons-and-mass-incarceration.

59 Ezra Klein and Evan Soltas, "Wonkbook: 11 Facts about America's Prison Population," *Wonkblog* (blog), August 13, 2013, https://www.washingtonpost.com/news/wonk/ wp/2013/08/13/wonkbook-11-facts-about-americas-prison-population/.

60 Cody Mason, "Too Good to Be True: Private Prisons in America," FollowTheMoney.org, January 13, 2012, http://beta.followthemoney.org/research/collaborations-and-outside-research/show/127/.

61 American Civil Liberties Union, *Banking on Bondage: Private Prisons and Mass Incarceration* (New York: American Civil Liberties Union, 2011), https://www.aclu.org/files/assets/ bankingonbondage_20111102.pdf.

62 Ibid.

63 Jon Schuppe, "Pennsylvania Seeks to Close Books on "Kids for Cash" Scandal," *NBC News*, August 12, 2015, http://www.nbcnews.com/news/us-news/pennsylvania-seeks-close-books-kids-cash-scandal-n408666.

64 American Civil Liberties Union, *Banking on Bondage: Private Prisons and Mass Incarceration* (New York: American Civil Liberties Union, 2011), https://www.aclu.org/files/assets/ bankingonbondage_20111102.pdf.

65 Stephanie Mencimer, "Florida Gov. Rakes in Campaign Cash from CEO Who Makes Millions Locking Up Immigrants," *Mother Jones*, July 18, 2014, http://www.motherjones. com/politics/2014/07/fundraiser-rick-scott-florida-geo-group.

66 "A Better Way to Treat Juvenile Offenders," *Broward Sheriff's Office*, November 19, 2013, http://www.sheriff.org/posts/post.cfm?id=75E776C8-CE6A-B7DC-6F57-3F24BDB498BF.

67 Mary Ellen Klas, "Miami-Dade a Leader in Use of Alternatives to Arrest for Under-Age Offenders," *Miami Herald*, July 15, 2015, http://www.miamiherald.com/news/local/ community/miami-dade/article27354157.html.

68 Ibid.

69 Ibid.

70 Stephanie Mencimer, "Florida Gov. Rakes in Campaign Cash from CEO Who Makes Millions Locking Up Immigrants," *Mother Jones*, July 18, 2014, http://www.motherjones. com/politics/2014/07/fundraiser-rick-scott-florida-geo-group.

71 Mary Ellen Klas, "The 'Cannibalizing' of Florida's Prison System," *Bradenton Herald*, March 2, 2015, http://www.bradenton.com/news/politics-government/state-politics/article34803480. html.

72 Ibid.

73 Ibid.

74 Ibid.

CHAPTER SIXTEEN: Marijuana Lobbyists—The Good, the Bad, and the Ugly

1 Katharine Q. Seelye, "Barack Obama, Asked about Drug History, Admits he Inhaled," *New York Times*, October 24, 2006, http://www.nytimes.com/2006/10/24/world/americas/24iht-dems.3272493.html?_r=0&mtrref=undefined&gwh=9636D247EF54410480CFFD7B9A53E EE6&gwt=pay.

2 Justin Sink, "Obama: Marijuana a 'Bad Habit and a Vice,' No More Dangerous than Alcohol," The Hill, January 19, 2014, http://thehill.com/blogs/blog-briefing-room/news/195896-obama-important-for-state-pot-laws-to-move-forward.

3 Leada Gore, "What Is an Executive Order? And How Many Has President Obama Issued?" AL.com, January 5, 2016, http://www.al.com/news/index.ssf/2016/01/what_is_an_executive_order_and.html.

4 Justin Sink, "Obama: Marijuana a 'Bad Habit and a Vice,' No More Dangerous than Alcohol," *The Hill*, January 19, 2014, http://thehill.com/blogs/blog-briefing-room/news/195896-obama-important-for-state-pot-laws-to-move-forward.

5 Radley Balko, "7 Ways the Obama Administration Has Accelerated Police Militarization," Huffpost Politics, *Huffington Post*, July 10, 2013, http://www.huffingtonpost.com/2013/07/10/obama-police-militarization_n_3566478.html.

6 http://cdn.ca9.uscourts.gov/datastore/opinions/2012/06/12/11-55004.pdf

7 Radley Balko, "7 Ways the Obama Administration Has Accelerated Police Militarization," Huffpost Politics, *Huffington Post*, July 10, 2013, http://www.huffingtonpost.com/2013/07/10/obama-police-militarization_n_3566478.html.

8 Andrew Becker, "Local Cops Ready for War With Homeland Security-Funded Military Weapons," *The Daily Beast*, December 21, 2011, http://www.thedailybeast.com/articles/2011/12/20/local-cops-ready-for-war-with-homeland-security-funded-military-weapons.html.

9 Ibid.

10 https://www.whitehouse.gov/sites/default/files/omb/budget/fy2016/assets/ap_23_drug_control.pdf

11 Phillip Smith, "The President's Budget: Drug War on Cruise Control," Drugs, *AlterNet*, February 2, 2015, http://www.alternet.org/drugs/presidents-budget-drug-war-cruise-control.

12 "The Federal Drug Control Budget: New Rhetoric, Same Failed Drug War," *Drug Policy Alliance*, February 2015, http://www.drugpolicy.org/sites/default/files/DPA_Fact_sheet_Drug_War_Budget_Feb2015.pdf.

13 Alexandra Jaffe, "Paul: Obama, Bush 'Lucky' Not to Be in Jail for Drug Use," *The Hill*, April 10, 2013, http://thehill.com/blogs/ballot-box/presidential-races/293083-paul-presidents-obama-bush-extraordinarily-lucky-not-to-be-in-jail-for-drug-use.

14 Richard L. Berke, "Bush to Seek $1.2 Million for a Bigger Drug War," *New York Times*, January 25, 1990, http://www.nytimes.com/1990/01/25/us/bush-to-seek-1.2-billion-for-a-bigger-drug-war.html.

15 Associated Press, "Bush: War on Drugs Aids War on Terror," *CBS News*, December 14, 2001, http://www.cbsnews.com/news/bush-war-on-drugs-aids-war-on-terror/.

16 Adam Cohen, "Fallout from a Midnight Ride," *TIME*, November 4, 2000, http://content.time.com/time/nation/article/0,8599,59739,00.html.

17 Elizabeth Chuck, "As Heroin Use Grows in US, Poppy Crops Thrive in Afghanistan," *NBC News*, July 7, 2015, http://www.nbcnews.com/news/world/heroin-use-grows-u-s-poppy-crops-thrive-afghanistan-n388081.

18 Ibid.

19 "Book: Bush Was Arrested for Cocaine in 1972," *Salon*, October 18, 1999, http://www.salon.com/1999/10/18/cocaine/.

20 Eliana Dockterman, "Clinton: I Never Denied Smoking Pot," *TIME*, December 3, 2013, http://swampland.time.com/2013/12/03/clinton-i-never-denied-smoking-pot/.

21 Jesse Ventura, interview by Larry King, *Larry King Live*, CNN, March 8, 2010, http://www. cnn.com/TRANSCRIPTS/1003/08/lkl.01.html.

22 Associated Press, "AP IMPACT: After 40 years, $1 trillion, US War on Drugs Has Failed to Meet Any of Its Goals," *Fox News*, May 13, 2010, http://www.foxnews.com/world/2010/05/13/ ap-impact-years-trillion-war-drugs-failed-meet-goals.html.

23 Reid J. Epstein, "Marijuana Industry Hires Lobbyists to Ease Bank Access," *Washington Wire* (blog), July 28, 2015, http://blogs.wsj.com/washwire/2015/07/28/marijuana-industry-hires-lobbyists-to-ease-bank-access/.

24 Ben Terris, "Big Pot Rising: The Marijuana Industry's First Full-Time Lobbyist Makes Rounds on Capitol Hill," *Washington Post*, March 24, 2014, https://www.washingtonpost. com/lifestyle/style/big-pot-rising-on-capitol-hill-nations-first-full-time-marijuana-lobbyist-makes-his-rounds/2014/03/24/dbc8c0c0-b07b-11e3-95e8-39bef8e9a48b_story.html.

25 Reid J. Epstein, "Marijuana Industry Hires Lobbyists to Ease Bank Access," *Washington Wire* (blog), July 28, 2015, http://blogs.wsj.com/washwire/2015/07/28/marijuana-industry-hires-lobbyists-to-ease-bank-access/.

26 "Overview," *Marijuana Policy Project*, accessed May 12, 2016, https://www.mpp.org/about/ overview/.

27 Brianna Gurciullo, "The Money in Marijuana: The Political Landscape," OpenSecrets.org, last modified November 2015, https://www.opensecrets.org/news/issues/marijuana/.

28 Brianna Gurciullo, "A Stash of Campaign Cash in Marijuana for Paul," OpenSecrets.org, October 23, 2015, https://www.opensecrets.org/news/2015/10/paul-holds-stash-of-campaign-cash-from-marijuana/.

29 "Ballot Initiative Campaigns," *Marijuana Policy Project*, accessed May 12, 2016, https://www. mpp.org/about/campaigns/.

30 www.regulatemarijuanainalaska.org

31 Kristen Wyatt, "Colorado Proposes Edible Pot Ban, Then Retreats," *Denver Post*, October 20, 2014, http://www.denverpost.com/ci_26763025/colorado-seeks-ban-most-edible-pot.

32 Ibid.

33 Joey Bunch, "Colorado Pot Lobby Loud, Clear on Regulations, as Government Listens," *The Cannabist*, December 26, 2014, http://www.thecannabist.co/2014/12/26/colorado-marijuana-lobbyist/26082/.

34 Kristen Wyatt, "Colorado Proposes Edible Pot Ban, Then Retreats," *Denver Post*, October 20, 2014, http://www.denverpost.com/ci_26763025/colorado-seeks-ban-most-edible-pot.

35 "NORML Advisory Board," *NORML*, accessed May 12, 2016, http://norml.org/advisory-board.

36 Joey Bunch, "Colorado Pot Lobby Loud, Clear on Regulations, as Government Listens," *The Cannabist*, December 26, 2014, http://www.thecannabist.co/2014/12/26/colorado-marijuana-lobbyist/26082/.

37 Brianna Gurciullo, "The Money in Marijuana: The Political Landscape," OpenSecrets.org, last modified November 2015, https://www.opensecrets.org/news/issues/marijuana/.

38 Brianna Gurciullo, "The Money in Marijuana: The Political Landscape," OpenSecrets.org, last modified November 2015, https://www.opensecrets.org/news/issues/marijuana/.

39 The Compassionate Access, Research Expansion, and Respect States Act of 2015, S. 683, 114th Cong. (2015), https://www.congress.gov/bill/114th-congress/senate-bill/683.

40 The Ending of Federal Marijuana Prohibition Act of 2015, S. 2237, 114th Cong. (2015), https://www.congress.gov/bill/114th-congress/senate-bill/2237.

41 Congress.gov, s.v. "Ending Federal Marijuana Prohibition Act," accessed May 12, 2016, https://www.congress.gov/search?q=%7B%22congress%22%3A%22all%22%2C%22source %22%3A%22legislation%22%2C%22search%22%3A%22%5C%22Ending+Federal+Mariju ana+Prohibition+Act%5C%22%22%7D.

42 The Veterans Equal Access Act of 2015, H. R. 667, 114th Cong. (2015), https://www.congress.gov/bill/114th-congress/house-bill/667.

43 The Respect State Marijuana Laws Act of 2015, H. R. 1940, 114th Cong. (2015), https://www.congress.gov/bill/114th-congress/house-bill/1940.

44 The Regulate Marijuana Like Alcohol Act of 2015, H. R. 1013, 114th Cong. (2015), https://www.congress.gov/bill/114th-congress/house-bill/1013.

45 The Marijuana Tax Revenue Act of 2015, H. R. 1014, 114th Cong. (2015), https://www.congress.gov/bill/114th-congress/house-bill/1014.

46 The States' Medical Marijuana Property Rights Protection Act of 2015, H. R. 262, 114th Cong. (2015), https://www.congress.gov/bill/114th-congress/house-bill/262.

47 Congress.gov, s.v. "Small Business Tax Equity Act," accessed May 12, 2016, https://www.congress.gov/search?q={%22congress%22%3A%22114%22%2C%22source%22%3A%22legislation%22%2C%22search%22%3A%22small%20business%20tax%20equity%20act%22}.

48 Congress.gov, s.v. "Marijuana Business Access to Banking Act," accessed May 12, 2016, https://www.congress.gov/search?q=%7B%22source%22%3A%22legislation%22%2C%22congress%22%3A%22114%22%2C%22search%22%3A%22/%22Marijuana+Business+Access+to+Banking+Act/%22%22%7D.

49 The Clean Slate for Marijuana Offenses Act of 2015, H. R. 3124, 114th Cong. (2015), https://www.congress.gov/bill/114th-congress/house-bill/3124.

50 Mike Liszewski, "Congress Set to Reauthorize the Rohrabacher-Farr Medical Cannabis Amendment," Americans for Safe Access, December 16, 2015, http://www.safeaccessnow.org/congress_set_to_reauthorize_the_rohrabacher_farr_medical_cannabis_amendment.

51 Ricardo Baca, "House Passes Bill to Prevent DOJ from Interfering in States' Medical Pot Laws," *The Cannabist*, June 3, 2015, http://www.thecannabist.co/2015/06/03/house-medical-pot-marijuana/35704/.

52 Brianna Gurciullo, "The Money in Marijuana: The Political Landscape," OpenSecrets.org, November 2015, https://www.opensecrets.org/news/issues/marijuana/.

53 Tim Cavanaugh, "The Golden State's Iron Bars," Reason.com, July 2011, http://reason.com/archives/2011/06/23/the-golden-states-iron-bars.

54 Brianna Gurciullo, "The Money in Marijuana: The Political Landscape," OpenSecrets.org, November 2015, https://www.opensecrets.org/news/issues/marijuana/.

55 Ibid.

56 "Pfizer Inc.," OpenSecrets.org, accessed May 12, 2016, https://www.opensecrets.org/lobby/clientsum.php?id=D000000138&year=2015.

57 Nadia Kounang, "Big Pharma's Big Donations to 2016 Presidential Candidates," *CNN*, February 11, 2016, http://www.cnn.com/2016/02/11/health/big-pharma-presidential-politics/.

58 Brianna Gurciullo, "The Money in Marijuana: The Political Landscape," OpenSecrets.org, November 2015, https://www.opensecrets.org/news/issues/marijuana/.

59 "Beer, Wine & Liquor," OpenSecrets.org, accessed May 12, 2016, https://www.opensecrets.org/lobby/indusclient.php?id=N02.

60 "Tobacco," OpenSecrets.org, accessed May 12, 2016, http://www.opensecrets.org/industries/contrib.php?cycle=2016&ind=a02.

CHAPTER SEVENTEEEN: Why Ohio's Corporate Marijuana Monopoly Failed

1 *BallotPedia*, s.v. "Ohio Marijuana Legalization Initiative, Issue 3 (2015)," accessed May 12, 2016, https://ballotpedia.org/Ohio_Marijuana_Legalization_Initiative,_Issue_3_(2015).

2 Ibid.

3 "Farmland Preservation," *Western Reserve Land Conservatory*, accessed May 12, 2016, http://www.wrlandconservancy.org/whatwedo/workingfarms/.

4 Jackie Borchardt, "4 Reasons Why Ohio Issue 3 Failed," Cleveland.com, November 5, 2015, http://www.cleveland.com/open/index.ssf/2015/11/4_reasons_why_ohio_issue_3_fai.html.

5 Mitch Smith and Sheryl Gay Stolberg, "On Ballot, Ohio Grapples With Specter of Marijuana Monopoly," *New York Times*, November 1, 2015, http://www.nytimes.com/2015/11/02/us/on-ballot-ohio-grapples-with-specter-of-marijuana-monopoly.html?_r=0&mtrref=undefined& gwh=4CEBF91F40795816145A4C538C9E3C70&gwt=pay&assetType=nyt_now.
6 Ibid.
7 Ibid.
8 http://www.cleveland.com/open/index.ssf/2016/05/ohio_senate_passes_medical_mar.html
9 "An Amendment for Individual Rights," *Grassroots Ohio*, accessed May 12, 2016, https://grassrootsoh.org/.
10 https://legalizeohio2016.org/qa-with-rob-kampia-mpp-executive-director/
11 http://www.dispatch.com/content/stories/local/2016/05/26/new-marijuana-law-could-lead-to-plants-growing-in-ohio-within-a-year.html#
12 http://www.dispatch.com/content/stories/local/2016/05/26/new-marijuana-law-could-lead-to-plants-growing-in-ohio-within-a-year.html#
13 https://legalizeohio2016.org/about/mission/
14 https://legalizeohio2016.org/amendment/

CHAPTER EIGHTEEN: *Hemp for Victory!*

1 "Look for 'Made in USA' before Buying Your American Flag," *BusinessWire*, May 27, 2015, http://www.businesswire.com/news/home/20150527005955/en/%E2%80%98Made-USA%E2%80%99-Buying-American-Flag.
2 Jacqueline Klimas, "That's No Ordinary Flag Flying over the Capital," *Washington Examiner*, November 11, 2015, http://www.washingtonexaminer.com/thats-no-ordinary-flag-flying-over-the-capitol/article/2576066.
3 Andrew Wright, *Wisconsin Agricultural Experiment Station Bulletin no. 293* (1918, Wisconsin's Hemp Industry), 13.
4 Sarah Haas, "2016 Could Be the Year for Industrial Hemp," *Boulder Weekly*, February 11, 2016, http://www.boulderweekly.com/boulderganic/2016-could-be-the-year-for-industrial-hemp/.
5 Andrea Miller, "Legalizing Weed: 4 Facts About the Industrial Hemp Farming Act," *Newsmax*, November 17, 2015, http://www.newsmax.com/FastFeatures/legalizing-weed-industrial-hemp-farming-act/2015/11/17/id/702575/.
6 Ibid.
7 Tim Devaney, "Hemp-Made Flag Flies over the US Capitol," *The Hill*, November 11, 2015, http://thehill.com/regulation/defense/259857-flying-high-hemp-made-flag-adorns-us-capitol.
8 Vote Hemp, "Congress Introduces Industrial Hemp Farming Act with Bi-partisan Support," news release, January 22, 2015, http://www.votehemp.com/PR/2015-1-22-congress-introduces-hemp-farming-acts.html.
9 Andrea Miller, "Legalizing Weed: 4 Facts About the Industrial Hemp Farming Act," *Newsmax*, November 17, 2015, http://www.newsmax.com/FastFeatures/legalizing-weed-industrial-hemp-farming-act/2015/11/17/id/702575/.
10 "2014 Farm Bill Section 7606," *Vote Hemp*, accessed May 12, 2016, http://www.votehemp.com/2014_farm_bill_section_7606.html.
11 Vote Hemp, "Kentucky Department of Agriculture Sues DEA in US District Court Over DEA's Refusal to Respect Farm Bill Hemp Provision," news release, May 15, 2014, http://votehemp.com/PR/2014-05-15-KentuckyDeptofAgriculture-suesDEA.html.
12 Ibid.
13 "State Industrial Hemp Statutes," *National Conference of State Legislatures*, March 4, 2016, http://www.ncsl.org/research/agriculture-and-rural-development/state-industrial-hemp-statutes.aspx.
14 "National Hemp Association (NHA) Introduces Hemp, Inc. as Its Newest Gold Member," *Yahoo! Finance*, December 1, 2015, http://finance.yahoo.com/news/national-hemp-association-nha-introduces-093000314.html.

15 Logan Yonavjak, "Industrial Hemp: A Win-Win for the Economy and the Environment," *Forbes*, May 29, 2013, http://www.forbes.com/sites/ashoka/2013/05/29/industrial-hemp-a-win-win-for-the-economy-and-the-environment/2/#5f6f0f8e6ad2.

16 Doug Fine, "A Tip for American Farmers: Grow Hemp, Make Money," Op-Ed, Los Angeles Times, June 25, 2014, http://www.latimes.com/opinion/op-ed/la-oe-fine-hemp-marijuana-legalize-20140626-story.html.

17 Lindsay Abrams, "Why America's Fired Up about Hemp," *Salon*, April 19, 2014, http://www.salon.com/2014/04/19/why_americas_fired_up_about_hemp/.

18 Ibid.

19 http://antiquecannabisbook.com/chap04/Virginia/VA_IndHempP2.htm

20 "Oilseed," *Vote Hemp*, accessed May 12, 2016, http://www.votehemp.com/markets_oilseed.html.

21 "Stalk," Vote Hemp, accessed May 12, 2016, http://www.votehemp.com/markets_stalk.html.

22 Ibid.

23 "Soybean Car," *The Henry Ford*, accessed May 12, 2016, https://www.thehenryford.org/research/soybeancar.aspx.

24 Rusty Davis, "Henry's Plastic Car: An Interview with Mr. Lowell E. Overly," *V8 Times*, 46–51.

25 Joseph Toomey, *An Unworthy Future: The Grim Reality of Obama's Green Energy Delusions*, (Richmond, BC: Archway Publishing, 2014), 312.

26 Ibid.

27 W. L. Faith, "Development of the Scholler Process in the United States," *Industrial and Engineering Chemistry* 37, no. 1 (1945): 9–11, http://pubs.acs.org/doi/abs/10.1021/ie50421a004.

28 "Welcome to BioWillie Biodiesel," *BioWillie.com*, accessed May 12, 2016, http://biowillie.com/bw/.

29 Michael Brick, "For Willie Nelson, a Biodiesel Dream Deferred," *Houston Chronicle*, October 30, 2014, http://www.houstonchronicle.com/business/energy/article/For-singer-a-biodiesel-dream-deferred-5859382.php#/0.

30 Thomas Prade, "Industrial Hemp (*Cannabis sativa* L.)—a High-Yielding Energy Crop" (doctoral dissertation, Swedish University of Agricultural Sciences, 2011), http://www.chicagomanualofstyle.org/16/ch14/ch14_sec224.html.

31 http://www.lotuscars.com/engineering/eco-elise#

32 Elaine Charkowski, "Hemp 'Eats' Chernobyl Waste, Offers Hope for Hanford," *Hemp.net*, January 10, 2014, http://web.archive.org/web/20140110154417/http://www.hemp.net/news/9901/06/hemp_eats_chernobyl_waste.html.

33 Patrick Reevell, "Chernobyl 30 Years Later: Those Who Live in Its Shadow Still Suffer," *ABC News*, April 26, 2016, http://abcnews.go.com/International/30-years-chernobyl-disaster-live-shadow-suffer-consequences/story?id=38678417.

34 Khalid Rehman Hakeem, Muhammad Sabir, Münir Öztürk, and Ahmet Ruhi Mermut, *Soil Remediation and Plants: Prospects and Challenges* (London: Elsevier, 2015), 243.

35 "Phytoremediation: Using Plants to Clean Soil," *Botany: Global Issues Map*, accessed May 12, 2016, https://www.mhhe.com/biosci/pae/botany/botany_map/articles/article_10.html.

36 P. Linger, J. Müssig, H. Fischer, and J. Kobert, "Industrial Hemp (*Cannabis sativa* L.) Growing on Heavy Metal Contaminated Soil: Fibre Quality and Phytoremediation Potential," *Industrial Crops and Products* 16, no. 1 (2002): 33–42, http://www.sciencedirect.com/science/article/pii/S0926669002000055.

37 http://www.chem.unep.ch/pops/pdf/lead/leadexp.pdf

38 I. Alkorta et al., "Recent Findings on the Phytoremediation of Soils Contaminated with Environmentally Toxic Heavy Metals and Metalloids Such as Zinc, Cadmium, Lead, and Arsenic," *Reviews in Environmental Science and Biotechnology* 3, no. 1 (2004): 71–90, http://link.springer.com/article/10.1023/B:RESB.0000040059.70899.3d.

39 Alex Bitter, "UH Could Lead Charge on Hemp Research," *Ka Leo*, March 31, 2014, http://www.kaleo.org/news/uh-could-lead-charge-on-hemp-research/article_7e591dd4-b8b1-11e3-b0e8-001a4bcf6878.html.

40 V. Angelova, R. Ivanova, V. Delibaltova, and K. Ivanov, "Bio-accumulation and Distribution of Heavy Metals in Fibre Crops (Flax, Cotton and Hemp)," *Industrial Crops and Products* 19, vol. 3 (2004): 197–205, http://www.sciencedirect.com/science/article/pii/S0926669003001110.

41 Jon Michael McPartland, Robert Connell, and David Paul Watson, *Hemp: Diseases and Pests: Management and Biological Control* (New York: CABI Publishing, 2000), 165.

42 Ibid.

43 Renée Johnson, "Hemp as an Agricultural Commodity," Congressional Research Service, February 2, 2015, http://www.fas.org/sgp/crs/misc/RL32725.pdf.

44 Alex Bitter, "UH Could Lead Charge on Hemp Research," *Ka Leo*, March 31, 2014, http://www.kaleo.org/news/uh-could-lead-charge-on-hemp-research/article_7e591dd4-b8b1-11e3-b0e8-001a4bcf6878.html.

45 Sonia Campbell, Daniel Paquin, Jonathan D. Awaya, and Qing X. Li, "Remediation of Benzo[a]pyrene and Chrysene-Contaminated Soil with Industrial Hemp (*Cannabis sativa*)," *International Journal of Phytoremediation* 4, no. 2 (2002): 157–168, http://www.tandfonline.com/doi/abs/10.1080/15226510208500080?src=recsys&.

46 Kathleen Gallagher, "A & B Hopeful Hemp Could Be a Replacement for Sugar," *Business News*, January 11, 2016, http://www.bizjournals.com/pacific/news/2016/01/11/a-b-hopeful-hemp-could-be-a-replacement-for-sugar.html.

47 Ibid.

48 "Hazardous Waste," *InfrastructureReportCard.org*, accessed May 12, 2016, http://www.infrastructurereportcard.org/hazardous-waste/.

49 Dewey & Merrill, *Bulletin #404. U.S. Dept. of Age. 1916*

50 Joe Martino, "Hemp vs. Cotton: The Ultimate Showdown," *Collective Evolution*, July 17, 2013, http://www.collective-evolution.com/2013/07/17/hemp-vs-cotton-the-ultimate-showdown/.

51 Brian Palmer, "High on Environmentalism," *Slate*, April 12, 2011, http://www.slate.com/articles/health_and_science/the_green_lantern/2011/04/high_on_environmentalism.html.

52 Nia Cherett et al., *Ecological Footprint and Water Analysis of Cotton, Hemp, and Polyester* (Stockholm: Stockholm Environment Institute, 2015), http://www.sei-international.org/mediamanager/documents/Publications/SEI-Report-EcologicalFootprintAndWaterAnalysisOfCottonHempAndPolyester-2005.pdf.

53 "General Hemp Information," *Hemp Basics*, May 12, 2016, http://www.hempbasics.com/shop/hemp-information.

54 Ibid.

55 Joe Martino, "Hemp vs. Cotton: The Ultimate Showdown," *Collective Evolution*, July 17, 2013, http://www.collective-evolution.com/2013/07/17/hemp-vs-cotton-the-ultimate-showdown/.

56 Logan Yonavjak, "Industrial Hemp: A Win-Win for the Economy and the Environment," *Forbes*, May 29, 2013, http://www.forbes.com/sites/ashoka/2013/05/29/industrial-hemp-a-win-win-for-the-economy-and-the-environment/2/#5cea26776ad2.

57 "Forest Fire Damage, Healed By Hemp" *Cannabis Health News*, August 2, 2012, http://cannabishealthnewsmagazine.com/legal/1875/forest-fire-damage-healed-by-hemp/.

58 Michael Karus, "European Hemp Industry 2002," *Journal of Industrial Hemp* 9, no. 2 (2004): 93–101, http://www.tandfonline.com/doi/abs/10.1300/J237v09n02_10.

59 Lyster H. Dewey, "Hemp," in *Yearbook of the United States Department of Agriculture 1913* (Washington, DC : United States Department of Agriculture, 1913), 283–346, http://www.votehemp.com/PDF/HEMP_Yearbook_of_Agriculture_1913.pdf.

60 B. B. Robinson, *Hemp: Farmer's Bulletin No. 1935* (Washington, DC: United States Department of Agriculture, 1952), http://www.votehemp.com/PDF/USDA_Bulletin_1935.pdf.

61 "Hemp for Victory," Global Hemp, accessed May 12, 2016, http://www.globalhemp.com/1942/01/hemp-for-victory.html.

CHAPTER NINETEEN: Hemp for Nutrition!

1 Cecille M. Protzman, "Bast, the Textile Fibers," in *The Yearbook of Agriculture 1964* (Washington, DC: United States Department of Agriculture, 1964), http://naldc.nal.usda.gov/naldc/download.xhtml?id=IND43861826&content=PDF.

2 "Hemp for Victory (1942)," *The Herb Museum*, May 24, 2014, http://www.herbmuseum.ca/content/hemp-victory-1942.

3 "Oregon Administrative Rules: Medical Marijuana," Oregon State *Archives*, accessed May 12, 2016, http://medicalmarijuana.procon.org/sourcefiles/oregon-ballot-measure-67.pdf.

4 http://norml.org/legal/item/oregon-hemp-law

5 Aaron Smith, "Recreational Pot Use Is Now Legal in Oregon," *CNN Money*, July 1, 2015, http://money.cnn.com/2015/07/01/news/oregon-marijuana-legalization/.

6 United States Drug Enforcement Administration, "Statement from the Drug Enforcement Administration on the Industrial Use of Hemp," news release, March 12, 1998, http://www.dea.gov/pubs/pressrel/pr980312.htm.

7 Ibid.

8 Renée Johnson, "Hemp as an Agricultural Commodity," Congressional Research Service, February 2, 2015, http://www.fas.org/sgp/crs/misc/RL32725.pdf.

9 Drew Walker, "Legalizing Weed: 8 Facts About Oregon's Legalization of Industrial Hemp Farming," *Newsmax*, February 19, 2016, http://www.newsmax.com/FastFeatures/oregon-industrial-hemp-legalizing-weed-facts/2016/02/19/id/715210/.

10 United States Drug Enforcement Administration, "Statement from the Drug Enforcement Administration on the Industrial Use of Hemp," news release, March 12, 1998, http://www.dea.gov/pubs/pressrel/pr980312.htm.

11 "DEA Form 225—New Application for Registration," *Office of Diversion Control*, accessed May 12, 2016, http://www.deadiversion.usdoj.gov/drugreg/reg_apps/225/225_instruct.htm.

12 Renée Johnson, "Hemp as an Agricultural Commodity," *Congressional Research Service*, February 2, 2015, http://www.fas.org/sgp/crs/misc/RL32725.pdf.

13 United States Drug Enforcement Administration, "Statement from the Drug Enforcement Administration on the Industrial Use of Hemp," news release, March 12, 1998, http://www.dea.gov/pubs/pressrel/pr980312.htm.

14 Renée Johnson, "Hemp as an Agricultural Commodity," *Congressional Research Service*, February 2, 2015, http://www.fas.org/sgp/crs/misc/RL32725.pdf.

15 "State Industrial Hemp Statutes," National Conference of State Legis*latures*, accessed May 12, 2016, http://www.ncsl.org/research/agriculture-and-rural-development/state-industrial-hemp-statutes.aspx.

16 Renée Johnson, "Hemp as an Agricultural Commodity," *Congressional Research Service*, February 2, 2015, http://www.fas.org/sgp/crs/misc/RL32725.pdf.

17 Renée Johnson, "Hemp as an Agricultural Commodity," *Congressional Research Service*, February 2, 2015, http://www.fas.org/sgp/crs/misc/RL32725.pdf.

18 Delfin Rodriguez-Leyva and Grant N. Pierce, "The Cardiac and Haemostatic Effects of Dietary Hempseed," *Nutrition & Metabolism* 7, no. 32 (2010), http://www.ncbi.nlm.nih.gov/pmc/articles/PMC2868018/.

19 Delfin Rodriguez-Leyva and Grant N. Pierce, "The Cardiac and Haemostatic Effects of Dietary Hempseed," *Nutrition & Metabolism* 7, no. 32 (2010), http://www.ncbi.nlm.nih.gov/pmc/articles/PMC2868018/.

20 Mike Roussell, "Ask the Diet Doctor: What's Up with the Hemp Seeds Hype?" Shape, accessed May 12, 2016, http://www.shape.com/healthy-eating/diet-tips/ask-diet-doctor-hemp-seeds-hype.

21 "Hemp Seed: Nutritional Value and Thoughts," The Nourishing Gourmet, March 11, 2009, http://www.thenourishinggourmet.com/2009/03/hemp-seed-nutritional-value-and-thoughts.html.

22 Monica Reinagel, "Chia vs. Hemp vs. Flax," QuickAndDirtyTips.com, February 27, 2013, http://www.quickanddirtytips.com/health-fitness/healthy-eating/chia-vs-hemp-vs-flax.

23 J. C. Callaway, "Hempseed as a Nutritional Resource: An Overview," *Euphytica* 140, no. 1 (2004): 65–72, http://link.springer.com/article/10.1007%2Fs10681-004-4811-6.

24 J. C. Callaway, "Hempseed as a Nutritional Resource: An Overview," *Euphytica* 140, no. 1 (2004): 65–72, http://link.springer.com/article/10.1007%2Fs10681-004-4811-6.

25 M. O. Weickert and A. F. Pfeiffer, "Metabolic Effects of Dietary Fiber Consumption and Prevention of Diabetes," *Journal of Nutrition* 138, no. 3 (2008): 439–442, http://www.ncbi.nlm.nih.gov/pubmed/18287346.

26 J. S. de Munter et al., "Whole Grain, Bran, and Germ Intake and Risk of Type 2 Diabetes: A Prospective Cohort Study and Systematic Review," *PLOS Medicine* 4, no. 8 (2007): e261, http://www.ncbi.nlm.nih.gov/pmc/articles/PMC1952203/.

27 J. Callaway et al., "Efficacy of Dietary Hempseed Oil in Patients with Atopic Dermatitis," *Journal of Dermatological Treatment*, 16, no. 2 (2005): 87–94, http://www.ncbi.nlm.nih.gov/pubmed/16019622.

28 E. A. Rocha Filho, J. C. Lima, J. S. Pinho Neto, and U. Motarroyos, "Essential Fatty Acids for Premenstrual Syndrome and Their Effect on Prolactin and Total Cholesterol Levels: A Randomized, Double Blind, Placebo-Controlled Study," *Reproductive Health* 8, no. 2 (2011), http://www.ncbi.nlm.nih.gov/pubmed/21241460.

29 D. F. Horrobin, "The Role of Essential Fatty Acids and Prostaglandins in the Premenstrual Syndrome," *Journal of Reproductive Medicine* 28, no. 7 (1983): 465–68, http://www.ncbi.nlm.nih.gov/pubmed/6350579.

30 A. Saberivand et al., "The Effects of Cannabis Sativa L. Seed (Hempseed) in the Ovariectomized Rad Model of Menopause," *Methods and Findings in Experimental Clinical Pharmacology* 32, no. 7 (2010): 467, http://www.ncbi.nlm.nih.gov/pubmed/21069097.

31 M. C. Kruger, "Calcium, Gamma-Linolenic Acid and Eicosapentaenoic Acid Supplementation in Senile Osteoporosis," *Aging* 10, no. 5 (1998): 385–394, http://www.ncbi.nlm.nih.gov/pubmed/9932142.

32 J. C. Callaway, "Hempseed as a Nutritional Resource: An Overview," *Euphytica* 140 (2004): 65–72, http://www.fao.org/fsnforum/sites/default/files/resources/Hempseed%20as%20a%20nutritional%20resource-%20An%20overview.pdf.

33 Ibid.

34 Lynn Osburn, "Hemp Seed: The Most Nutritionally Complete Food Source in the World," *Hemp Line Journal* 1, no. 1 (1992): 14–15.

35 J. C. Callaway, "Hempseed as a Nutritional Resource: An Overview," *Euphytica* 140 (2004): 65–72, http://www.fao.org/fsnforum/sites/default/files/resources/Hempseed%20as%20a%20nutritional%20resource-%20An%20overview.pdf.

36 Ibid.

37 Pavlo Holoborod'ko, "Hemp Research and Growing in Ukraine," *Institute of Bast Crops, Hlukhiv, Ukraine*, accessed May 12, 2016, http://www.aginukraine.com/bast/bast01.htm.

38 Jennifer D'Angelo, "3 Reasons to Try Hemp Milk (Dr. Oz Loves It!)" Self, May 3, 2011, http://www.self.com/flash/nutritionnews/2011/05/hemp-milk/.

CHAPTER TWENTY: Cooking with Cannabis—Hemp and Marijuana
1 Steven Wishnia, "Smoke vs. Snack: Why Edible Marijuana Is Stronger than Smoking," *The Daily Beast*, June 13, 2014, http://www.thedailybeast.com/articles/2014/06/13/smoke-vs-snack-why-edible-marijuana-is-stronger-than-smoking.html.
2 Bailey Rahn, "Ingest or Inhale? 5 Differences Between Marijuana Edibles and Flowers," Leafly, July 17, 2014, https://www.leafly.com/news/cannabis-101/ingest-or-inhale-5-differences-between-marijuana-edibles-and-flow.
3 Steven Wishnia, "Smoke vs. Snack: Why Edible Marijuana Is Stronger than Smoking," *The Daily Beast*, June 13, 2014, http://www.thedailybeast.com/articles/2014/06/13/smoke-vs-snack-why-edible-marijuana-is-stronger-than-smoking.html.
4 Bailey Rahn, "Ingest or Inhale? 5 Differences Between Marijuana Edibles and Flowers," *Leafly*, July 17, 2014, https://www.leafly.com/news/cannabis-101/ingest-or-inhale-5-differences-between-marijuana-edibles-and-flow.
5 Roni Cayn Rabin, "The Drug Dose Gender Gap," *New York Times*, January 28, 2013, http://well.blogs.nytimes.com/2013/01/28/the-drug-dose-gender-gap/?_r=1&mtrref=undefined&gwh=C58FE1681BBB478108DBD102E263158E&gwt=pay.
6 FDA Drug Safety Communication: Risk of Next-Morning Impairment after Use of Insomnia Drugs; FDA Requires Lower Recommended Doses for Certain Drugs Containing Zolpidem (Ambien, Ambien CR, Edluar, and Zolpimist)," *US Food and Drug Administration*, accessed May 12, 2016, http://www.fda.gov/Drugs/DrugSafety/ucm334033.htm.
7 Roni Cayn Rabin, "The Drug Dose Gender Gap," *New York Times*, January 28, 2013, http://well.blogs.nytimes.com/2013/01/28/the-drug-dose-gender-gap/?_r=1&mtrref=undefined&gwh=C58FE1681BBB478108DBD102E263158E&gwt=pay.
8 Susan Squibb, "How to Calculate THC Dosage in Recipes for Marijuana Edibles," *The Cannabist*, July 7, 2014, http://www.thecannabist.co/2014/07/07/marijuana-recipes-calculating-thc-dosage-cannabutter-canna-oils-marijuana-infused/15457/.
9 Ibid.
10 Robyn Griggs Lawrence, *The Cannabis Kitchen Cookbook* (New York: Skyhorse Publishing, 2015), 78.
11 "Decarboxylation," *Herb*, accessed May 12, 2016, http://herb.co/decarboxylation/.
12 Robyn Griggs Lawrence, *The Cannabis Kitchen Cookbook*, 2015 Skyhorse Publishing NYC, pg 34.

AFTERWORD: It's High Time to End Prohibition
1 *This Day in History*, s.v. "December 5: 1933, Prohibition Ends," *History*, accessed May 12, 2016, http://www.history.com/this-day-in-history/prohibition-ends.
2 https://books.google.com/books?id=OigDAAAAMBAJ&pg=PA19&dq=1930+plane+%22Popular&hl=en&ei=UoKOTpXcNMOUtwfE1sSLDA&sa=X&oi=book_result&ct=result&resnum=3&ved=0CDwQ6AEwAjgK#v=onepage&q=1930%20plane%20%22Popular&f=true
3 *The American Presidency Project*, s.v. "Franklin D. Roosevelt," accessed May 12, 2016, http://www.presidency.ucsb.edu/ws/?pid=88395.
4 Will Carless, "Uruguay's Year in Marijuana: 3 Successes, 3 Burning Questions," NBC News, January 7, 2015, http://www.nbcnews.com/news/latino/uruguays-year-marijuana-3-successes-3-burning-questions-n281311.
5 "Uruguay," *The Global Initiative for Drug Policy Reform*, accessed May 12, 2016, http://reformdrugpolicy.com/beckley-main-content/new-approaches/future-directions-for-drug-policy-reform/latin-america/uruguay/.
6 "Jose Mujica: 'I Earn More than I Need," Talk to Aljazeera, October 26, 2013, http://www.aljazeera.com/programmes/talktojazeera/2013/10/jose-mujica-i-earn-more-than-i-need-2013102294729420734.html.

7 Manuel Rueda, "Uruguayan President: Yes, We'll Have Legal Weed, but Love Is All You Need," *ABC News*, August 15, 2013, http://abcnews.go.com/ABC_Univision/uruguayan-president-legal-weed-love/story?id=19972551.

8 Matt Thompson, "The Mysterious History of 'Marijuana,'" *Code Switch: Word Watch*, July 22, 2013, http://www.npr.org/sections/codeswitch/2013/07/14/201981025/the-mysterious-history-of-marijuana.

9 *The American Presidency Project*, s.v. "Jimmy Carter," accessed May 12, 2016, http://www.presidency.ucsb.edu/ws/?pid=7908.

10 Ian Bickis, "Canada's Hemp Industry Is Growing Fast, but Competition Looms," Business, *The Star*, July 10, 2015, https://www.thestar.com/business/2015/07/10/canadas-hemp-industry-is-growing-fast-but-competition-looms.html.

About the Author

JESSE VENTURA is the former Independent governor of Minnesota. He is also a former US Navy frogman, a professional wrestler, a movie actor, a visiting fellow at Harvard Kennedy School of Government, and the *New York Times* best-selling author of seven books, including *American Conspiracies*, *63 Documents the Government Doesn't Want You to Read*, and *Don't Start the Revolution Without Me*. He was the host and executive producer of truTV's *Conspiracy Theory with Jesse Ventura*, which won the Stony Award from *High Times* magazine in 2010. He was also the host of the political talk show *Off The Grid*, which aired on RT America and online at Ora.tv. He has a reputation as a rebel and a freethinker; he also has no qualms about questioning authority. He spends half the year in Baja, Mexico, and the other half in his home state of Minnesota.

As a publicity consultant, **JEN HOBBS** has represented Oscar and Emmy award–winning clients as well as politicians and authors. Her family owns and operates Hobbs Greenery, a California medical cannabis collective that buys, sells, cultivates, and distributes cannabis and cannabis-infused products. Her short stories and articles have been featured in literary journals and on websites such as *Cafe Mom*. She has worked behind the scenes with Governor Jesse Ventura since 2007 and shares his enthusiasm for searching for the truth, no matter where it leads. She lives in Anaheim Hills, California.